Chronic Care—Science and Practice

Daniela Schmitz · Manfred Fiedler ·
Heike Becker · Simone Hatebur ·
Jan-Hendrik Ortloff
Editors

Chronic Care—Science and Practice

Springer

Editors
Daniela Schmitz
Department of human medicine
Witten/Herdecke University
Witten, Germany

Manfred Fiedler
Department of human medicine
Witten/Herdecke University
Witten, Germany

Heike Becker
Faculty of Health
Witten/Herdecke University
Witten, Germany

Simone Hatebur
Faculty of Health
Witten/Herdecke University
Witten, Germany

Jan-Hendrik Ortloff
Department of human medicine
Witten/Herdecke University
Witten, Germany

ISBN 978-3-662-72297-8 ISBN 978-3-662-72298-5 (eBook)
https://doi.org/10.1007/978-3-662-72298-5

Translation from the German language edition: "Chronic Care—Wissenschaft und Praxis" by Daniela Schmitz et al., © Der/die Herausgeber bzw. der/die Autor(en), exklusiv lizenziert an Springer-Verlag GmbH, DE, ein Teil von Springer Nature 2024. Published by Springer Berlin Heidelberg. All Rights Reserved.

This book is a translation of the original German edition "Chronic Care—Wissenschaft und Praxis" by Daniela Schmitz et al., published by Springer-Verlag GmbH, DE in 2024. The translation was done with the help of an artificial intelligence machine translation tool. A subsequent human revision was done primarily in terms of content, so that the book will read stylistically differently from a conventional translation. Springer Nature works continuously to further the development of tools for the production of books and on the related technologies to support the authors.

This Springer imprint is published by the registered company Springer-Verlag GmbH, DE, part of Springer Nature.
The registered company address is: Heidelberger Platz 3, 14197 Berlin, Germany

Contents

List of Editors and Authors

About the Editors

Heike Becker, M.A., Dipl.-Soc. Ped. UAS Heike Becker is a pharmaceutical-technical assistant (PTA), holds a diploma in social pedagogy (FH), a Master of Arts, is a lecturer for special assignments at the University of Applied Sciences Düsseldorf, as well as a research associate and doctoral candidate at the University of Witten/Herdecke. From 2011 to 2022, she worked as a research associate in the practice office at the University of Applied Sciences Düsseldorf; in addition, since 2019 she has been working as a research associate at the University of Witten/Herdecke. Since 2023, she has also been a lecturer for special assignments at the University of Applied Sciences Düsseldorf. Her areas of focus are: methods of social work with an emphasis on multiprofessional approaches in innovative senior citizen work and social medicine.

Manfred Fiedler, Dipl. rer. soc. Manfred Fiedler is a research associate at the Department of Human Medicine at Witten/Herdecke University. For years, he has been conducting research and teaching with a focus on multiprofessional care for people with dementia and chronic impairments. He holds a degree in social sciences with specializations in health economics, business administration, and social policy. For a long time, he worked in management positions in various contexts within associations and healthcare organizations, especially hospitals. His professional focus therefore lies in interdisciplinary teaching, as well as in interprofessional collaboration in healthcare and, finally, in the transfer between science and practice.

Simone Hatebur, M.Sc. Simone Hatebur is an orthoptist and has worked in both inpatient and outpatient settings. She studied interprofessional healthcare as well as health services research and implementation sciences (M.Sc.). She then gained experience in quality and risk management at a tertiary care hospital. Since 2021, she has been a research associate at the Junior Professorship for Digital and Innovative Teaching and Learning Methods in Multiprofessional Healthcare, as well as a doctoral candidate at the Chair for the Development of Personal and Interpersonal Competencies in Healthcare at Witten/Herdecke University. Her areas of focus are: (medical) communication, multiprofessional collaboration between health and non-health professions, and patient empowerment.

Jan-Hendrik Ortloff, M.A. Jan-Hendrik Ortloff is an occupational therapist and specialist therapist for dementia with many years of practical experience in advising and supporting people with chronic illnesses in the clinical specialties of geriatrics and psychiatry. Since 2018, he has been a lecturer at DIPLOMA University of Applied Sciences, focusing on conceptual health promotion and prevention, clinical reasoning, and evidence-based practice. Since 2021, he has also been working as a research associate at the University of Witten/Herdecke in the interprofessional education and competency development of health professions. As part of a research project funded by the Federal Ministry of Education and Research, he is pursuing a doctorate on the influencing factors of new didactic teaching and learning concepts for the inclusion of complementary medicine.

Jun.-Prof. Dr. Phil Daniela Schmitz, Dipl.-Ped. Daniela Schmitz studied for a diploma in Educational Science with a focus on Social Pedagogy and earned her doctorate at TU Dortmund in the Faculty of Educational Science and Sociology on images of aging in intergenerational knowledge transfer. Alongside her doctoral studies, she worked as a research associate at TU Dortmund, initially in technology didactics and later in higher education didactics. After completing her doctorate, she moved to the Chair of Multiprofessional Care for the Chronically Ill at the Faculty of Health, UW/H, as a research associate. Since 2021, she has held a junior professorship for Innovative and Digital Teaching and Learning Methods in Multiprofessional Health Care, Faculty of Health, Department of Human Medicine, Witten/Herdecke University. She leads the master's program "Multiprofessional Care for People with Dementia and Chronic Impairments." Her main areas of work include multiprofessional teaching and learning, strategies for establishing common ground in multiprofessional learning groups, as well as the possibilities and limitations of digital learning in this field.

About the Authors

Dr. Galia Assadi Galia Assadi studied Social Work and Sociology and earned her doctorate in Philosophy on the modern concept of responsibility. She is a research associate at the Evangelische Hochschule Nürnberg, and her research areas are in medical ethics as well as the ethics of human-technology relations.

Kirsten Balcerzak, B.Sc., M.Sc. Kirsten Balcerzak holds a bachelor's degree in social sciences and a master's degree in clinical gerontopsychology. She works in the social services department of a psychiatric hospital and has completed further training as a systemic counselor (SG-certified) alongside her job. As part of a self-help group, she volunteers to support relatives of people with dementia.

Dr. Heike Baranzke Heike Baranzke is an ethicist and Catholic theologian at the University of Wuppertal. From 2016 to 2019, together with Dr. Helen Güther, she developed, coordinated, and researched the DFG-funded project "Habitus in Long-Term Residential Care for People with Dementia" (HALT).

Dr. med. dent. Korbinian Benz, MHBA He is a specialist in oral surgery working in private dental practice, a faculty member at the Faculty of Health at Witten/Herdecke University, and part of the Department of Dental Surgery and Outpatient Clinic (Head: Univ.-Prof. Dr. Jochen Jackowski) at the Department of Dental, Oral, and Maxillofacial Medicine. His clinical and scientific work focuses on oral surgical and oral medical care for patients with complex systemic diseases and patients with rare diseases.

Prof. Dr. phil. Christian Bleck Christian Bleck holds a degree in social work and is a professor of social work science at the University of Applied Sciences Düsseldorf. He is co-founder and spokesperson of the specialist group "Social Work in Contexts of Aging" of the German Association for Social Work. His main areas of work include: social work with older people; community-based approaches and the promotion of participation in elderly care; community-based action research, evaluation, and impact research in social work.

Prof. Dr. PH Patrick Brzoska, MSc, EMPH Patrick Brzoska holds the Chair of Health Services Research at the Faculty of Health at Witten/Herdecke University. His main areas of research and teaching include managing diversity in healthcare, rehabilitation research, international public health, epidemiology, and quantitative research methods.

Dr. rer. medic. Theresa Sophie, RN Theresa Sophie Busse is a health scientist employed in the Department of General Medicine, Faculty of Medicine, at Ruhr University Bochum. Her research focuses on the intersection of digitalization and palliative care, with an emphasis on participatory development.

Dipl.-Des. Diana Cürlis Diana Cürlis is a design researcher working in the context of social design and societal issues. Her current focus is on participatory design with people with cognitive impairments.

Prof. Dr. Wolfgang Deiters Wolfgang Deiters holds a professorship in Health Technologies at the University of Applied Sciences for Health in Bochum. There, he has, among other things, co-initiated a degree program on health data and digitalization. In addition, he is involved part-time at the Fraunhofer ISST in Dortmund.

Daniel Diehl Daniel Diehl is a senior physician at the Department of Periodontology and a postdoctoral researcher at the Department of Pharmacology at Witten/Herdecke University, where he teaches geriatric dentistry, periodontology, and pharmacology, among other subjects. His research focuses on post-translational modifications in inflammatory diseases.

Christine Dunger, Ph.D. Christine Dunger is Deputy Program Director of the Ph.D. Nursing & Allied Health Sciences at the Institute of Nursing Science and Practice at Paracelsus Medical University Salzburg and a research associate at the Chair of Social Philosophy and Ethics in Health Care at Witten/Herdecke University.

Dr. Helen Güther Helen Güther is a remedial teacher, health and nursing scientist. She earned her doctorate at the Chair of Gerontological Nursing (PTHV) and, together with Dr. Heike Baranzke, developed, coordinated, and researched the DFG-funded project "Habitus in Long-Term Institutional Care of People with Dementia" (HALT). Since 2018, she has been working as a research associate in the degree program "Multiprofessional Care for People with Dementia and Chronic Impairments" at UW/H.

Dr. med. Martin Haas Martin Haas is Director of the Medical Clinic at Klinikum Westfalen, Lütgendortmund location. Specialist in Internal Medicine, Geriatrics, and Diabetology. Chief Physician of the Geriatric Department, Head of Geriatric Traumatology with 3 certified trauma surgery departments.

Jun.-Prof. Dr. Dennis Häckl Dennis Häckl is Junior Professor of Health Economics and Management at the Faculty of Economics and Management Science at Leipzig University, as well as founder and director of the WIG2 Institute in Leipzig. He earned his doctorate at HHL Leipzig Graduate School of Management and subsequently conducted research and taught at the Technical University of Dresden. His research focuses on the financing of healthcare systems and the economic significance of lifestyle diseases.

Patrizia Held, M. Sc. Patrizia Held is a research associate at the Institute for People, Technology and Participation at Furtwangen University, with a background in health sciences. Her research focuses on the use of technology in nursing as well as user-oriented and participatory research.

Prof. Dr. Felix Hoffmann Felix Hoffmann is the initiator and chairman of the Purpose:Health e.V. network. After completing his specialist training in orthopedics and trauma surgery, he shifted his professional focus and has been working for several years in corporate development at various hospitals. He is currently a Professor of Digital Health at APOLLON University in Bremen.

Prof. Dr. Ulrike Höhmann, Ulrike Höhmann, Witten/Herdecke University, Faculty of Health, until 2020 Chair of Multiprofessional Care for People with Chronic Illnesses. Research and expertise since 1993: care-related and multiprofessional care concepts for people with chronic illnesses, professionalization of nursing and health professions, personnel and organizational development in healthcare institutions, participatory practice development, policy consulting.

Univ.-Prof. Dr. med. dent. Jochen Jackowski He is a specialist dentist in oral surgery, holds a chair, and is head of the Department of Dental Surgery and Outpatient Clinic at the Department of Dental, Oral, and Maxillofacial Medicine of the Faculty of Health at

Witten/Herdecke University. The focus of his clinical and scientific work is the oral surgical and oral medical care of patients with complex systemic diseases (acute or chronic) and patients with rare diseases.

Prof. Dr. med. Detmar Jobst Detmar Jobst is a lecturer at the Chair of General Medicine I and Interprofessional Care at the Institute of General Medicine and Outpatient Health Care at Witten/Herdecke University.

Dr.-Ing. Julia Kirch In her practice-based postdoc, Julia Kirch combines practical experience and research in hospital construction. In this capacity, she works at the architecture firm alsh sander.hofrichter architekten and at the Frankfurt University of Applied Sciences. Before leading corporate communications at alsh architekten, she completed her doctorate at TU Dresden on dementia-sensitive hospital architecture.

Prof. Christiane Knecht, Ph.D. Christiane Knecht is a Professor of Acute Care Nursing at FH Münster, a registered nurse, and a nursing scientist. After completing her diploma and master's studies, she earned her doctorate at the research college "Family Health Across the Life Course" at Witten/Herdecke University. Following an interim professorship there, she became a professor at the Protestant University of Applied Sciences Bochum RWL. Her research focuses include family-centered care, acute care, and advanced nursing practice.

Hans Lemke Physician specializing in trauma surgery, emergency, and intensive care medicine. Chief physician of the Center for Severe Burn Injuries and the Central Emergency Department at the supraregional trauma center of Klinikum Dortmund. At the same time, for over 20 years, medical director of the emergency medical services of the city of Dortmund and spokesperson for the Federal Association of Medical Directors of Emergency Services (ÄLRD e.V.) on the TraumaNetwork Advisory Board of the DGU. Retired since 01.07.2020.

Ulrike Lindwedel, M.Sc. Ulrike Lindwedel is a research associate at the Institute for People, Technology and Participation at Furtwangen University. She is a nursing and health scientist. Her research focuses on the use of technology in nursing as well as the care of people with dementia in both national and international contexts.

Prof. Dr. theol. habil. Arne Manzeschke Arne Manzeschke has been Professor of Anthropology and Ethics for Health Professions at the Protestant University of Nuremberg since 2012. In 2012, he led the BMBF project MEESTAR; from 2017 to 2020, he was head of the project "ComplexEthics—Ethical Orientation in Complex Digital Worlds" (funded by the BMBF), and from 2021 to 2024, he has led the subcluster 'Digitalized Living Environments' within the BMBF-funded cluster "Integrated Research".

Prof. Dr. Sven Meister Sven Meister holds the Chair of Health Informatics at Witten/Herdecke University. He is also affiliated with the Fraunhofer ISST, Department of Healthcare. He serves on the advisory board of various health start-ups and is a board member of several health-related associations.

Prof. Dr. oec. troph. Eva Münster, MPH postgraduate. Eva Münster holds the Chair of General Practice Health Services Research in Vulnerable Population Groups at the Department of General Practice I and Interprofessional Care, Institute of General Practice and Outpatient Health Care at the University of Witten/Herdecke.

Prof. Dr. sc. med. Ina Carola Otte Ina Carola Otte is a health services researcher with an academic background in sociology and medical ethics. As part of her junior professorship in health services research at the Department of General Practice at Ruhr University Bochum, she is particularly interested in the potential of digital innovations for the health and autonomy of older adults.

Prof. Dr. Ulrike Pfannes She studied and earned her doctorate at the University of Giessen in the field of Household and Nutritional Sciences. She subsequently held management positions in various social institutions. Since 2007, she has been teaching and conducting research at the Hamburg University of Applied Sciences in the field of Supply and Catering.

Dr. Beate Radzey The PhD home economist heads the LANDaufwärts business unit at Vinzenz von Paul gGmbH. For many years, she has been engaged with the support potential of technical aids and assistance systems, particularly in supporting people with dementia.

Prof. Dr.-Ing. Dr. rer. medic. Peter Rasche He is Professor of Digital Health at the Niederrhein University of Applied Sciences. His research focuses on the digital transformation of healthcare, with an emphasis on mobile devices.

Prof. Dr. Lisa Schmidt Lisa Schmidt is a registered nurse, holds a diploma in nursing management, and an M.Sc. in Public Health. In 2022, she earned her doctorate at the Philosophical-Theological University of Vallendar with a dissertation on metaphorical concepts of geriatric nurses in the field of nursing science. Since 2012, she has been involved in a variety of nursing-related research projects and currently holds an interim professorship at the Frankfurt University of Applied Sciences.

Tobias Schäffer, M.Sc. He is a research associate and doctoral candidate at the Chair of Health Economics and Management at the University of Leipzig and has several years of experience in health policy consulting. He is currently conducting research on data-driven, objective measurement of quality of life.

Prof. Dr. Pirjo Susanne She studied and earned her doctorate in Oecotrophology with a focus on Household Science at the University of Giessen. Since 2012, she has been teaching and conducting research at the FH Münster and heads the Competence Center for Household Science. Her main areas of focus are household-related services and sustainability in social institutions.

Prof. Carolin Schreiber She is a graduate designer and professor at the Münster School of Design, among other roles, specializing in Social (Product) Design. As a visiting professor at the Folkwang University of the Arts in Essen, she was, among other things, responsible for the design-scientific direction of the project "Dementia Things."

Kirstin Schütz, M.A. She is a health scientist specializing in multiprofessional care for people with dementia and chronic impairments. Among other roles, she works in the areas of social law consulting and project coordination at the regional association of the German Rheumatism League NRW e.V.

Jun.-Prof. Dr. Michaela Stratmann She is a psychologist specializing in interprofessional and collaborative didactics in medical and health professions at the Faculty of Health, Department of Human Medicine, Witten/Herdecke University. Her research focuses on the development of professional identity in the context of interprofessional practice requirements, decision-making in the selection processes for human medicine, psychology, and dentistry, as well as the digital transformation in the health sciences.

PD Dr. Christine Thomas She is a neurologist, psychiatrist, and geriatrician, and completed her habilitation on delirium and dementia at the University of Münster in the field of psychiatry and psychotherapy. Since April 2014, she has been the medical director of the Clinic for Psychiatry and Psychotherapy for the Elderly at Klinikum Stuttgart and teaches in Tübingen., She is actively involved on the board of the European Delirium Association and the German Society for Gerontopsychiatry and Psychotherapy, and, together with Prof. G. Eschweiler, Tübingen, successfully conducted the largest European delirium prevention study (PAWEL).

Prof. Dr. med. Horst Christian Vollmar, MPH He heads the Department of General Practice (AM RUB) at Ruhr University Bochum. His research focuses on the digital transformation of healthcare, age-related diseases such as dementia, as well as implementation and health services research.

Prof. Dr. med. Klaus Weckbecker He is the holder of the Chair of General Medicine I and Interprofessional Care at the Institute of General Medicine and Outpatient Health Care at the University of Witten/Herdecke (Director).

Prof. Dr. Werner Vogd He is Professor of Sociology at the Faculty of Health at Witten/Herdecke University. His main areas of focus include: systems theory and reconstructive social research, organization and decision-making processes, hospital research, and sociological perspectives on (psycho-)therapy.

Univ.-Prof. Dr. Frank Weidner He is the acting head of the Institute for Nursing Science at the University of Koblenz and Director of the German Institute for Applied Nursing Research (DIP) in Cologne.

Sarah Weller, B.A., M.Sc. She is a social worker (B.A.) and gerontologist (M.Sc.) at Klinikum Stuttgart, Clinic for Psychiatry and Psychotherapy for the Elderly. She has many years of experience in social psychiatry through direct contact with patients and relatives, as well as extensive expertise in the fields of health and mental illness in old age, as well as delirium and quality of life, which she explored in greater depth in her recently submitted dissertation at Heidelberg University.

Dr. PH Yüce Yilmaz-Aslan, Dipl.-Soc., Dipl.-Ed. She is a research associate at the Chair of Health Services Research in the Faculty of Health at Witten/Herdecke University. Her research and teaching focus on the areas of diversity and health, chronic diseases, nursing and rehabilitation, as well as qualitative research methods.

Part I

Introduction

1 Why a Handbook on Chronic Care?

Daniela Schmitz, Manfred Fiedler, Heike Becker,
Simone Hatebur and Jan-Hendrik Ortloff

Contents

1.1 Idea and Background of the Handbook

Dear readers, we are pleased that you have picked up this book. The idea for this book—to present, for the first time, the fundamentals of care for people with chronic diseases in a comprehensive, multi-perspective manner—arose from our teaching and research

D. Schmitz (✉) · M. Fiedler · J.-H. Ortloff
Department of human medicine, Witten/Herdecke University, Witten, Germany
e-mail: daniela.schmitz@uni-wh.de

M. Fiedler
e-mail: manfred.fiedler@uni-wh.de

J.-H Ortloff
e-mail: jan-hendrik.ortloff@uni-wh.de

H. Becker · S. Hatebur
Faculty of Health, Witten/Herdecke University, Witten, Germany
e-mail: heike.becker@uni-wh.de

S. Hatebur
e-mail: simone.hatebur@uni-wh.de

D. Schmitz et al. (eds.), *Chronic Care—Science and Practice*,
https://doi.org/10.1007/978-3-662-72298-5_1

practice. The term "Chronic Care," which cannot be adequately translated into German, is best described as follows: *chronic* refers to the care of chronically ill, often multimorbid elderly people and all the resulting tasks and consequences of appropriate care; *care* highlights that different professional groups are addressed, each contributing their knowledge and skills accordingly.

In higher education, our team—composed of various disciplines—has gathered many years of experience in the care of chronically ill people and in multiprofessional learning groups, experiencing the manifold added value of joint learning and perspective shifts. Research, too, demonstrates the necessity of thinking beyond one's own discipline. These experiences contributed to the idea of considering and publishing care issues in a transdisciplinary way.

The content focus of the handbook therefore encompasses the challenges of caring for people with chronic illnesses from inter-institutional and transdisciplinary perspectives, seeking to integrate and discuss solution approaches from individual disciplines across sectors in a solution-oriented manner. Every professional group involved in the care process will thus find points of connection beyond their own disciplinary knowledge—on the one hand as a science-based field of practice, and on the other as a practice-oriented field of health services research. Thus, it is not only health professions that are addressed, but also non-health professions working in contexts where they help shape the political, legal, economic, and other framework conditions of care.

1.2 Chronic Care and Societal Development Trends

Chronic diseases are and will remain the challenge of our healthcare system. This is due, on the one hand, to the continuously increasing life expectancy of the population and, on the other, to advances in diagnostic and therapeutic capabilities within the health system. For the individual, this means that more or less long phases of life are influenced by one or more persistent illnesses, which affect the ability to manage daily activities and experiences to varying degrees. To enable those affected to participate in all areas of society, a more comprehensive understanding of illness is required—one that goes beyond an organ-centered perspective to include social and environmental factors. In addition, preventive measures are being used to minimize comorbidities and secondary diseases and to strengthen resilience (see contribution 18). All of this is provided by various professional groups, which, however, are increasingly shrinking due to a declining pool of skilled workers in care. In medicine and nursing in particular, about half of the current workforce is over 50 years old. In contrast, there is a growing number of chronically ill and care-dependent people with complex needs, who are multimorbid and/or have complicating secondary diagnoses. Current statistics on this can be found in the Federal Health Reporting Information System (GBE) of the Federal Statistical Office.

The Covid-19 pandemic has also highlighted further perspectives and desiderata in the care of people with chronic illnesses. From the perspective of those affected, these include new chronic impairments such as Long Covid or the increase in mental health disorders. Furthermore, the pandemic revealed an undersupply of care for chronic conditions or acute illnesses with the potential to become chronic. In times of societal crisis and beyond, it is therefore especially important to consider people with chronic illnesses in healthcare provision.

1.3 Objectives and Target Audience of this Handbook

As editors, our aim is to bring together multidisciplinary approaches to the care of people with chronic diseases—beyond monodisciplinary boundaries—in a single handbook, thereby providing insights into the scientific foundations and practical issues of caring for people with chronic diseases. The goal is to consider both practical perspectives and to classify and make them manageable from a scientific standpoint. This handbook also establishes a shared knowledge base for the professional groups involved in care, which can serve as a foundation for collaboration and mutual understanding. The underlying objective is to ensure compatibility for all disciplines directly and indirectly involved in care and care design.

The target audience is therefore broad and open—essentially anyone who wishes to contribute to Chronic Care, in both science and practice: researchers, teachers, and learners in the field of Chronic Care Sciences and its related disciplines, such as medicine, nursing science, therapy sciences, as well as other related fields like social work, sociology, psychology, law, political science, business, and cultural studies, and finally, practitioners involved in the care and care planning for people with chronic diseases.

The increasing importance of chronic conditions for the design of healthcare requires, on the one hand, a cross-disciplinary perspective and, on the other, a multiprofessional context for care provision to people with chronic limitations. The significance of chronic diseases lies in their relevance to everyday life, which determines both the design dimension of care services and direct practical interventions. The life-world or everyday relevance of Chronic Care calls for the strengthening of inter-institutional and interprofessional cooperation. The structuring perspectives underlying this handbook serve as points of reference for the various target groups: first, the individual level; second, the organizational level; and third, a societal perspective (explanations of these levels can be found in contribution 02). Due to the handbook can be used as a subject-specific book with content that builds on itself. The strictly modular structure allows it to be used as a reference work for practice and as an interdisciplinary textbook to support teaching and learning. Depending on the context, different terms are used in the handbook—for example, "patients" in medical contexts, "clients" in advisory settings, and "service recipients" in contexts with an economic focus. For orientation in transdisciplinary fields, correct use of terminology is essential and helps readers to properly classify phenomena.

1.4 Brief Overview of the Handbook's Contributions

The handbook is divided into five main sections: introductory contributions, contributions from the action level of individuals, contributions from the perspective of service-providing organizations, contributions on the system level, and concluding contributions on aspects of the implementation of chronic care.

At the outset, the four introductory contributions examine chronic care from the perspectives of science, research, teaching, and practice. First, the term is defined in more detail and distinguished from related concepts. Building on this, transdisciplinary approaches are explained and requirements for multiprofessional collaboration are highlighted.

The first substantive focus is on the individual level, which is divided into medical, theoretical, and conceptual approaches to care from the perspective of the affected person and their relatives. Fundamental knowledge about the development, causes, course, and impact of chronic diseases is presented from a medical perspective. Theoretical references are drawn from key related disciplines and provide sociological, social science, psychological, and environmental explanations for living with chronic diseases. Practical concepts also originate from various related disciplines and offer practical guidance for person- and patient-centered care, for example from a technical perspective.

The organizational level, as the second substantive focus, brings together fundamental aspects from the perspective of care-providing organizations. In addition to questions of migration and cultural sensitivity, structural aspects of segmented care and the resulting interfaces play a role. This is followed by contributions addressing issues of institutional forms of care, which cover the development of personnel, competencies, knowledge, and the organization itself, as well as digital processes. Ultimately, perspectives on self-determined living are included, exploring how this is possible with chronic diseases and how it can be supportively accompanied.

The third substantive focus is the system level. This section first addresses the social law and health policy framework conditions and explains economic aspects of the organization of the healthcare system. Furthermore, approaches to public health care and community health care are presented with regard to the care of people with chronic diseases. This perspective is rounded off by insights into the field of digital health as a social innovation. The three concluding contributions of the handbook deal with guidance on the implementation of chronic care in teaching, research, and practice. Fixed terms and functional titles, where the gender of the person is not the focus, are excluded from gendering for the sake of clarity.

What is Chronic Care? Perspectives from Science, Research, Teaching, and Practice

2

Manfred Fiedler, Simone Hatebur and Daniela Schmitz

Contents

2.1 On the Concept of Care

The Latin word *curare* is the root for both the English word *cure* (to heal) and *care* (to care for, to look after). With this etymological background, the concept of care can be professionally assigned to healthcare, although in the form of care work it is also significant in other fields of social support and provision.

In German translation, it is often rendered as *pflegen* (to nurse), although the German term *Pflege* in contemporary health-related usage is mostly associated with the nursing profession and thus with nursing-specific activities, which does not do justice to the

M. Fiedler (✉) · D. Schmitz
Department of human medicine, Witten/Herdecke University, Witten, Germany
e-mail: manfred.fiedler@uni-wh.de

D. Schmitz
e-mail: daniela.schmitz@uni-wh.de

S. Hatebur
Faculty of Health, Witten/Herdecke University, Witten, Germany
e-mail: simone.hatebur@uni-wh.de

D. Schmitz et al. (eds.), *Chronic Care—Science and Practice*,
https://doi.org/10.1007/978-3-662-72298-5_2

actual meaning of the term care. In the English-speaking context, there is a technical distinction between *Care* as a comprehensive, and in this sense, cross-disciplinary and thus multiprofessional concept of healthcare, whereas *Nursing* is understood as a nursing-specific concept of healthcare.

This becomes clear in the differentiation between *Public Health Care* and *Public Health Nursing* (see contribution 48). While the former emerged in Germany as early as the mid-19th century as public health care—a population-based applied science for safeguarding health, particularly in the context of communicable diseases—Public Health Nursing developed around 1900 in the USA as a nursing-led concept to ensure healthcare provision for underserved population groups or neighborhoods.

In German, the term Pflege (nursing/care) is marked by linguistic ambiguities regarding the scope of the subject of care. Therefore, the term care is used for general healthcare concepts to express an understanding of concepts and methods of (health) care that is both interprofessional in practice and interdisciplinary in teaching and research.

2.2 Chronic Care—Conceptual Approaches and Definitions

Chronic care refers to the comprehensive care of individuals with persistent physical, mental, or psychological impairments or risks that may lead to a long-term need for help and support. It encompasses all aspects of care, from disease prevention, treatment, health maintenance and restoration, to everyday support and care, as well as ensuring participation and (re-)inclusion.

When a condition is referred to as a *chronic disease*, the definition is not as clear-cut in professional discourse as everyday language might suggest, making a conceptual classification necessary. The following section will therefore explicate and discuss contextual factors associated with chronic illness or impairment.

- Permanence—Incurability

One of the seemingly clearest characteristics of a chronic disease is the criterion of permanence, usually linked to incurability. In this sense, we speak of a chronic disease when it is incurable and thus has a lifelong course. However, this perspective becomes blurred in the case of acute illnesses that lead to death within a short to medium period in a clinical context or shortly thereafter. Therefore, permanence is often described as a minimum duration of three or six months that a disease must last. This also limits the criterion of incurability, as long-lasting but curable diseases are also defined as such. Conversely, lifelong, incurable conditions are sometimes not considered chronic, such as people with visual impairments who, apart from adjusting their visual aids, require no care services for much of the course of their condition.

- Restriction of daily living—Need for assistance—Need for care

A particular contextual factor of a disease is the illness-related restriction of daily living, which leads to the need for support services, either from informal caregivers (such as family members) or professional staff, as well as material support. This aspect is reflected in long-term nursing care, which is legally defined as the need for care.

- Progressive course—Life-limiting

An important factor is the course of a disease. We speak of a progressive course when the severity of the disease and the associated limitations increase over the life course. This is generally, though not necessarily, associated with being life-limiting. This means that a disease directly or as a consequence shortens the life expectancy of the affected person compared to those without the disease. The disease itself may be the cause of death, or death may result from limitations caused by the disease.

- Therapeutic—Interventional Interaction

Chronic diseases affect both the effectiveness and feasibility of therapies and interventions. For example, people at risk of thrombosis are particularly vulnerable during surgical procedures, as they must discontinue anticoagulants preoperatively, resulting in an increased risk of complications during this period, especially intraoperatively. Osteoarthritis, as a degenerative, wear-related joint disease, can lead to chronic pain, making therapeutic exercise and gait training more difficult. In acute as well as other persistent diseases, interventions can also interact, reinforce, diminish, or produce various known and unknown side effects.

- Comorbidities—Secondary diseases—Multimorbidity

On this basis, chronic diseases can be understood as comorbidities in the presence of other diseases, which, even independently of treatment, affect the manifestation in terms of disease probability (prevalence), severity, consequences, and coping. An example is dementia, which affects both the treatment and coping with other diseases.

Of particular importance are secondary diseases that arise from the limitations of a chronic illness, but can also result directly or indirectly from trauma or an acute illness. Examples include post-traumatic stress disorder or chronic wounds in people with diabetes mellitus.

Consequently, we speak of people with multiple chronic conditions (multimorbidity), which influences and complicates both the treatment and management of the various diseases.

- Risk factor model

Risk factors are of outstanding importance both for the development (see contribution 07) and for the influence and management of chronic diseases. For a wide range of chronic diseases, risk factor models have been developed that can be described as disease-categorical risk models. At their core, three general factors can be identified:

- Health behavior, which manifests as lifestyle in the form of ingrained habits or socially conditioned behaviors. Especially with regard to prevention and coping, health literacy as well as intellectual, mental, cognitive, and physical abilities are of paramount importance in this context.
- Living environment conditions or circumstances in which a person grows up and lives are decisive factors, which can also form the basis for health behavior.
- Genetic predisposition increases the likelihood of developing a disease. A related concept is that of familial predisposition, i.e., the clustering of diseases within a family relationship, which may be genetically determined or due to family-learned behaviors that are passed on to growing family members.

An overarching concept of a complex risk factor model is that of the social determinants of health (see contribution 16). A related concept with significant overlaps is the concept of disability, which primarily refers to the social, physical, mental, and psychological limitations of participation in social institutions in the broadest sense. Here, too, a distinction can be made between congenital and acquired disabilities over the life course.

- Social and everyday life contexts

Chronic diseases are not only influenced by the social and everyday life contexts of those affected, but also influence these contexts in turn. This is particularly true in three areas of action:

- Chronic diseases are a family matter. They affect family life, relationships, and stability within the family and among relatives, as well as the quality and intensity of family members' external relationships.
- The living environment responds very differently to chronic diseases. It can respond with care and support, but also with stigmatization and rejection.
- The world of *labor* can be a cause of illness in the form of work-related diseases. Conversely, a chronic illness restricts access to the labor market. Thus, a chronic disease always has the potential for exclusion from *professional* life.

2.3 Care Setting and Care Arrangement in Chronic Diseases

The diversity of phenomena associated with chronic diseases points to the variety of institutional contexts in which the care of people with chronic illnesses takes place. In this context, we refer to *care settings*, which relates to the institutional and contextual framework of care. It is described as:

- the institutional space of care, that is, whether care takes place in an outpatient or inpatient facility, or, for example, in the home of people with chronic illnesses,
- the facility's relation to the reason for care, that is, whether it is an acute care facility or a long-term care facility,
- finally, the professional-institutional context of care, whether care is provided in an intensive care facility or in an emergency care facility (see Contribution 23).

Specifying the care setting is a prerequisite for care design. This refers to the organization of care with reference to a particular care setting. Typically, we refer to this as a care arrangement. At times, this term is seen as a broader concept compared to the care arrangement, because in the context of care research and practice, it encompasses not only the organization of direct nursing services but also medical, therapeutic, domestic, or other everyday support services. However, arrangements of nursing can often also form the basis of a care arrangement, from which other services are defined and the integration of other professions is carried out.

In the context of chronic care, however, we refer to the conceptual understanding of the care arrangement, since in practice this always includes the concept of the arrangement of nursing, but fundamentally also addresses the various service relationships relevant to people with chronic illnesses. In addition, it enables a scientific, cross-disciplinary comparison of perspectives on the design of person-centered care.

With regard to care arrangements, the classic questions arise: who, where, what, why, and how. We translate these questions into three perspectives: those of the actors involved in care; the goals of care; and, finally, care planning.

Basically, three groups of participants can be distinguished. On the one hand, there are the people affected by illness and their relatives, and on the other, the professionals directly and indirectly involved in care. This distinction is fundamentally important because a continuous negotiation process regarding the care arrangement must be organized between these three groups throughout the care process.

The subject of this negotiation process is the goals of care, that is, the question of the desired outcomes of care, which are reflected in forms of care such as prevention, rehabilitation, quality of life, but also end-of-life care. Finally, the negotiation processes among the participants in the care arrangement also include care planning, as is particularly evident in consultative and supportive health planning (advance care planning), especially for people in existential phases of life.

Further Reading

Güthlin C, Köhler S, Dieckelmann M (2020) Chronisch krank sein in Deutschland: Zahlen Fakten und Versorgungserfahrungen. Robert-Bosch-Stiftung, Institut für Allgemeinmedizin der Goethe-Universität Frankfurt am Main. http://publikationen.ub.uni-frankfurt.de/frontdoor/index/index/docId/55045. Accessed 21. Juli 2023

Hackmann T, Huschik G, Maetzel J, Schmutz S, Sulzer L, Vollmer J (2018) Pflege- und Unterstützungsbedarf sogenannter vulnerabler Gruppen: Schlussbericht. https://www.prognos.com/sites/default/files/2021-01/vulnerable_gruppen_schlussbericht_final_2018_04_26.pdf. Zugegriffen am 21. Juli 2023

Transdisciplinarity—Chronic Care as a Transdiscipline

3

Manfred Fiedler and Daniela Schmitz

Contents

3.1 Background—Problem Statement

For more than half a century, there has been a general scientific discussion about interdisciplinarity and transdisciplinarity. Contrary to what one might expect, the starting point of this discussion was not the humanities, but rather the natural sciences, which, particularly in light of the emerging sustainability debate, began to focus on the limitations of monodisciplinary perspectives. Historically, scientific disciplines have differentiated themselves, evolving from universal scholarship, or polyhistory—which, through Leibniz, acquired universal scientific thought structures and fundamental principles—

M. Fiedler (✉) · D. Schmitz
Department of human medicine, Witten/Herdecke University, Witten, Germany
e-mail: manfred.fiedler@uni-wh.de

D. Schmitz
e-mail: daniela.schmitz@uni-wh.de

D. Schmitz et al. (eds.), *Chronic Care—Science and Practice*,
https://doi.org/10.1007/978-3-662-72298-5_3

into a multitude of individual disciplines, each with its own methods and theoretical foundations, yet all directed at a scientific subject. The current discussion on interdisciplinarity and transdisciplinarity does not represent a return to universal science, but rather accepts the significance of each discipline and seeks to overcome or supplement the disciplinary perspective in the face of increasingly complex questions.

The conceptual understanding remains inconsistent, with regard to the definition of the terms, their practical scientific significance, and their distinction from inter- and multiprofessionality, which are sometimes used synonymously (see Contribution 04). Understandably, this is especially true where primary qualifying degree programs also serve as a source of professional identity. The health sciences in particular are increasingly confronted with complex issues that can no longer be addressed monodisciplinarily. This is especially evident in the field of chronic diseases. The following will therefore clarify the understanding and various references for teaching and research, concluding with a reference to the science and practice of chronic care.

3.2 On the Terminology of Disciplinarity

Historically, the emergence of scientific disciplines and fields of study is due to differentiation, separation, and thus specialization. Based on Defila and Di Giulio (1998), five characteristics of disciplines can be identified:

1. a relatively uniform language within an identity-forming scientific group,
2. shared theories and a common body of knowledge,
3. recognized research questions or a relevant domain of knowledge acquisition,
4. a unified set of methods and methodological forms for problem-solving and resolution, and finally
5. a specifically structured career path as access to the respective scientific community.

The term *disciplinarity* itself concerns the organization of fields of study. It involves both the classification of disciplines and their structure and relationships, as well as their boundaries and interfaces with one another. The suffixes 'mono', 'multi', or 'inter' thus express the internal organization (especially the degree of closure or openness of subject matter, methods, and theories to other disciplines) and the external relationships between scientific fields. As early as the 1970s, Jantsch (1970) presented a comprehensive concept of disciplinary classification, which we will refer to below.

(Mono-)disciplinarity refers to the isolated development of a field without substantive or methodological reference to other fields, with an increasing degree of specialization.

Multidisciplinarity refers to addressing a question from different disciplines without cooperation, i.e., the problem or question is addressed exclusively monodisciplinarily in each case, without cross-disciplinary exchange. Research and publications consider a question from, for example, an economic, medical, or nursing science perspective, without a shared comparison of perspectives.

In *pluridisciplinarity*, such cooperation does occur, but it is situational and not structured. Connections between the individual disciplines are established, but ultimately remain uncoordinated in terms of problem-solving competence and thus revert to the perspective of each respective discipline. An example of this is pluralist economics.

Interdisciplinarity is understood as the disciplinary, equally weighted, temporary, problem-centered approach to a question. This requires agreement on the forms and content of collaboration and a shared understanding of the issue to be solved that integrates the individual disciplines. This includes, for example, research projects conducted by different subject specialists, where the research result is subsequently formulated as a joint outcome.

Between pluridisciplinarity and interdisciplinarity, Jantsch (1970) also identifies what he calls *crossdisciplinarity*, which, in terms of substantive and methodological coordination, features a lead discipline that determines the involvement of cooperating disciplines. It is surprising that this form of disciplinarity has received little attention in later literature, even though the concept of a lead discipline is frequently found in scientific practice and in the transfer between science and practice. In this context, research projects are organized by a lead discipline, and participating disciplines are only involved in a supporting role. The result, however, is evaluated and presented from the perspective of the lead discipline, such as medicine.

The most intensive form of disciplinary relationship is transdisciplinarity, as a comprehensive scientific cooperation and coordination that can lead, through substantive and axiomatic development, to a new, shared paradigmatic understanding. While many authors, in distinguishing between interdisciplinarity and transdisciplinarity, focus primarily on the durability of (interdisciplinary) collaboration, Jantsch, Piaget, and later Luhmann see a new scientific quality that can be understood as a transdiscipline or as a path toward scientific universality.

Behind the above definitions lie very different scientific perspectives on disciplinary collaboration in research and teaching, which will be discussed further below.

3.3 Inter- and Transdisciplinarity as Method

While the aforementioned definitions fundamentally focus on the relationship between disciplines, an important aspect of the discussion centers on transdisciplinarity as a method, whereby the distinction between inter- and transdisciplinarity becomes blurred. At its core, transdisciplinarity as a method in research and teaching is oriented toward the scientific subject area in its real-world manifestation. To use Piaget's words (1972), it is praxeological and seeks to achieve an ideal understanding of the phenomenon itself from a transdisciplinary perspective unrestricted by disciplinary boundaries. According to Defila and Di Giulio (2019), transdisciplinary research as a *practice science* is both participatory and, in particular, transformative, thus going beyond mere knowledge acquisition and positioning itself as both problem- and solution-oriented. Mittelstraß (2005) highlights the argumentative strength of such practical transdisciplinarity, which emulsifies the perspectives of the participating disciplines into a supra-disciplinary view.

There are many fundamental concepts. One significant concept is that of 'Real World Labs', which in Germany are primarily known as 'Reallabore' and in other countries are usually associated with the concept of 'Living Labs'. Research takes place directly in the relevant environment or in the health sector within a related setting, potentially as a permanent research structure. This environment may well be scientifically modified, but it is generally designed so that knowledge acquisition and production always occur participatively, incorporating the perspectives of real-world actors, and are accompanied by the mutual transformation of practice into knowledge and knowledge into practice. Fundamental research approaches can be found in ethnographic methods, in 'Action Research', and other participatory research methods. Related participatory research approaches include Community Based Research or *Practitioner Research* (Wright 2021).

In recent years, interdisciplinary teaching methods have become increasingly established in academic education, initially focusing on reflecting on the shared future field of practice and therefore often defined as interprofessional teaching. These include problem-centered or case-based learning, simulations of setting-specific care processes, or shadowing in the shared field of practice. In addition, inter-/transdisciplinary teaching and learning formats are increasingly being developed, often organized on the basis of 'Problem Based Learning' (PBL). In PBL, complex *real-life* questions are central, but are usually addressed within the protected learning environment of the university/college and, in contrast to real-world labs, tend to address problems more theoretically and without practical transfer. According to Stentoft (2017), characteristics of PBL include self-generated knowledge gain through independent problem-solving, student-centered or student-directed teaching/learning formats, a focus on reflective, critical thinking and construction, as well as learning in cross-disciplinary study groups. The role of instructors shifts toward learning facilitation, which, instead of emphasizing expert knowledge, foregrounds the forms and pathways of knowledge acquisition within the interdisciplinary thinking model, thereby aiming to strengthen students' cognitive abilities for problem analysis and solution.

3.4 Transdisciplinarity as Scientific Competence

Whereas Mittelstraß (2005) sees interdisciplinary competence as a prerequisite for interdisciplinarity or as a long-term cooperation (transdisciplinarity), other authors refer to transdisciplinarity as an individual and also disciplinary competence that enables interdisciplinarity in the first place. Wille (2005) defines transdisciplinarity in this sense as the competence of a discipline to make its own scientific perspectives *rationally comprehensible* beyond disciplinary boundaries in order to solve practical problems that cannot be exhaustively addressed monodisciplinarily. Wille calls for an understanding of general science, by which he primarily means the communication of one's own scientific developments and methods to the scientific community at large, as well as the ongoing disciplinary discourse about goals, procedures, values, and claims to validity.

3.5 Transdisciplinarity as Scientific Structure

The different perspectives on transdisciplinarity respect disciplinary viewpoints, require open forms of cooperation, and distinguish between their intensity, structures, and permanence, as well as the necessary competencies to enable them. They encompass methods in research and teaching, with the boundary between inter- and transdisciplinarity not being clearly defined. According to Jantsch and Piaget, transdisciplinarity is a new scientific quality in which the participating disciplines emulsify and virtually transcend into a new discipline. This new scientific structure does not represent a specialization that becomes independent as a subdiscipline and develops its own structures. Rather, a permanent scientific cooperation focused on a subject area evolves into its own disciplinary field with its own self-concept and perspectives. In addition to shared research questions, this structure is characterized by fundamental properties;

- Methodological plurality: diversity of scientific instruments in research and teaching.
- Plurality of perspectives: the participating disciplines do not disappear, but remain as disciplinary bridgeheads or as subdisciplines.
- Integrative scientific concept as a new paradigm or explanatory approach.

Even though this understanding, with reference to Jantsch, was developed early on, this form of scientific structure actually remains an exception in science. Nevertheless, examples can be found where such a new scientific structure with its own defined subject area exists. One of the oldest fields is ergonomics, which, originating from engineering sciences, has integrated other disciplines such as medicine, business and organizational sociology, and psychology. Another example is gerontology, which, with connections to medicine, social work, psychology, and sociology, among others, has become an independent science.

3.6 Chronic Care as Transdiscipline?

The subject of this handbook is the sciences and practice of chronic care. From a future perspective, they represent a permanent interdisciplinary reference field in terms of problem identification and solution, which at least aims to integrate the various scientific perspectives—and perhaps must do so. In this shared scientific endeavor, the aforementioned aspects of methodological diversity, plurality of perspectives, and also the development of general scientific competencies can be found. Whether this will result in an independent scientific structure in the sense of a transdiscipline remains to be seen. Given the outstanding importance of the subject area and the fact that solutions are ultimately only conceivable in a transdisciplinary way, the foundations have been laid. In this handbook, the multitude of reference sciences and practice disciplines—be it therapy sciences, medicine, nursing science, psychology, but also design, social work, economics, sociology, and many more—are brought together in a conclusive and coherent understanding. They are intended to serve as a basis for a shared cross-disciplinary understanding, for knowledge acquisition, and for problem analysis and solution.

References

Defila R, Di Giulio A (1998) Interdisziplinarität und Disziplinarität. In: Olbertz J-H (Hrsg) Zwischen den Fächern—über den Dingen? VS Verlag für Sozialwissenschaften, Wiesbaden, S 111–137

Defila R, Di Giulio A (2019) Wie Reallabore für Herausforderungen und Expertise in der Gestaltung transdisziplinären und transformativen Forschens sensibilisieren—eine Einführung. In: Defila R, Di Giulio A (Hrsg) Transdisziplinär und transformativ forschen, Bd 2, S 1–30. Heidelberg, Springer VS, Wiesbaden

Jantsch E (1970) Inter- and transdisciplinary university: a systems approach to education and innovation. Policy Sci 1(1):403–428. https://doi.org/10.1007/BF00145222.O

Piaget J (1972) The epistemology of interdisciplinary relationship. In: Organisation for Economic Cooperation and Development, Centre ICBR Educational Research and Innovation (CERI) (Hrsg) Interdisciplinarity: problems of teaching and research in universities. Seminar on interdisciplinarity in universities. Nice, 7th–12th Sept 1970. OECD/CERI

Stentoft D (2017) From saying to doing interdisciplinary learning: is problem-based learning the answer? Act Learn High Educ 18(1):51–61. https://doi.org/10.1177/1469787417693510

Wille R (2005). Allgemeine Wissenschaft und transdisziplinäre Methodologie. Technikfolgenabschätzung—Theorie und Praxis 14(2):57–62

Wright MT (2021) Partizipative Gesundheitsforschung: Ursprünge und heutiger Stand. Bundesgesundheitsbl Gesundheitsforsch Gesundheitsschutz 64(2):140–145. https://doi.org/10.1007/s00103-020-03264-y

Chronic Care as a Multiprofessional Field of Practice with Profession-Specific Approaches

4

Daniela Schmitz, Heike Becker and Manfred Fiedler

Contents

4.1 Understanding Multiprofessional Collaboration

Chronic care requires a cross-professional approach and a shared understanding of tasks and problem-solving strategies. The intensities of cross-professional collaboration are addressed differently and inconsistently in the literature. Here, we address the concept of multiprofessional collaboration. Multiprofessional emphasizes the multitude of professional groups involved and often occurs on a case-by-case basis for specific topics, problems, or care occasions, as well as ad hoc and solution-oriented, aiming to overcome

D. Schmitz (✉) · M. Fiedler
Department of human medicine, Witten/Herdecke University, Witten, Germany
e-mail: daniela.schmitz@uni-wh.de

M. Fiedler
e-mail: manfred.fiedler@uni-wh.de

H. Becker
Faculty of Health, Witten/Herdecke University, Witten, Germany
e-mail: heike.becker@uni-wh.de

D. Schmitz et al. (eds.), *Chronic Care—Science and Practice*,
https://doi.org/10.1007/978-3-662-72298-5_4

institutional or conceptual interfaces (see Contribution 31). In contrast to regular and ongoing interprofessional collaboration (see Contribution 33), which usually takes place within an organization, the professional groups involved in multiprofessional collaboration work alongside and largely independently of each other. Multiprofessionality is a particular form of professionalism and has a different meaning than multidisciplinarity, which refers to the interaction of different disciplines (see Contribution 3). A *profession* is characterized by systematic, scientifically based, and methodically controlled knowledge, has an academic education, and its own professional ethics. *Professionalism* describes a particular quality of a person-centered service and is not tied to a single profession. Thus, multiprofessionality implies that each of the professional groups involved purposefully contributes its skills and knowledge to achieve a shared quality of person-centered service.

Social forms of multiprofessional collaboration can include teams, networks, or integration into an existing organization. Each professional group brings its own professional routines and profession-specific ways of thinking into practice and maintains them. This inevitably leads to the coming together of more than two professional groups, requiring detailed coordination of actions for specific work tasks and continuous professional exchange, with each group bringing a high degree of specialization (Speck et al. 2011). Difficulties particularly arise in the coordination processes of the different logics and routines of a care facility, i.e., when and how information is shared (see Contribution 34). This is further exacerbated by profession-specific routines and a lack of knowledge about the professional approaches of the other groups involved.

4.2 Negotiation and Overcoming of Boundaries in Joint Action

Multiprofessional care, which aims to ensure seamless continuum of care for those affected, pursues two goals: first, overcoming institutional barriers that arise from the perspective of those affected due to transitions between care facilities (see Contribution 11), and second, overcoming conceptual barriers rooted in the routines and knowledge bases of the professional groups involved as described at the outset. The latter is further complicated by the value each professional group places on multiprofessional collaboration. Lützenkirchen (2005) examined the assessment of collaboration among the professions of medicine, nursing, psychology, economics, and social work, and concluded that collaboration crossing professional boundaries is more often perceived as a threat than as an enrichment. For respondents from the professions of psychology, nursing, and social work, multiprofessional collaboration is important and self-evident, but in practice, it is sometimes problematic due to framework conditions. Social work, due to its integration/embedding in its reference sciences, already sees itself as a mediating profession (Lützenkirchen 2005; Schumacher 2011). A look at other fields of action provides more positive insights into multiprofessional collaboration. For example, in child and youth welfare, school education, school social work, and all-day school care, various models and forms of collaboration have already been established.

However, multiprofessional collaboration is based on boundary work (Bauer 2014). Boundary work describes the negotiation of areas of responsibility and the effort to maintain these boundaries. This involves implicit processes of reinforcing one's own profession by drawing on profession-inherent concepts and theories to preserve and strengthen one's professional identity. Each profession claims, based on its own body of knowledge, sole responsibility for the well-being of its clients, which, in professional relationships and in the responsibility for shaping these relationships, is not easily shared. From this perspective, the willingness to relinquish competencies and responsibility appears problematic. From a cross-boundary perspective, cooperation requires that tasks and responsibilities must be repeatedly renegotiated and legitimized, sometimes even in opposition to each other, which can ultimately lead to a shift in the boundaries that have been painstakingly established. New tasks and areas of responsibility must be distributed and assigned according to previous implicit and explicit or hierarchy-mediated task allocations. Boundary work is not inherently negative, as it serves to define responsibilities and maintain identity. For multiprofessional collaboration, it is beneficial as long as so-called 'tacit agreements' (Bauer 2014) are observed. Tacit agreements are unspoken agreements between the professions involved. They consist of implicit task assignments that regulate responsibilities—i.e., 'who does what'—as well as define responsibilities or hierarchies in terms of 'who has a say when and where.' This enables established routines in collaboration that do not have to be renegotiated constantly.

In everyday care, multiprofessional collaboration always takes place when the appropriate framework conditions and so-called 'programs' (Luhmann 1973) make this possible and provide for it. Luhmann outlines with his programmatic character of help that helping, in its various forms, only occurs when the necessary structures for such help exist and help can also be expected. Especially in modern societies, organizations have emerged that specialize in helping through personnel and corresponding programs. For example, these programs regulate when a chronically ill person can be admitted to a suitable disease management program and according to which procedures forms of help are then provided. This implies that decisions about help are made twice: once in the form of developing and maintaining programs, and again in each individual case as to whether and when a person fits the program and how the program is implemented. This makes intrinsically motivated action based on motives of charity or reciprocity outside of programs unattractive and unlikely (Luhmann 1973), especially since the refinancing of professional action with limited working hours would otherwise lack any basis. With regard to multiprofessional collaboration, this always takes place when appropriate programs exist and, through the alignment of the problem and program components, joint collaboration is provided for.

4.3 Profession-Specific Language and Categories of Problem Assignment and Processing

When a person with chronic diseases encounters the different professions in the respective care facilities, they will quickly notice that the professions interpret the problem differently, each with its own focus. This is because each profession refers to a reference science, which is linked to corresponding standards that set the benchmarks for daily practice, without individual practical experiences diminishing the importance of these standards (Gieseke-Schmelzle 1984). The reference sciences can also be identity-forming as a member of a profession, along with internalized values and norms. This also shapes a profession-specific language for describing each case, using categories derived from the reference science. Thus, categories are derived from scientific knowledge that enable systematic recording and classification of the problem, as well as corresponding diagnostic, treatment, and interpretive abilities (Gieseke-Schmelzle 1984).

These languages and categories are shared and used within each profession to facilitate internal communication. Other professional groups do not initially have access to these categories and language. An illustrative example is a person receiving assistance, who is referred to from an economic perspective as a beneficiary, from social science reference disciplines as a client, and from health science perspectives as a patient. In addition to their own discipline-specific terms, there are also concepts that can have different meanings in the reference sciences, such as resistance, which in physics refers to electrical resistance in a component, or in sociology to opposition against certain programs or individuals. Similarly, the German term cross-section refers in medicine to a spinal cord injury, in engineering to the thickness of pipes or cables, and in statistics to a specific value. The term care also has different meanings in healthcare than in the energy sector. For multiprofessional collaboration to succeed without misunderstandings and linguistic exclusion of individual professions, a common understanding must first be established on the basis of a so-called common ground.

4.4 Common Ground as the Goal of Joint Action

The common ground is a shared knowledge base that is established situationally in communication and serves further mutual understanding. In this sense, this handbook is also intended to serve as a common ground, providing a shared understanding of chronic care in both science and practice, on the basis of which interfaces with other professional groups and points of contact for joint action become apparent.

The common ground is established within the framework of expert-layperson communication. Expert-layperson communication assumes a systematic knowledge asymmetry between experts and laypersons (Bromme et al. 2004). In this model, experts are professionals with specialized knowledge, while laypersons are those who, due to their need for information, consult experts in order to make informed decisions. An example of this is a doctor-patient conversation in which the diagnosis and treatment options are explained.

Interdisciplinary expert-layperson communication is considered a special case of the model, in which the roles of expert and layperson within the multiprofessional team can shift situationally, depending on the topic being addressed. In order to transfer professional knowledge within the framework of the model, the expert must adopt or anticipate the perspective of the layperson and adapt their own communication accordingly from this perspective. The task, therefore, is to take on the perspective and translate the statements of the layperson. Since experts and laypersons are equipped with different cognitive reference systems and bodies of knowledge, establishing a common basis for subsequent joint action is all the more important. The results of these two processes—anticipation and adaptation—flow into the common ground. This is created through verbal confirmation that information and word meanings have been understood, as well as nonverbally through nodding in agreement, regular speaker changes, and the asking of follow-up questions. Only when a statement has been accepted by both conversation partners does it become part of the common ground (Bromme et al. 2004). In multiprofessional practice fields, it is particularly important to establish a common ground for collaborative work processes in the field of chronic care.

References

Bauer P (2014) Kooperation als Herausforderung in multiprofessionellen Handlungsfeldern. In: Faas S, Zipperle M (Eds) Sozialer Wandel. Springer, Berlin, pp 173–286

Bromme R, Jucks R, Rambow R (2004) Experten-Laien-Kommunikation im Wissensmanagement. In: Reinmann G, Mandl H (Eds) Psychologie des Wissensmanagements. Hogrefe, Göttingen, pp 176–188

Gieseke-Schmelzle W (1984) Die Professionalisierungsdiskussion und ihre Relevanz für pädagogische Berufe. Bild Erzieh 37(4):365–381

Luhmann N (1973) Formen des Helfens im Wandel gesellschaftlicher Bedingungen. In: Otto H-U, Schneider S (Eds) Gesellschaftliche Perspektiven der Sozialarbeit 1. Luchterhand, München, pp 21–43

Lützenkirchen A (2005) Interdisziplinäre Kooperation und Vernetzung im Gesundheitswesen – eine aktuelle Bestandsaufnahme. Gruppe. Interaktion. Organisation. Z Angew Organisationspsychol 36:311–324

Schumacher T (2011) Die Soziale Arbeit und ihre Bezugswissenschaften. Lucius & Lucius, Stuttgart

Speck K, Olk T, Stimpel T (2011) Auf dem Weg zu multiprofessionellen Organisationen. In: Helsper W, Tippelt R (Eds) Pädagogische Professionalität. Beltz, Weinheim, pp 184–201

Part II

Individual Level: Medical Aspects, Theories of Illness and Diseases, Illness Experience, Coping with Illness, and Practical Concepts

Morphology of Chronic Diseases

5

Martin Haas

Contents

Morphology describes the appearance, i.e., the symptomatology of a disease.

5.1 The Genetically Determined Course

When a disease manifests, it takes on a form that can be categorized and diagnosed based on characteristic symptoms. The cause of this pathological development often remains unknown, sometimes rooted in genetic makeup or environmental exposures. Genetic predispositions have been identified for a wide range of chronic diseases that only manifest as morphologically detectable illnesses during certain phases of life. For example, type 2 diabetes (diabetes mellitus type 2) is almost always genetically determined and, due to its many organ complications, is a clearly defined chronic disease. In this context, the morphology, as reflected in the respective organ damage, is dominant

M. Haas (✉)
Knappschaft Kliniken Lütgendortmund, Dortmund, Germany
e-mail: martin.haas@knappschaft-kliniken.de

D. Schmitz et al. (eds.), *Chronic Care—Science and Practice*,
https://doi.org/10.1007/978-3-662-72298-5_5

for the suffering of patients, so that the chronic disease diabetes mellitus type 2 can have a very different impact on individual quality of life. Furthermore, at the onset of a determined disease, it is crucial that additional patterns of damage may still go undetected and that further symptoms may be added to the initially dominant ones, which can significantly worsen the disease experience. In diabetes, mild symptoms such as increased thirst are initially predominant, and the diagnosis can be easily made with a few laboratory values. Through lifestyle changes (diet, exercise, weight optimization), the disease with its first morphologically detectable symptoms can seemingly be brought to a standstill. However, more precise diagnostics are required to detect still inapparent morphological disease patterns at an early stage. Thus, a discrepancy between the perception of a cure from the patient's perspective and a defined, progressive, chronic disease is a core component of patient education and professional support, as it is essential for compliance and understanding of the ongoing disease process. By the time the first elevated blood glucose value is detected, years of beta cell loss in the pancreas have already occurred, initial patterns of vascular damage are already apparent, and the risk of heart attack and stroke is significantly increased—yet patients can hardly comprehend this during the asymptomatic honeymoon phase of the disease. The clinical picture in the advanced stage of the disease differs significantly, and increasing organ complications define quality of life. However, if certain therapies are effective at the time of diagnosis (which is not the same as the onset of the disease, which is rooted in genetic predisposition), a largely complication-free course is possible. As with many chronic diseases, trained management and therapeutic support are essential. These measures can delay the disease by years, but even in slim and physically fit patients, further beta cell loss occurs; only the organ changes that cause complications become morphologically limiting only at an advanced age. In this way, good quality of life in terms of independent living can be significantly extended.

Summary: *Asymptomatic* diseases, from which patients are affected without noticing, are often only detected and diagnosed at an advanced stage. Modern laboratory diagnostics can identify these genetic constellations as risk factors and classify them individually before the onset of typical symptoms. In this respect, the onset of a disease is timed with the diagnosis and not necessarily with the appearance of symptoms experienced by the patient. This silent *pre-phase* probably precedes many chronic diseases. The threshold at which disease perception begins varies greatly from individual to individual (Fig. 5.1).

5.2 The Initial Disease with an Undulating Course

A fundamentally different disease mechanism can be distinguished from the course described above. Using the example of a herpes infection, a chronologically different process is evident, which is initiated by an initial disease that only progresses over decades and manifests in eruptive, changing symptoms. Typical of this pattern is that the first viral infection usually occurs in adolescence or young adulthood, presents locally

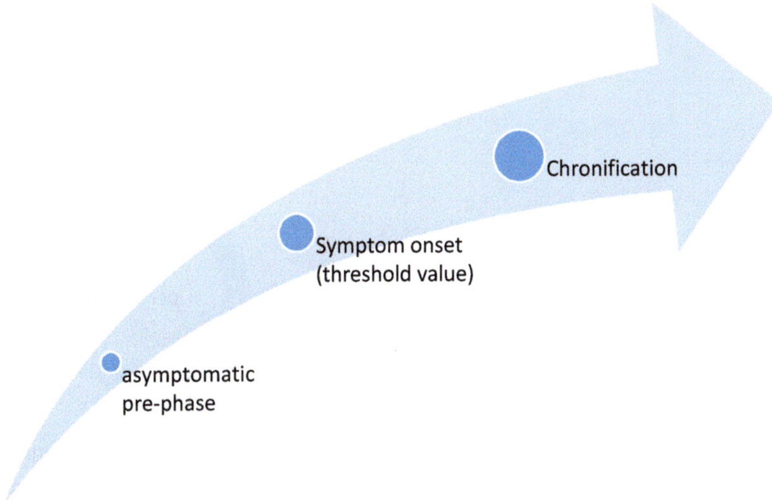

Fig. 5.1 Individual threshold for the onset of symptoms of a disease (own illustration)

with mild symptoms, and appears to heal *apparently*. However, it is characterized by active viral components that remain dormant in nerve cells, only to be reactivated by certain stimuli and cause very painful skin and organ changes along the nerve fibers. This herpes zoster infection (shingles) thus dates back decades when it triggers these chronic foci and dominates the morphology from the patient's perspective. Here, too, with appropriate laboratory diagnostics, this colonization can be detected or, with adapted vaccination techniques, even fixed in an asymptomatic dormant state.

Summary: An *acute disease* can also progress to a chronic course, often beginning with severe initial symptoms that then persist as ongoing symptomatology. This chronification maintains a process of varying intensity with phases of activation. Often, the triggering acute disease cannot be clearly identified in the patient's history. Examples include viral infections that, sometimes years or decades later, trigger immune processes and whose symptoms are not obviously related to the initial disease (Fig. 5.2).

After an acute illness, a chronic course is initiated, known as an undulating process (sometimes with significant fluctuations in symptom severity).

5.3 The Chronic Degenerative Course

Until now, mechanical joint stress was thought to cause wear and tear, ultimately leading to changes in form and accompanied by inflammatory irritation, such as the formation of fluid deposits. This *mechanical worldview* has become significantly more complex in recent years: the static bone/joint framework is subject to highly precise regulation of formation and resorption. Thus, the supporting skeleton is constantly undergoing

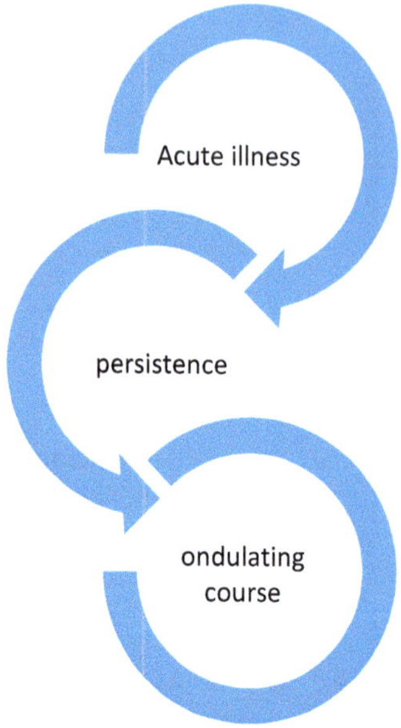

Fig. 5.2 Undulating process (own illustration)

remodeling processes that adapt to mechanical load. In addition to vital bone remodeling, there is also a synthetic performance in the connective tissue area, which has only recently been given the necessary importance: fasciae and ligamentous structures. The category of *pre-arthrosis* constitutions also includes micro-injuries (e.g., sports overuse), traumatic misloading (e.g., ligament tears, fractures), post-inflammatory structural damage (e.g., femoral head necrosis), and genetic predispositions (e.g., chromosomal defects, hip dysplasia). From this highly differentiated individual framework, environmental influences lead to biographically distinct morphological manifestations and rates of disease progression. As a result, the first symptom is usually not temporally linked to the triggering mechanism, and the damage patterns only become clinically apparent through chronic pain accompanied by additional muscle loss. An example is degenerative spinal changes (e.g., spondyloarthrosis, intervertebral disc degeneration), which first become apparent with additional muscle loss when, due to immobility, the deep back muscles lose their supporting effect: sarcopenia. The isolated view at the osseous level is a historically outdated interpretation. Therefore, chronic degenerative osteoarthritis must be classified and treated in the context of other organ findings. With early diagnosis and appropriately stage-adapted therapies, the pre-arthrosis phase can be prolonged, so that, for example, joint replacement procedures need only be used at a later stage. Training, dietary recommendations, and pain-relieving movement therapies are necessary for this. In geriatric frailty situations, these aforementioned procedures are essential components in maintaining independence and safer mobility (Fig. 5.3).

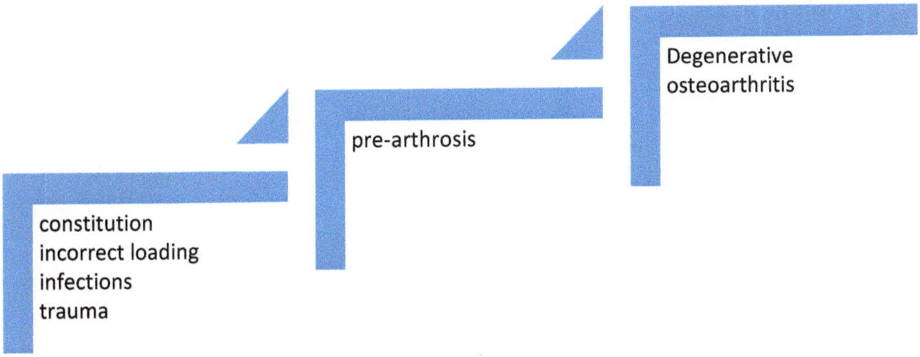

Fig. 5.3 Different initial situations of osteoarthritis (own illustration)

From different starting points, a chronic degenerative change develops via an initial stage (pre-arthrosis), which becomes morphologically dominant for the symptoms as the disease progresses.

5.4 Frailty

This term, which is only inadequately translated as frailty, describes a vulnerable risk constellation, usually in elderly patients, in which the convergence of individual low-threshold disorders triggers a downward spiral for survival. The resulting damage patterns are extremely complex, and successful treatment can only be achieved through a multiprofessional approach. Usually, a single event (e.g., a fall resulting in a fracture) pushes the previously fragile constitution into a life-threatening phase.

The starting point is biological aging with reduced regenerative capacity due to cellular aging (including stress adaptation, damage to macromolecules in cellular synthesis deficits, protease activities, oxidation processes, limited metabolism, epigenetics), osteo-sarcopenia (simultaneous degradation processes of muscular and osseous regenerative capacity). In addition, inflammatory processes, usually triggered by bacteria, parasitically exploit the limited cellular immune response and cause severe complications. These self-reinforcing processes shift the previous *at-risk situation* into a frequently fatal imbalance. Ultimately, even counterproductive therapeutic attempts (e.g., resistance-promoting antibiotics) contribute to harm in this tragic physical state. Also noteworthy are the deteriorating nutritional situation with dysphagia, cognitive impairments due to delirious states, and progressive muscle loss due to immobility (see Chapter 9). Previously unnoticed cardiac, renal, and hepatic organ damage complete the morphological downward spiral (Fig. 5.4).

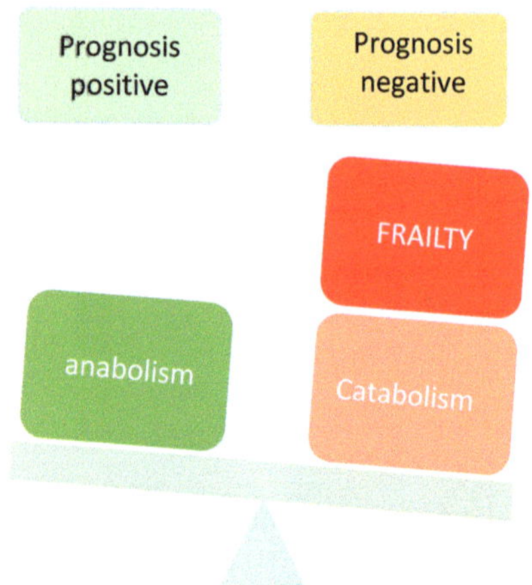

Fig. 5.4 The frailty balance (own illustration)

The balance between anabolic and catabolic processes (anabolism vs. catabolism) is shifted by frailty into a prognostically unfavorable position, preventing complete restitution.

5.5 Degenerative Diseases of Organs and Skeletal Systems

Due to aging processes and varying mechanical stresses on the musculoskeletal system, reaction zones develop at the contact points in the joint area, characterized by remodeling and resorption processes. In cases of overload, micro-injuries followed by inflammatory reactions occur, resulting in structural deformities and functional limitations. Occupational exposures involving strong vibration trauma, such as jackhammer work, are exemplary and can lead to significant mechanical destruction around affected joint areas and microfractures.

Through activation of the muscular system, physiological loading provides stimuli for stabilization and metabolically active buildup of periarticular structures, as physical adaptation to external stimuli triggers an anabolic response. The intensity and frequency of the stimulus are decisive. If excessive demands are placed here, deformities and premature arthrotic remodeling formations develop—beyond natural aging processes.

In the context of aging, muscular degradation processes are described by the term sarcopenia. This is usually the result of immobility and nutritional deficits in acute and exacerbated chronic diseases. In addition to muscle loss, bone-related degradation processes (e.g., osteoporosis) are collectively referred to as osteo-sarcopenia.

Necessary stimuli for maintaining muscular and osseous functions are isometric and isotonic movement patterns, with short and frequent stimuli eliciting a higher cellular response.

In general, aging processes in the musculoskeletal system are determined by genetic predisposition. This physiological remodeling must be distinguished from pathological damage patterns. The multifactorial degenerative remodeling in the musculoskeletal system, as a complex adaptation to changing needs in old age, is a biologically predetermined course that can at best be modified and delayed by training measures. In addition, cardiac, pulmonary, and hormonal aging processes increasingly limit physical resilience.

Summary: Sarcopenia and osteosarcopenia describe age-related degradation processes in the muscle and bone system. Joint deformities and adaptation processes to physical stress situations are dynamically developed bodily reactions. At the same time, multifactorial physiological aging occurs, which must be distinguished from pathological degeneration.

Prevalence of Chronic Diseases

6

Detmar Jobst, Klaus Weckbecker and Eva Münster

Contents

6.1 Chronic Diseases and Prevalence—Basic Concepts

Chronic diseases (ChD) are long-lasting and often slowly progressing illnesses, which, however, do not necessarily have to be incurable. Chronic diseases entail long-term effects on a person's health and daily life and can represent psychosocial stress

D. Jobst (✉)
Lehrstuhl für Allgemeinmedizin I und Interprofessionelle Versorgung, Universität Witten/Herdecke, Witten/Herdecke, Germany
e-mail: Detmar.Jobst@uni-wh.de

K. Weckbecker
Lehrstuhl für Allgemeinmedizin I und Interprofessionelle Versorgung, Universität Witten/Herdecke, Witten, Germany
e-mail: klaus.weckbecker@uni-wh.de

E. Münster
Fakultät für Gesundheit (Department für Humanmedizin), Lehrstuhl für Allgemeinmedizin I und Interprofessionelle Versorgung, Universität Witten/Herdecke, Witten, Germany
e-mail: eva.muenster@uni-wh.de

D. Schmitz et al. (eds.), *Chronic Care—Science and Practice*,
https://doi.org/10.1007/978-3-662-72298-5_6

situations. One or more areas of the body are affected on a permanent basis. Examples of chronic diseases include diabetes mellitus, heart failure, chronic respiratory diseases such as chronic obstructive pulmonary disease (COPD) or asthma, rheumatoid arthritis, chronic pain syndromes, certain types of cancer, mental illnesses such as depression or anxiety disorders, and many others. Almost always, they require long-term medical care, appropriate treatment, and support in coping with symptoms in order to improve the quality of life of those affected and to prevent complications. Chronic diseases can have a significant impact on the daily lives of those affected, limiting their activities and their physical, emotional, and social capabilities (see Contribution 10).

In addition to the individual suffering of patients, the management and coping with chronic diseases represent a considerable burden for the healthcare system and society as a whole.

The Federal Joint Committee (Gemeinsamer Bundeausschuss im Gesundheitswesen, G-BA) defines, as an example in the so-called Chronic Disease Guideline according to Paragraph 62 of the German Social Code Book V, that a disease is considered severely chronic if it has been treated by a physician at least once per quarter for at least one year. In addition to the continuous need for medical care, a care level of 3 to 5 or a degree of disability of at least 60% must be determined. (Federal Joint Committee 2004). In medical understanding, the chronicity of a disease can also be derived from the diagnosis itself, without specifying a duration. This applies, for example, to multiple sclerosis, hypertension, rheumatoid arthritis, or Crohn's disease.

The determination of the frequency (prevalence) of chronic diseases is carried out through epidemiological studies, health surveys, and secondary data analyses, for example, based on health insurance data. A distinction is made between the frequency of a disease at a specific point in time (point prevalence) or within a specific time window (period prevalence). Epidemiological findings and study results on chronic diseases should be critically examined with regard to the definition of disease chronicity.

The Robert Koch Institute, as a federal authority in Germany, regularly conducts nationwide surveys among children, adolescents, and adults. This so-called health monitoring of the population also provides information on the prevalence of chronic diseases.

The surveys often include questions about chronic diseases and their prevalence, with self-assessments predominating. A period of illness as mentioned above can be used to determine chronicity. The monitoring data are considered representative of the residential population in Germany, even though subgroups such as people with a migration background or people admitted to institutions (e.g., hospitals, nursing homes, prisons) are underrepresented or not represented at all.

The large-scale study "Health in Germany Current" (GEDA study, see below) supplements other examination and survey studies among adults and children, such as the Study on the Health of Children and Adolescents in Germany (KiGGS study, see below). The GEDA study is/was conducted by telephone in various years (survey waves). These surveys should always be discussed with regard to selection effects due to voluntary participation.

In addition to epidemiological primary surveys, health insurance funds can provide important information. They have extensive data on the insured and their illnesses. The data, primarily from statutory health insurance funds, can be used to determine the prevalence of chronic diseases as well as for scientific purposes. However, it should be noted that not all people in Germany are insured with a statutory health insurance fund and that not all diseases are adequately recorded in the data, as they are influenced and possibly distorted by the billing practices of physicians. Different studies and data sources yield different results. Prevalence varies over time, as new cases occur and existing cases may be cured or have died. It also differs by country and by population group, as well as according to risk factors. A reliable determination of the prevalence of ChD therefore requires the most robust data possible, sufficiently large samples, clear definitions of ChD, and data collection in defined areas or at several locations at the same time.

6.2 Prevalence of Chronic Diseases

In general, chronic diseases are on the rise worldwide. A publication on multimorbidity in Germany (Schmitz et al. 2023) reports the prevalence of chronic diseases in Germany by age and gender. The data are derived from 67 million statutory health insurance records from 2014. The various diagnoses were assigned based on an existing list of 46 defined morbidities (van den Bussche et al. 2011), (see Fig. 6.1). A wave-like increase can be observed, starting at just under 10% among infants and preschool children and rising with age. From the age of 80, over 90% of the individuals recorded are chronically ill. When considering the genders separately, girls and women show an earlier increase in prevalence between the ages of 15 and 19, which levels off again at age 24. The higher disease burden may be related to diseases of the reproductive organs. With increasing age, the number of chronic diseases rises for both genders. In the 55–59 age group, half of women and men already have an average of three chronic diseases (Schmitz et al. 2023)

More recent findings than the 2014 data are provided by the health monitoring of the Robert Koch Institute through a telephone survey wave 2019/2020-EHIS within the study Health in Germany Current (GEDA). In total, about 23,000 people participated in telephone interviews between April 2019 and September 2020 (Heidemann et al. 2021). The following question and explanation were used to record the presence of a chronic disease or a long-lasting health problem: (Gutsche et al. 2021) "Do you have a chronic disease or a long-lasting health problem? This refers to diseases or health problems that have lasted or are expected to last at least 6 months." (Gutsche et al. 2021, p. 5). In total, 49.2% (95% confidence interval (CI) 48.2–50.2%) of participants answered yes to this question, with women at 51.9% more frequently than men at 46.4%. As expected, self-reported prevalence also increases with age. It is 33.8% among 18–29-year-olds and 61.9% among those aged 80 and older. (Heidemann et al. 2021)

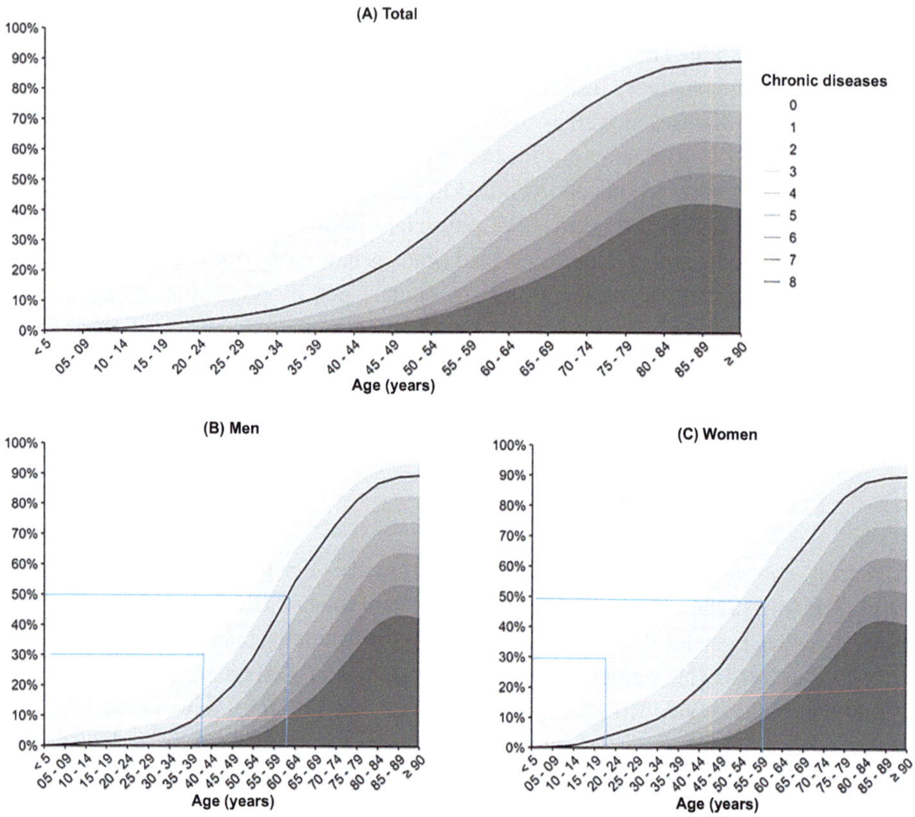

Fig. 6.1 Relative Proportion of chronic diseases per age groups and number of chronic diseases (Schmitz et al. 2023)

Significant differences in prevalence between the statutory health insurance data and the GEDA study are evident. This can be explained, among other things, by selection bias in participation: The statutory health insurance data also include information from insured individuals who do not wish to participate in a study or are unable to take part in a telephone survey.

The cause-of-death statistics from the Federal Statistical Office (Federal Health Reporting 2023) can also provide insight into the relevance of chronic diseases: The leading cause of death is chronic ischemic heart disease or coronary heart disease (CHD) (ICD-10: I25), which claims the lives of around 75,000 people in Germany each year. This number has decreased from 93,000 in 2001 (Federal Health Reporting 2023). This reflects the success of treatment methods and the avoidance of risk factors. In general, the prevalence of coronary heart disease, according to calculations by the Robert Koch Institute, has decreased among women (Gößwald et al. 2013): In the earlier survey, the lifetime prevalence of CHD was 10.4% of all respondents (95% CI 9.3–11.7%), with men at 12.1% (95% CI 10.8–13.6%) and women at 8.9% (95% CI 7.4–10.6%), while in the more recent survey, the prevalence of CHD was lower in the overall cohort and among women: 9.3% in the overall cohort (95% CI 8.4–10.3%) and 6.4% among women (95% CI 5.4–7.6%). In the male cohort, no change in prevalence was observed in the more recent survey, with 12.3% (95% CI 10.8–14.0%) compared to the earlier survey. (Gößwald et al. 2013)

In addition to studies on adults, the Robert Koch Institute also conducts surveys among children and adolescents. The German Health Interview and Examination Survey for Children and Adolescents (KiGGS) collects important data on health problems in this target group. In the first wave (2009–2011), a prevalence of chronic diseases or long-lasting health problems of 16.2% among children and adolescents aged 0–17 years was determined via self-reports from parents or the child during telephone interviews. Boys show a higher prevalence of chronic diseases or health problems at 17.9% compared to girls at 14.3% (Neuhauser and Poethko-Müller 2014). They are more often overweight and more frequently suffer from ADHD, although selection bias due to different willingness to participate must also be discussed here. Heart disease was recorded in 2.0% of 0- to 6-year-olds (girls 2.1%, boys 1.9%).

6.3 On the Significance of High Prevalence of Chronic Diseases

1. Personal Suffering

While affected patients usually strive to maintain composure and cope, making their suffering less obvious to others, (caregiving) relatives can provide very authentic accounts of the depression, pain, and existential questions that torment people with chronic illnesses, as they often witness the full spectrum of symptoms (see DEGAM Guideline No. 6, Caregiving Relatives). Not every chronic illness requires nursing care, but at the end of 2021, 4.96 million people in Germany were in need of care as defined by statutory health insurance (DeStatis). More than two-thirds of them are cared for at home. In 2023, about 1.3 million people are employed in nursing care. The burdens caused by chronically ill people in need of care can be very pronounced, making it necessary to distribute care and support tasks across several shoulders/pillars. Here, general practice, human and psychological support, inclusive thinking, and medication play the most significant roles.

What contribution can people with chronic illnesses make themselves? "More than half of the respondents with chronic diseases stated that they have their illness largely under control." (Health Knowledge Foundation (Stiftung Gesundheitswissen) 2022, Sec. 6.1). 55% of respondents without limitations said they could manage their illness well, but only 27% of those with significant limitations. "Both healthy individuals (53%) and people with chronic illnesses overall (48%) attribute by far the greatest influence on disease risk to their own lifestyle." (Stiftung Gesundheitswissen 2022, Sec. 6.2) Chronically ill people live significantly healthier lives than those without illness, but they exercise less and take more medication (Stiftung Gesundheitswissen 2022).

How do people with chronic illnesses feel best supported and cared for? This is examined in a study by the Robert Bosch Foundation (Güthlin et al. 2020). Using the example of patients with heart failure, the following findings emerged:

- Good care provides orientation, supports self-management and acceptance of the chronic illness, offers security through supervision, and responds individually. The effectiveness of medication also conveys a sense of security.
- Good care offers timely assistance and is sensibly organized, so that at the very least there are no errors or deficiencies. Good care rests on many pillars.
- Good care treats people, not cases. It is evident in reciprocal conversations without time pressure and in a forward-looking and equal relationship. The chemistry must be right. (Güthlin et al. 2020)

2. On the Care Situation

The German insurance system enables the comprehensive care of chronically ill, including severely ill, individuals. The travel burden alone for dialysis patients could plunge many families into financial hardship—the thrice-weekly dialysis sessions would be unaffordable. Extensive statutory support services, also reflected in the solidarity-based long-term care insurance, are supplemented by labor law relief for caregiving relatives and those with long-term illnesses, and by elements of day care and short-term residential care in the Social Code. Chronically ill people can obtain support and specialized knowledge in specific self-help groups; people with dementia are entitled to dementia assistants; for a number of chronic diseases, rehabilitation services are available every three to four years; and for six chronic diseases, there are disease management programs. Medical and psychotherapeutic care are fully covered by the statutory health insurance system, and even very expensive medications cost patients a maximum of €10 per 100 tablets. People with low incomes often cannot afford these co-payments, which the insurance system imposes on everyone. They can apply for an exemption.

However, the large and growing number of chronically ill people is leading to noticeable and, in some cases, difficult-to-overcome bottlenecks. This applies, for example, to the availability of specialists in orthopedics, neurology/psychiatry, or gastroenterology, to radiological imaging, to outpatient nursing services, and to appointments for physiotherapy and psychotherapy. In some districts, the care situation is even inadequate, while in university cities it is usually exceptionally good.

3. Societal and Economic Impacts

The above-mentioned study by Güthlin et al. (2020) also addresses the disease burden and lost healthy life years. According to this, about 26 million healthy life years were lost in Germany in 2017 (see Fig. 6.2). More than 2 million people died prematurely from coronary heart disease and about 180,000 from diabetes mellitus. Back pain accounted for 1.7 million years of illness (see Fig. 6.3) (Güthlin et al. 2020). Behind these shockingly high numbers stand not only the great suffering of those affected, not only the efforts to alleviate and care for them, but also, implicitly, the pressure to reduce and prevent lost healthy life years in the future—thus, a call for more prevention and chronic care!

In addition to individual suffering, there is the economic burden on society. Dementia, diseases of the spine and back, cerebral vessels, as well as hypertension and depression, caused costs of €54.9 billion in 2015 (Federal Statistical Office 2015). In 2019, more than one fifth of sick leave was due to musculoskeletal disorders (22.4%), followed by mental illnesses (11.9%). 40% of long-term unemployment is attributable to these two areas (Meyer and Buschle 2020). Mental illnesses account for the majority of disability pensions. All periods of absence together reduce economic value creation and require additional expenditure for the recovery and rehabilitation of the sick. Early retirement applications weaken the solidarity community and indirectly demand more from those in employment.

People with chronic illnesses regularly and sometimes for decades take medication. Medication use increases with age up to about 85 years. The economic burdens are matched by ecological ones. Human excretion of pharmaceuticals, for example, poses challenges not only for wastewater treatment, which must keep rivers free of (still active) drug metabolites. Drinking water suppliers also register micro-contaminations from pharmaceuticals in raw drinking water and, if necessary, must ensure their removal from drinking water.

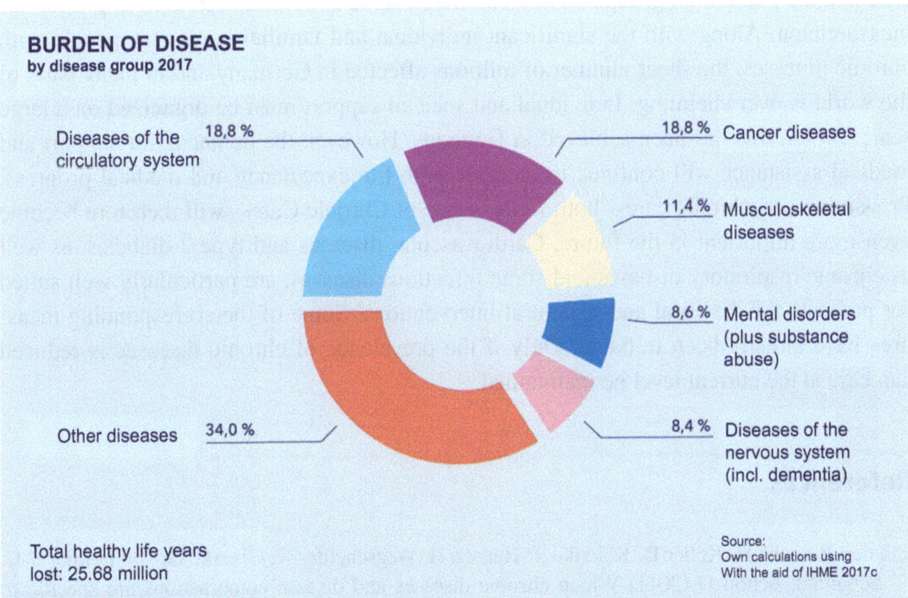

Fig. 6.2 Prevalence of disease burden for selected chronic diseases. (Güthlin et al. 2020)

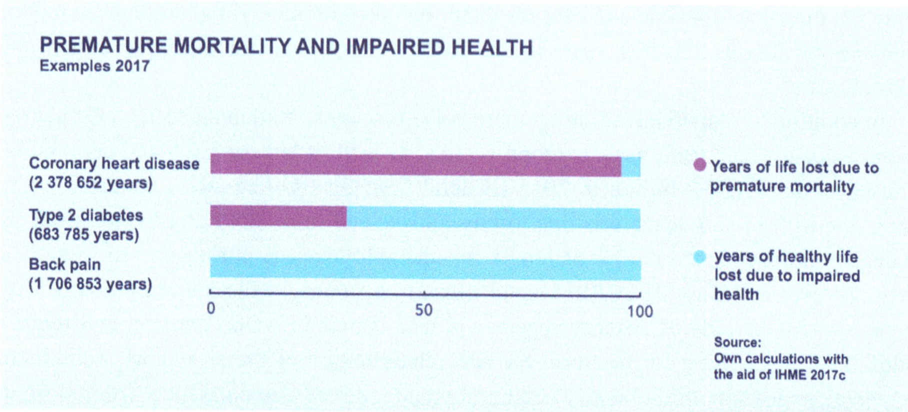

Fig. 6.3 Premature mortality and impaired health. (Güthlin et al. 2020)

6.4 Conclusion

In summary, it can be stated that the occurrence of chronic diseases depends on psychosocial and socioeconomic factors, lifestyles, genetic predispositions, environmental factors, and medical care. Variables at the individual, societal, and scientific levels influence the determination of the prevalence of chronic diseases, so that, depending on the disease and the population group considered, there can be extreme differences in prevalence measurement. Along with the significant individual and familial burden on people with chronic illnesses, the sheer number of millions affected in Germany and in many parts of the world is overwhelming. Individual and societal support must be organized on a large scale. So far, this has been achieved in Germany. However, the demands for support and medical assistance will continue to increase with life expectancy and medical progress. Prevention and chronic care—both in the sense of Chronic Care—will therefore become even more important in the future. Cardiovascular diseases and type 2 diabetes, as well as chronic respiratory diseases and some infectious diseases, are particularly well suited for preventive behavioral and structural interventions. Some of the corresponding measures have already been initiated. Only if the prevalence of chronic diseases is reduced can care at the current level be maintained.

References

van den Bussche H, Koller D, Kolonko T, Hansen H, Wegscheider K, Glaeske G, von Leitner E-C, Schäfer I, Schön G (2011) Which chronic diseases and disease combinations are specific to multimorbidity in the elderly? Results of a claims data based cross-sectional study in Germany. BMC Pub Health 11:101. https://doi.org/10.1186/1471-2458-11-101. Accessed 10. Feb. 2024

Gemeinsamer Bundesausschuss (2004) Richtlinie des Gemeinsamen Bundesausschusses zur Umsetzung der Regelungen in § 62 für schwerwiegend chronisch Erkrankte: („Chroniker-Richtlinie"). https://www.g-ba.de/richtlinien/8. Accessed 10. Feb. 2024

Gesundheitsberichterstattung des Bundes (09. Aug 2023) Sterbefälle (absolut, Sterbeziffer, Ränge, Anteile) für die 10/20/50/100 häufigsten Todesursachen (ab 1998) Gliederungsmerkmale: Jahre, Region, Alter, Geschlecht, ICD-10. https://www.gbe-bund.de/gbe/pkg_isgbe5.prc_menu_olap?p_uid=gast&p_aid=81538905&p_sprache=D&p_help=0&p_indnr=517&p_indsp=&p_ityp=H&p_fid=. Accessed 10. Feb. 2024

Gößwald A, Schienkiewitz A, Nowossadeck E, Busch MA (2013) Prävalenz von Herzinfarkt und koronarer Herzkrankheit bei Erwachsenen im Alter von 40 bis 79 Jahren in Deutschland: Ergebnisse der Studie zur Gesundheit Erwachsener in Deutschland (DEGS1) [Prevalence of myocardial infarction and coronary heart disease in adults aged 40–79 years in Germany: results of the German Health Interview and Examination Survey for Adults (DEGS1)]. Bundesgesundheitsbl Gesundheitsforsch Gesundheitsschutz 56(5–6):650–655. https://doi.org/10.1007/s00103-013-1666-9. Accessed 10. Feb. 2024

Güthlin C, Köhler S, Dieckelmann M (2020) Chronisch krank sein in Deutschland: Zahlen, Fakten und Versorgungserfahrungen. Goethe-Universität, Frankfurt am Main, Institut für Allgemeinmedizin. https://publikationen.ub.uni-frankfurt.de/frontdoor/index/index/docId/55045. Accessed 10. Feb. 2024

Gutsche J, Hintzpeter B, Prütz F, Rabenberg M, Rommel A, Ryl L, Saß A-C, Seeling S, Ziese T (2021) Journal of Health Monitoring, Fragebogen zur Studie Gesundheit in Deutschland aktuell: GEDA 2019/2020-EHIS: GESUNDHEITSBERICHTERSTATTUNG DES BUNDES GEMEINSAM GETRAGEN VON RKI UND DESTATIS. Robert Koch-Institut. https://www.rki.de/DE/Content/Gesundheitsmonitoring/Gesundheitsberichterstattung/GBEDownloadsJ/Supplement/JoHM_03_2021_Fragebogen_GEDA_2019_2020_EHIS.pdf?__blob=publicationFile. Accessed 10. Feb. 2024

Heidemann C, Scheidt-Nave C, Beyer A-K, Baumert J, Thamm, R, Maier B, Neuhauser H [Hannelore], Fuchs J, Kuhnert R, Hapke U (2021) Gesundheitliche Lage von Erwachsenen in Deutschland—Ergebnisse zu ausgewählten Indikatoren der Studie GEDA 2019/2020-EHIS. https://edoc.rki.de/handle/176904/8749. Accessed 10. Feb. 2024

Meyer N, Buschle Ch (2020) Soziale Arbeit in der Corona-Pandemie (2020): Zwischen Überforderung und Marginalisierung. IUBH Discussion Papers, Reihe: Sozialwissenschaften 1:4. https://eproofing.springer.com/ePb/books/dmuZi0ev4zJulSOcHW6h2bITqk8kzgt_gClE26yY-3OUVzAnh0FvniOCRnGLevG2DH_xZfaoGQw8BruiobW4gd5yGcOQVRySLmhP0DH-h8EPv1XN0UBMD6z0mZOTqlnz8xwHj6lgQnLb6uLcuXItCIw==?lang=2. Accessed 14. Feb. 2024

Neuhauser H [H.], Poethko-Müller C (2014) Chronische Erkrankungen und impfpräventable Infektionserkrankungen bei Kindern und Jugendlichen in Deutschland: Ergebnisse der KiGGS-Studie—Erste Folgebefragung (KiGGS Welle 1) [Chronic and vaccine-preventable diseases in children and adolescents in Germany: results of the KiGGS study: first follow up (KiGGS wave 1)]. Bundesgesundheitsbl Gesundheitsforsch Gesundheitsschutz 57(7):779–788. https://doi.org/10.1007/s00103-014-1976-6. Accessed 10. Feb. 2024

Schmitz M-T, Just JM, Weckbecker K, Schmid M, Münster E (2023) Multimorbidität in Deutschland und ihre Bedeutung für die Versorgung der Zukunft—eine Sekundärdatenanalyse basierend auf 67 Mio. Versichertendaten [Multimorbidity and its Importance in Future Health Care in Germany: a Secondary Data Analysis Based on 67 Million Health Insurance Policy Holders]. Gesundheitswesen (Bundesverband der Arzte des Öffentlichen Gesundheitsdienstes (Germany)). Vorab-Onlinepublikation. https://doi.org/10.1055/a-2011-5423. Accessed 10. Feb. 2024

Statistisches Bundesamt (2015) Statistisches Jahrbuch 2015: Deutschland und Internationales. Statistisches Bundesamt. https://www.statistischebibliothek.de/mir/servlets/MCRFileNodeServlet/DEAusgabe_derivate_00000229/StatistischesJahrbuch2015.pdf. Accessed 10. Feb. 2024

Stiftung Gesundheitswissen (2022) Chronisch Kranke: Je stärker die Einschränkungen, desto geringer der Glauben an die Selbstwirksamkeit. Stiftung Gesundheitswissen. https://www.stiftung-gesundheitswissen.de/projekte/chronisch-kranke-je-staerker-die-einschraenkungen-desto-geringer-glauben-an-selbstwirksamkeit. Accessed 10. Feb. 2024

Etiology of Chronic Diseases

7

Detmar Jobst, Klaus Weckbecker and Eva Münster

Contents

7.1 Cause Clusters

Etiology, as the study of the causes of diseases, can be divided into modifiable and non-modifiable causes in the context of chronic diseases. The following distinctions can be made

D. Jobst (✉)
Fakultät für Gesundheit (Department für Humanmedizin), Lehrstuhl für Allgemeinmedizin I und Interprofessionelle Versorgung, Universität Witten-Herdecke, Witten-Herdecke, Germany
e-mail: Detmar.Jobst@uni-wh.de

K. Weckbecker
Fakultät für Gesundheit (Department für Humanmedizin), Lehrstuhl für Allgemeinmedizin I und Interprofessionelle Versorgung, Universität Witten/Herdecke, Witten, Germany
e-mail: klaus.weckbecker@uni-wh.de

D. Schmitz et al. (eds.), *Chronic Care—Science and Practice*,
https://doi.org/10.1007/978-3-662-72298-5_7

- Lifestyles and psychosocial factors
- Accidents, chronic infections, environmental noxae (environmental damage, e.g., due to heat, smoke, radon radiation)
- Genetics and genetic predispositions
- Unclear causes of disease (e.g., in functional disorders)

Factors from these clusters, also in combination, are essentially responsible for the development of chronic diseases. Knowledge of individual causes and their interactions is necessary in order to develop targeted measures for prevention and risk reduction. Especially in disease courses that appear to be a matter of fate, early etiological classification facilitates a *Chronic Care Model*. The following attempts to provide examples for the specified cause clusters—both those for which a preventive or curative approach appears promising, as well as examples where *chronic* care is required due to a lack of prospects for a cure. But first, a brief look at the history.

1. **History**

Until recent modern times, there were imaginative, often incorrect ideas about the causes of diseases. For example, until the 1950s, asthma bronchiale, migraine, and chronic inflammatory bowel diseases were considered to be psychosomatically caused. Other diseases were described as primary, essential, or idiopathic, such as arterial hypertension, which meant that the unknown cause of the disease was dismissed with a foreign word. Significantly improved diagnostic procedures have since allowed not only more precise diagnoses but often also the identification of the underlying etiology. For example, a disease previously described as *pernicious* (incurable) could be traced back to a vitamin B12 deficiency, *cretinism* (permanent impairment of physical and mental development) to an early childhood deficiency of thyroid hormone, and chronic lower leg ulcers to an arterio-venous nutritional disorder of the skin.

7.2 Cardiovascular Diseases

1. **Coronary Heart Disease (CHD)**

Despite different genetic predispositions of those affected and a tendency toward chronicity, coronary perfusion disorders appear promising for a preventive-curative approach. Thus, in the early stages of the disease, they do not require Chronic Care concepts.

E. Münster
Fakultät für Gesundheit (Department für Humanmedizin), Lehrstuhl für Allgemeinmedizin I und Interprofessionelle Versorgung, Universität Witten/Herdecke, Witten, Germany
e-mail: eva.muenster@uni-wh.de

Coronary Risks The ARRIBA Heart, PROCAM, or ESC scores have become established for estimating coronary cardiac risk. These scores combine lifestyle factors (diet, cigarette smoking), a family history of early heart attacks or high blood pressure, age, as well as laboratory findings for cholesterol and blood sugar. These parameters allow reliable predictions for the occurrence of a heart attack, expressed as a percentage in a 10-year risk. Patients can learn at the doctor's office computer how much at risk they are and how effective behavioral changes or medications can be, demonstrated by the reduction of their risk. The ARRIBA score allows the calculation of risk reductions immediately after entering these parameters.

Etiologically caused by inflammation of the inner vessel wall (endothelium) and arteriosclerosis, the vessel-narrowing disease often begins in early adulthood and can progress chronically. Those affected usually do not experience a disease burden, except for the need to follow medical recommendations to avoid becoming manifestly ill at an early stage.

Patients and physicians partially control the chronicity and course of the disease. The attention both sides devote to the problem determines the success of prevention (annual check-ups, Disease Management Program (DMP CHD), cardiac exercise, if necessary, medications, and avoidance of risky behaviors). Rapid progression due to unfavorable genetic lipoprotein profiles in the blood additionally requires long-term medication or intermittent plasmapheresis (mechanical blood purification).

2. **Status Post Heart Attack/Myocardial Infarction**

For heart attacks (MI, myocardial infarction) or cerebral infarctions with comparable etiology, established emergency and early mobilization procedures exist. Afterwards, the situation changes, and the outcome depends on early diagnosis and the speed of intervention. Since the timely use of stents, it has been possible to restore an almost status quo ante after heart attacks—thus, there is a low disease burden, but with a more concrete and already experienced threat to life. Chronic Care subsequently focuses on so-called secondary prevention: the aim is to prevent another infarction using the same measures as before—now carried out more reliably, usually including several long-term medications and often maintained for a longer period (patient self-management).

3. **Heart Failure**

Structural damage after an MI or with chronically poor coronary perfusion (chronic ischemic heart disease, CHD) is associated with reduced cardiac output. The diagnosis is heart failure (HF, cardiac insufficiency). In addition to MI, other diseases are etiologically possible, e.g., high blood pressure, heart valve defects, chronic atrial fibrillation, or cardiomyopathies (chronic disorders of muscle and electrophysiological functions). The causes of these diseases lie in congenital or acquired valvular defects or in chronic damage to the working myocardium/conduction system due to pressure-related, alcohol-toxic, infectious, allergic, or autoimmune attacks and stresses.

The symptoms of HF are similar for all the causes mentioned: reduced physical performance, exertional shortness of breath, ankle or leg edema, fluid in the lungs, kidney dysfunction, and digestive problems indicate heart weakness. The heart loses contractile strength, remains dilated and filled even in systole, the heart valves no longer close properly, and the blood volume can no longer be adequately circulated.

More severe HF significantly shortens life expectancy. It requires a Chronic Care model, polypharmacy, and a DMP HF. This is available to all statutory insured persons throughout Germany, but has not yet been implemented.

4. **Arterial Hypertension**

For arterial hypertension, which is also etiologically significant for HF, ongoing attention and treatment are required. Hypertension is a very common, well-treatable chronic disease of mixed etiology. Blood pressure is increased by adrenergic stimulation due to our lifestyle with time pressure, lack of physical activity, noise, sleep deprivation or disturbances, and other stressors. Hypertension often occurs together with overweight and type 2 diabetes. In many adults, this etiological bundle coincides with a family predisposition. The result is persistently elevated blood pressure values. In people over 65, the loss of elasticity in arterial vessels leads to further increases in blood pressure and greater cardiac strain. Hypertension is treated predominantly with medication—lifestyle changes are only partially successful. Relaxation techniques, weight loss, and endurance sports are essential supportive measures that help reduce the need for medication. Since 2021, there has been a special "Hypertension" contract between health insurers and the Association of Statutory Health Insurance Physicians of Westphalia-Lippe. It is similar to a DMP.

7.3 Chronic Joint Pain

1. **Osteoarthritis**

When focusing on the chronicity of joint pain, osteoarthritis is epidemiologically (and economically) at the forefront. Like coronary heart disease, it increases inevitably with age, thus representing a biological life risk. In contrast to arteriosclerotic vascular narrowing, osteoarthritis is more associated with the term *wear and tear* than with undesirable deposits. Both diseases appear to share a long-lasting, sluggish inflammatory component as a contributing factor.

2. **Cartilage Damage**

The (wear-and-tear) processes in the joint that occur without acute inflammation primarily involve the cartilage. As a tissue without its own blood supply, it can suffer irreversible damage from repeated microtraumas (e.g., from contact sports), accidents, or misaligned joint axes. Body weight and the upright gait place stress on the joints of the lower body at every age. With increasing load and age, cartilage damage becomes more common. Most frequently, the knee and hip joints as well as the small vertebral joints of the lumbar spine become symptomatic.

3. **Genetic and Autoimmune Joint Inflammations**
Joint pain overall presents with etiologically different disease variants, including chronic inflammatory forms with subsequent joint changes. The most common variants are rheumatoid arthritis, polyosteoarthritis of the finger joints, and ankylosing spondylitis. In these genetically determined diseases, persistent inflammatory infiltrates of the synovial membranes cause the symptoms and complaints: swelling, pain on movement and loading, (radiological) joint deformities within months, and irreversible loss of function in the affected joints.

4. **Therapy**
To treat chronic joint complaints, medicine offers all available options. Physiotherapy and structured self-exercises, herbal topical agents, anti-inflammatory analgesics (antirheumatics/NSAIDs), X-ray therapy, radiosynoviorthesis, proliferation-inhibiting cytostatics, biologics, and surgical interventions up to and including joint replacement are used. Close and individualized contact with treating physicians is required in every case. Chronic care concepts exist for surgical joint replacement and for rheumatoid arthritis.

5. **Epidemiology and Prevention**
The burden on those affected and on the healthcare system can be estimated from a Dutch study from 1989 (Van Saase et al. 1989): Women between the ages of 55 and 64 already showed *radiologically* 61.5% distal interphalangeal joint osteoarthritis, 29% wrist osteoarthritis, 18.6% knee osteoarthritis, and 3.1% hip osteoarthritis (men 7.8%, women aged 65 to 74 years 12.5% hip osteoarthritis). Fortunately, not all radiologically detected osteoarthritis becomes painful or limiting—for example, less than 50% of all radiologically diagnosed knee osteoarthritis cases become symptomatic and require treatment. (Hannan et al. 2000)

Prevention of joint complaints is significantly less popular than, for example, the prevention of cardiac risks. Preventive measures include avoiding high-risk sports and overweight—an almost ineffective recommendation for young people and adults up to 40 years of age.

7.4 Chronic Viral Inflammations

1. **Viral Pathophysiology**
Viruses represent precursors of independent life. These tiny protein particles, measuring 0.02 to 0.3 μm, can survive for long periods outside a host organism without their own

metabolism. They force the infected organism to reproduce them by creating vast numbers of identical viral copies. To do this, viruses infiltrate host cells and take over protein production. The infected individual becomes ill, for example, at the moment when the cloned progeny are released into the bloodstream. This is often accompanied by chills and fever as a result of the body's immune response. Alleviation of such inflammatory reactions is possible and is part of acute medical care.

Usually, after the acute phase of illness, viral chromosomes remain in the cell. Occasionally, they become part of the cell's own DNA. The generative production of viruses continues either continuously (viral hepatitis B or C, AIDS) or in bursts (herpes labialis). It can also temporarily cease (varicella virus). The chronic presence of viruses leads to a permanent immune response in infected organisms, depletion of organ cells, damage up to organ failure or malignant transformation (as in chronic hepatitis), later secondary diseases (e.g., varicella-zoster), or death (AIDS).

2. **Immune Defense**

In vertebrates and humans, antibody production plays a central role in immune defense. Specialized leukocytes scan the viral surface and relay the information. B lymphocytes produce precisely fitting antibodies (specific globulins) that attach to the viruses, inhibit their activity, or destroy them. An acute viral infection can be mitigated or halted with specific globulins from pooled serum of other people (e.g., tetanus, hepatitis B). Because viral DNA remains intracellular, viruses can only be completely eliminated if the cell dies. This type of healing occurs, for example, in gastrointestinal infections and sometimes in respiratory infections—the dying body cells are excreted or coughed out. Virus eradication is only successful in a few chronic diseases, such as hepatitis C in > 90% of cases using protease and polymerase inhibitors. In other viral diseases, it is only possible to keep the blood free of viruses—the infected cells cannot become virus-free (e.g., HIV infection).

For repeated attacks by the same viral strain, immunological memory in T and B lymphocytes retains matching cytotoxic receptors as well as a minimum level of antibodies (antibody titer) and their blueprint. Both specialized lymphocytes and antibodies are produced in large quantities within hours, allowing a renewed viral infection to proceed almost without symptoms (Schulze and Aschenbrenner 2021).

3. **Prevention**

Careful general hygiene, sexual hygiene, handwashing, and wearing face masks can effectively prevent viral infections. However, efforts to maintain cleanliness and hygiene regularly fail due to adverse living conditions and events. Fortunately, there is another pillar of prevention through active immunization/vaccination: In response to the subcutaneous administration of a virus-like substrate, our immune system forms antibodies and specialized lymphocytes without causing disease symptoms. The mostly positive experiences with vaccinations have led to increasingly extensive vaccination recommendations. These begin in infants during the first year of life with a six- or seven-fold vaccination. If boosted twice, this vaccination package lasts until school age, when it is boosted again. Additional protective vaccinations are recommended for long-distance travel. Since vaccinations are generally intended for healthy individuals, there is an obligation to describe inherent, albeit low, vaccination risks in detail. Chronic care is not required if this type of primary prevention is observed and continued in a timely manner.

7.5 Chronic Metabolic Disorders

Endocrinological, often glandular (gland-related) diseases are considered to be partly acquired, partly genetically determined, and in some cases of unknown etiology. Examples of diseases of the incretory or hormonal glands include type 1 diabetes, hyperthyroidism, Cushing's disease, Conn syndrome, acromegaly, among others. Only a few chronic metabolic disorders (CMDs) are acquired despite a healthy lifestyle. Epidemiologically, for those affected and for the economy, type 2 diabetes mellitus (DM 2) is highly problematic. It occurs much more frequently than the aforementioned gland-related CMDs.

In contrast, inherited severe CMDs such as phenylketonuria, maple syrup urine disease, homocystinuria, and a large number of other CMDs (approx. 3,000) are rare. They usually require lifelong attention and treatment. Some of them are incompatible with life, while a few cause only minor burden to carriers (e.g., Gilbert-Meulengracht disease).

The prevention of acquired CMDs depends heavily on societal circumstances. Chronic nutritional deficiencies, physical overexertion, accidental or insidious poisoning, malnutrition or overnutrition, intake and overdose of supplements, or government-mandated measures can lead to metabolic damage, e.g., hypo- or hyperthyroidism due to iodization, lead in tap water or vehicle exhaust, mercury in incinerator ash, obesity with endocrine effects, chronic alcohol abuse, avitaminoses, less commonly hypervitaminoses, working under exposure to radioactivity. The pathogenic influences mentioned are known, but are not taken into account in all countries or working conditions. In addition to body glands, other sensitive structures such as bone marrow, intestinal epithelium, nerve functions, or (childhood) growth are also damaged. Since most pathogenic influences are medically well known, they should be generally considered in order to promote effective prevention, or better yet, to develop programs for this purpose.

7.6 Chronic Bronchitis/COPD (Chronic Obstructive Pulmonary Disease)

Chronic bronchitis can be seen as a model of a monocausal progressive disease caused by smoke inhalation: Persistent cigarette use (as well as prolonged occupational exposure to cooking on open fires) leads to inflammation of all mucous membranes exposed to smoke. This results in redness, soreness, deposits, and mucus formation from the pharynx to the bronchioles. Soot particles and reactive condensates enter the body via the alveoli.

After years of exposure, initially minor damage becomes irreversible. Even if smoking ceases or there is no further exposure to smoke, the so-called remodeling of the lung continues: the alveolar membrane remains chronically inflamed and thickens, and the surface area for air exchange is significantly reduced. This results in delayed, and later insufficient, gas exchange, chronic production of bronchial mucus, and a tendency toward bronchospasm. Cough (attacks), exertional dyspnea, and emphysema formation (severely thinned and overinflated lung tissue) increasingly burden patients with slowly intensifying severity. Patients and their internal organs become less efficient. Debilitation with only limited mobility, the need for oxygen therapy, increased respiratory infections requiring ventilation, and ultimately death from heart failure or suffocation are the inevitable consequences of COPD.

7.7 Chronic Diseases with Unknown or Suspected Etiology

At the beginning of the chapter on etiologies, past misjudgments were mentioned. Today, large-scale research protects humanity from further misinterpretations and errors. Most often, international working groups and national research consortia with modern equipment focus on chronic diseases whose etiology remains puzzling, no matter how frequently they occur. This applies, for example, to chronic fatigue syndrome, somatoform disorders, and irritable bowel syndrome, which remain etiologically unexplained (Oka et al. 2020). For the latter condition, four international conferences have been held in Rome (1992, 1998, 2006, 2016). Their definitions and diagnostic criteria have influenced the assessment, classification, and medical management of the symptom complex of abdominal pain, constipation, and diarrhea for decades. To this day, there is no clear understanding of the origin of irritable bowel syndrome.

Some characteristics apply to the three examples mentioned: there are no or very few specific blood markers. Many indications point to psychogenic triggers and/or individual misinterpretation of bodily signals. Other research findings suggest possible multicausality or the realization that the diagnosis may actually encompass different diseases. In fact, research efforts are gradually making progress—with each new insight, therapeutic understanding also grows. In particular, this has increased for somatoform disorders, see the S3 guideline *Functional Somatic Symptoms* (2018). Chronic care is not easy in these and other cases, as there is no targeted prevention or evidence-based care available.

7.8 Etiology of Chronic Diseases, Summary

Chronic disorders do not necessarily mean disease or chronic suffering. Some diseases can be completely prevented through preventive behavior or preventive measures. These include, for example, applied basic health knowledge, adequate good nutrition, as well as newborn metabolic screening and vaccinations. The nature of some chronic disorders and diseases lies in smoldering inflammatory processes (chronic dermatitis, arthritis/arthrosis, arteriosclerosis, as well as bacterial (tuberculosis) or viral (chronic hepatitis) diseases). Here, good diagnostics and therapeutic intervention can be curative, while support, including chronic care, can be palliative and disease-delaying. Early recognition of symptoms leads in many other cases to alleviating (dietetics, physiotherapy), postponing (antibodies, plasmapheresis), or definitive medical measures (vascular catheter, joint replacement).

In the end, all chronically ill as well as very elderly people always require more help and care in all areas of life. If this helps to alleviate suffering and bridge the gap to death, it was the last good chapter of chronic care.

References

Hannan MT, Felson DT, Pincus T (2000) Analysis of the discordance between radiographic changes and knee pain in osteoarthritis of the knee. J Rheumatol 27:1513–1517

Oka P, Parr H, Barberio B, Black CJ, Savarino EV, Ford AC (2020) Global prevalence of irritable bowel syndrome according to Rome III or IV criteria. Lancet Gastroenterol Hepatol 5(10):908–917

Schulze J, Aschenbrenner A (2021) COVID-19 and the human innate immune system. Cell 184(7):1671–1692

Van Saase J, Van Romunde L, Cats A, Vandenbroucke P, Valkenburget HA (1989) Epidemiology of osteoarthritis: Zoetermeer survey. Comparison of radiological osteoarthritis in a Dutch population with that in 10 other populations. Ann Rheumat Dis 48:271–280

The Masticatory Organ and Chronic Diseases

8

Jochen Jackowski and Korbinian Benz

Contents

8.1 Introduction

Demographic change, increased life expectancy, and advances in dentistry have brought challenges but also new diagnostic and therapeutic opportunities for the care of the masticatory system and the maintenance of oral health. Oral health can be particularly

J. Jackowski (✉)
Universität Witten/Herdecke, Witten, Germany
e-mail: Jochen.Jackowski@uni-wh.de

K. Benz
Fakultät für Gesundheit, Department für Zahn-, Mund- und Kieferheilkunde, Universität Witten/Herdecke, Witten, Germany
e-mail: Korbinian.Benz@uni-wh.de

D. Schmitz et al. (eds.), *Chronic Care—Science and Practice*,
https://doi.org/10.1007/978-3-662-72298-5_8

threatened or impaired by the consequences of acute and chronic diseases and sometimes by the aging process itself.

Oral and systemic health influence each other. Both epidemiological and clinical studies as well as in vitro and animal studies underscore the significant importance of oral health for systemic health. Certain at-risk populations exhibit a bidirectional relationship between oral and systemic health.

There is potential for multiple comorbidities (multimodal relationships) because periodontal diseases can involve the most important organ systems and conditions (kidney, liver, heart, gastrointestinal tract, respiratory system, adipose tissue, brain, neuroendocrine system/stress, reproductive system, skeletal system/joints, aging, cancer).

Known mechanisms mediating this connection between oral and systemic health include predispositions, behaviors, and other mechanisms such as genetic factors (gene polymorphisms), environmental factors (stress, habits—e.g., smoking and dietary habits such as high-fat diets/consumption of highly processed foods), medications, microbial dysbiosis and bacteremia, as well as an altered host immune response/reaction (Kapila 2021).

Since many systemic diseases have significant direct and indirect effects on oral health, it must be an integral part of the management of chronic diseases.

The most widespread oral diseases, caries and periodontitis, are largely preventable (Jepsen et al. 2017). Caries is the most common chronic disease in childhood and continues into adulthood. In addition to primary prevention, the progression of the disease in its early stages can be prevented by efficient oral hygiene, fluoridation, sealing of teeth, and dietary modification.

8.2 Oral Health and Chronic Diseases

Burning Mouth Syndrome (BMS) is defined in the International Classification of Orofacial Pain as idiopathic orofacial pain with intraoral burning or dysesthesia that occurs daily for more than two hours and persists for longer than three months, without identifiable causative lesions, with or without somatosensory changes (International Classification of Orofacial Pain 2020). The prevalence of BMS ranges from 0.1% to 3.9% and occurs mainly in postmenopausal women aged between 50 and 70 years (Bergdahl and Bergdahl 1999; Kohorst et al. 2015). A distinction is made between glossodynia, glossopyrosis, stomatodynia, and stomatopyrosis.

BMS typically presents as burning, tingling, prickling, itching, or numbness affecting the tongue, lips, palate, gums, and other areas of the oral mucosa (Scala et al. 2003). Pain intensity increases over the course of the day, peaking in the late evening (Forssell et al. 2012). Patients report dysgeusia (taste disturbance: metallic, bitter), a sensation of xerostomia (dry mouth), and psychological problems such as anxiety and depression. The pathogenesis of BMS has also been linked to psychological disorders (Schiavone et al. 2012) and peripheral and central neuropathy (Jaaskelainen and Woda 2017).

The diagnosis and treatment of patients with BMS remains a challenge for clinicians, as the pathogenesis is insufficiently understood. Complete resolution of symptoms cannot be expected; the prevalence of spontaneous remission is low at 3–4% five to six years after diagnosis (Sardella et al. 2006). There are no universally accepted guidelines for BMS treatment, and published review articles generally include clinical studies with limited follow-up periods (< 2 months) (de Souza et al. 2018; Liu et al. 2018; McMillan et al. 2016). Clinically controlled studies with larger patient cohorts are needed to demonstrate the analgesic benefit of topical clonazepam and alternative drugs with neurodegenerative preventive potential. Likewise, the therapeutic effect of psychological support in the treatment of this syndrome needs further clarification. Secondary BMS can occur as a consequence of chronic diseases such as Sjögren's syndrome, systemic lupus erythematosus, systemic scleroderma, granulomatosis with polyangiitis, giant cell arteritis, fibromyalgia, rheumatogenic oral aphthae, and ulcerations.

Chronic kidney disease (CKD) can, among other things, be closely associated with cardiovascular diseases. It is associated with an increased risk of thromboembolism and may therefore require anticoagulant therapies, which are associated with an increased risk of bleeding.

Platelet hyperreactivity in the early stages is compensated by reduced platelet activity and decreased platelet–vessel wall interaction. This is due to changes in platelet-dependent mechanisms involved in physiological hemostasis (Limdi et al. 2015; Ng et al. 2013; Potpara et al. 2018). Hemorrhage is exacerbated by CKD-related anemia, extrinsic iatrogenic factors (nonsteroidal anti-inflammatory drugs, antithrombotic medications, antibiotics, invasive procedures, dialysis procedures), and gastrointestinal lesions (Lau et al. 2016).

Several studies have demonstrated a close association between periodontal diseases and chronic kidney disease. The main mechanisms underlying this association are malnutrition, vitamin dysregulation, especially of B-group vitamins as well as vitamins C and D, oxidative stress, metabolic acidosis, and low-grade inflammation (Ausavarungnirun et al. 2016; Bastos Jdo et al. 2013; Clase et al. 2013; Noce et al. 2016, 2019, 2021; Raimann et al. 2013). These may be related to the stage of CKD and worsen particularly in ESRD (End Stage Renal Disease), the terminal stage of CKD, which often requires renal replacement therapy such as dialysis or kidney transplantation (Hashmi et al. 2023). In particular, in adult hemodialysis patients, impairment of nutritional status has been observed, not only due to the hemodialysis procedures themselves but also as a result of numerous CKD-related comorbidities. Malnutrition leads to systemic manifestations that affect oral health, such as dysbiosis of the oral microbiota, delayed wound healing due to hypovitaminosis C, and changes in the bone structures of the oral cavity associated with metabolic acidosis and vitamin D deficiency. Periodontal diseases can also manifest as low-grade inflammation, with an interaction between CKD and periodontal diseases being assumed. Patients with CKD and oral diseases must be cared for by a multiprofessional team in order to demonstrate the coincidence of these two diseases in a patient-stratified manner and subsequently develop therapeutic strategies.

These patients should be included in a follow-up program that provides for regular check-ups to ensure accurate documentation of disease progression.

In end-stage kidney disease, the progression of untreated periodontitis leads to tooth loss (Han and Park 2021; Limeres et al. 2016). This can impair chewing, masticatory behavior, phonetics, and aesthetics, and may result in loss of self-esteem and a reduction in quality of life. A cross-sectional study investigated the relationship between periodontitis and health-related quality of life (HRQoL) in hemodialysis patients. The results showed that HRQoL decreased in these patients with severe periodontitis (Iwasaki et al. 2017).

In addition to renal replacement therapy, metabolic acidosis and vitamin deficiency also contribute to the development of periodontitis. Treatment of periodontal disease can reduce the systemic inflammatory burden caused by oral pathology and decrease the risk of atherosclerotic vascular disease and mortality in hemodialysis patients.

Biological, psychological, sociodemographic, clinical, and therapeutic factors influence the health-related quality of life of patients with chronic liver diseases. Low health-related quality of life in these patients has been associated with depression (Bianchi et al. 2000) and cirrhosis complications such as hepatic encephalopathy, ascites, spontaneous bacterial peritonitis, and bleeding due to esophageal varices (Dan et al. 2007; Younossi et al. 2001).

Oral manifestations in patients with chronic liver diseases have been described. These patients often have reduced salivary flow (Lins et al. 2011), making them more susceptible to caries and periodontal diseases. These oral manifestations can, in turn, trigger severe complications such as hepatic encephalopathy or a pyogenic liver abscess (Ohyama et al. 2009). A systematic review (Gronkjaer 2015) found only a few published studies on the association between periodontal disease and liver cirrhosis. In a cohort study, mortality was lower in patients who received dental treatment compared to those who were not treated (Lins et al. 2011). Another study reported an association between reduced work ability and diseases of the teeth/periodontium in patients with chronic liver disease (Aguiar et al. 2016). The results underscore the need for specialized dental care for patients with chronic liver diseases.

A meta-analysis showed that in patients with respiratory diseases such as asthma and COPD (chronic obstructive pulmonary disease), an association with the presence of periodontal diseases can be assumed (Gomes-Filho et al. 2020). In this context, medications—such as asthma drugs like bronchodilators, corticosteroids, or anticholinergics that are inhaled by patients—can also increase the risk of dry mouth, carious lesions, dental erosion, periodontal diseases, and oral candidiasis (Gani et al. 2020; Thomas et al. 2010). Especially in severely ill patients, such as those with cystic fibrosis or COPD, oral pathogenic bacteria associated with dental and periodontal diseases can also colonize the lungs and increase the risk of complications (Bansal et al. 2013; Coffey et al. 2020). The complex relationship between oral and respiratory health is multifactorial, with oral diseases potentially playing a significant role due to the anatomical proximity between the oropharyngeal and respiratory tracts.

Patients with chronic respiratory diseases may have a lower oral health-related quality of life (OHRQoL). To maintain this oral health-related quality of life, patients with chronic respiratory diseases should undergo regular check-ups of the masticatory system.

Inflammatory bowel diseases (IBD) are chronic conditions that affect the gastrointestinal tract, including the oral cavity. Genetic predispositions, immunological disorders, and environmental conditions are potential etiopathogenetic factors (Kaplan 2015). Crohn's disease (CD) and ulcerative colitis (UC) exhibit similar clinical symptoms. However, they differ in the extent of inflammatory processes and their reflection in biochemical parameters of blood and saliva (Nijakowski et al. 2021). The course of the disease is associated with disturbances in the immune system, leading to an imbalance with predominance of proinflammatory cytokines and an increase in markers indicating a higher risk of oxidative stress (Nijakowski and Surdacka 2020). Oral Crohn's manifestations characteristically present as erythema, edematous swelling, granulation or erosion of the oral mucosa, aphthous lesions, persistent linear ulcerations, or as localized areas of inflammatory swelling with fissuring (*cobblestone appearance*). In addition to lymphadenopathy, facial changes such as swelling of the face and lips may occur. Pyostomatitis vegetans can also develop in association with ulcerative colitis (Lauritano et al. 2019).

The most common oral comorbidities include caries and periodontitis. Carious lesions arise from changes in the biofilm and thus from disturbances in the neutral environment of the oral cavity, leading to demineralization of the dental enamel (Marsh 2010).

Both in the progression of chronic inflammatory bowel diseases and in periodontitis, immunoinflammatory processes involving cytokines play a decisive role (Brandtzaeg 2001; Indriolo et al. 2011). Periodontal pathogenic bacteria can alter the composition of the gut microflora, intensify inflammatory processes, and disrupt host defense (Said et al. 2014; Van Dyke et al. 1986).

When considering the relationship between oral health status and inflammatory bowel diseases, sociodemographic aspects and environmental factors must also be taken into account.

The most common cause of death worldwide is coronary heart disease (CHD) (Mathers et al. 2009). Oral health, for example impaired by periodontal diseases, is associated with an increased risk of CHD (Blaizot et al. 2009; Granados-Principal et al. 2012; Kebschull et al. 2010; Meurman et al. 2004; Persson and Persson 2008). Whether there is a direct causal relationship between periodontitis and CHD, or whether both entities are due to a common underlying condition such as inflammation, is the subject of research (Friedewald et al. 2009). Many of the potential pathogenetic effects of periodontal diseases on CHD have been postulated, including that they are due to the entry of bacteria or bacterial products into the bloodstream (Kebschull et al. 2010). A common periodontitis-associated bacterium, Porphyromonas gingivalis, can invade both endothelial cells (Deshpande et al. 1998) and atheromatous tissue (Chiu 1999; Haraszthy et al. 2000). This is one of the pathogenetic links between periodontal diseases and CHD, as can be shown in pathway 5-23-P. gingivalis in an integrated model (Mathews et al. 2015).

Diabetes mellitus leads to numerous complications, which increase if patients' blood glucose control is inadequate.

Two mechanisms are involved in the development of diabetic complications. First, via the sorbitol-aldose reductase pathway, glucose is reduced to sorbitol, which is subsequently oxidized to fructose. This leads to tissue damage and other diabetic complications. Second, glycation reaction products are formed, known as advanced glycation endproducts (AGEs). Glycation refers to the irreversible reaction of proteins, lipids, and nucleic acids with carbohydrates (Mealey 2000).

AGEs are involved in the development of various chronic inflammatory diseases such as type II diabetes mellitus, vascular and cardiovascular diseases, osteoporosis, and arthritis. The underlying cause is considered to be that glycation disrupts the functionality of important regulatory enzymes and membrane systems on the one hand, and on the other, the AGEs themselves also influence key metabolic processes.

Glycation of neuronal myelin promotes neuropathies, which can occur in diabetes mellitus or in Alzheimer's disease. Foods and beverages containing high concentrations of AGEs can also acutely impair blood vessel function, with the long-term damaging effect being of primary concern. The broad negative effects on metabolism are mainly explained by the fact that numerous, especially short-lived substances such as lipids, amino acids, enzymes, hormones (e.g., insulin), or growth factors are structurally and functionally damaged by glycation (Christ-Crain et al. 2019).

It has been shown that diabetes has a bidirectional relationship with periodontitis and can also lead to other oral pathologies. For this reason, physicians and dentists must be thoroughly familiar with the various oral manifestations of diabetes mellitus in order to intervene therapeutically at an early stage and to act preventively. Comprehensive awareness and understanding of the pathophysiology, manifestations, and management of the various diabetes-induced orofacial changes by endocrinologists and dentists are essential for optimizing the care of diabetic patients (Mauri-Obradors et al. 2017; Poudel et al. 2018).

Oral manifestations associated with diabetes mellitus present as periodontal diseases (Arrieta-Blanco et al. 2003), periapical pathologies (Lopez-Lopez et al. 2011), caries (Bharateesh et al. 2012), hyposalivation or xerostomia (Ivanovski et al. 2012), taste disorders/burning mouth syndrome (Stolbova et al. 1999), and pathological oral mucosal changes (Cristina de Lima et al. 2008).

8.3 Oral Surgery and Chronic Diseases

Oral health affects both general medical condition and various other aspects such as social interaction, self-esteem, and health-related quality of life (Nam et al. 2018). Alterations in the oral cavity can occur as a concomitant symptom of chronic diseases, but can also result from the use of medications to treat systemic/chronic diseases.

The German Society for General and Family Medicine defines multimorbidity as "the simultaneous presence of at least three chronic diseases. None of the diseases needs to be of central importance" (DEGAM 2017).

None of the definitions of multimorbidity refer to oral diseases, but it is known that caries, periodontitis, and other oral diseases (e.g., oral mucosal changes) can be chronic and long-lasting, affecting a significant proportion of adults and especially the elderly population (Kassebaum et al. 2017). Against this background, the therapy of oral pathological alterations in people with chronic (multiple) diseases resulting in polypharmacy requires a patient-stratified approach.

8.4 Interaction of Polypharmacy and Oral Health

Many studies have demonstrated the relationship between general and oral health. Three factors play a significant role here: infection, inflammation, and adaptive immunity. In its further course, persistent local inflammation in the periodontal tissue can trigger a systemic inflammatory response, which may contribute to the pathogenesis of certain systemic diseases such as diabetes, cardiovascular diseases, and rheumatoid arthritis (Cekici et al. 2014; Mankia et al. 2019). The individual immune response is influenced by behavioral, environmental, and other risk factors such as diet (e.g., high in sugar/salt), tobacco and alcohol consumption, as well as social factors such as socioeconomic status, psychosocial factors, and access to medical care (Barnett et al. 2012).

While studies on the relationships between oral and systemic diseases exist, there are currently no evidence-based longitudinal studies that have examined the relationship between oral health and multimorbidity/polypharmacy.

8.5 Polypharmacy

In general, polypharmacy (synonyms: polymedication, multimedication, multiple prescriptions) is understood as the cumulative prescription of five or more medications per quarter (Holt et al. 2010). In this context, it is also important to consider the possibility of acquiring over-the-counter medications, the so-called "over-the-counter" (OTC) drugs. The negative assessment of prescription and non-prescription medications due to their unfavorable benefit-risk ratio and their comparatively high potential for harm is described by the term "potentially inappropriate medications" (PIM) (Neuner-Jehle 2013). PIM medications are listed in the PRISCUS (Beers and Ouslander 1989) and FORTA lists (Wehling 2009). The prevalence of polypharmacy in Germany is about 42% among those over 65 years of age, with a rising trend (Moßhammer et al. 2016). Polypharmacy results from the use of different medications required to treat several coexisting diseases. In addition, it can result from the insufficient effect of an otherwise appropriate and indicated medication that does not provide adequate therapeutic effectiveness. The desired therapeutic effect thus requires the administration of another or several medications with a similar spectrum of action. Polypharmacy can also arise when the adverse effects of a medication necessitate the prescription of one or a series of additional medications (typical examples are the prescriptions of various drugs for hypertension, bronchial asthma, chronic obstructive pulmonary disease, Parkinson's disease).

Complications in the context of polypharmacy arise from inadequate therapy adherence as well as disease- or therapy-related changes in absorption, distribution, metabolism, and elimination. Medication errors are often associated with age-related disorders [e.g., impairments of vision and fine motor skills, depression, cognitive disorders (including dementia)]. Changes in receptor density or receptor sensitivity can lead to a decreased or increased response of the target organ (e.g., paradoxical reaction to benzodiazepines). In addition, age-related physiological limitations in compensatory mechanisms may exist (e.g., use of antihypertensives can lead to a risk of hypotension). The greatest age-associated pharmacokinetic influence is a reduced renal excretion (decrease in glomerular filtration rate). In older people, there is also a significantly increased risk of delirium due to polypharmacy and fluid deficit (Clegg et al. 2013).

8.6 Interactions of Pharmaceuticals and Consequences for Oral Surgical Procedures

Oral surgical procedures in patients using antithrombotic medications require careful preparation to prevent bleeding or postoperative hemorrhage. For this reason alone, preoperative coordination with the treating physicians is very important, during which the general resilience of the patients, in light of the underlying condition that indicates the use of one or more antithrombotic agents (platelet aggregation inhibitors and/or anticoagulants), should also be discussed. In addition, interactions of these medications with other pharmaceuticals must be considered. The use of certain anti-inflammatory drugs and analgesics (e.g., salicylic acid derivatives, piroxicam), some anti-infectives (e.g., ciprofloxacin, erythromycin, metronidazole), as well as various other medications (e.g., omeprazole, citalopram) and some foods or herbs (e.g., fenugreek, mango, fish oil) can increase the risk of bleeding by enhancing the effect of coumarins, while the use of adrenaline or epinephrine, atropine, multivitamin preparations containing vitamin K, barbiturates, or certain psychotropic drugs can increase the risk of thrombosis by reducing the effect of coumarins (Halling 2016; Weber 2013). Increasingly, non-vitamin K-dependent anticoagulants with antagonistic effects on thrombin or factor Xa (also known as NOACs) are being used (Lutz and Wille 2016). Due to their direct action on one of the aforementioned coagulation factors, these are also referred to as direct oral anticoagulants (DOACs). These agents also carry an increased risk of bleeding (Graham et al. 2015; Larsen et al. 2013; Southworth et al. 2013).

It must also be noted that these medications, due to their thrombin- or factor Xa-antagonistic effects, differ not only in terms of elimination and antagonization, but apparently also present an increased risk of postoperative bleeding during and after dental surgical procedures. Therefore, surgical intervention should only be performed up to 24 hours after the last dose. In patients with renal dysfunction, depending on the preparation, longer withdrawal periods may be necessary (up to 72 hours after the last dose), and, depending on the medication, different recommendations exist regarding pausing the medication based on once- or twice-daily dosing. There are also various recommendations regarding the resumption of DOAC medication after an oral surgical procedure. If discontinuation is not feasible, minor dental surgical procedures should be performed at the trough level (depending on the prescription pattern, 12 to 18 hours after the last dose), and—the shorter the withdrawal interval after the last dose—the more carefully local hemostatic measures should be implemented (Wahl 2014).

That drug interactions due to self-medication resulting from lack of information can have negative consequences is illustrated by the example of taking St. John's wort preparations, for which even life-threatening interactions have been reported. These include a significant reduction in plasma levels of numerous drugs such as ciclosporin, digoxin, indinavir, phenprocoumon, simvastatin, and warfarin (By the American Geriatrics Society Beers Criteria Update Expert 2015; Holt et al. 2010; Lohse 2016).

The use of antiresorptive medications increases the risk of jawbone necrosis—depending on the indication, medication, and dosage. To minimize risk, perioperative systemic anti-infective therapy with antibiotics is recommended, for which interactions with other medications must again be considered (DGMKG and DGZMK 2018).

In general, antibiotics and analgesics or anti-inflammatory drugs are among the most frequently prescribed medications in the context of dental procedures (Halling 2016).

For local anesthetics, which are also used in dental surgery—usually in combination with vasoconstrictors—in addition to the relative risks associated with underlying systemic diseases (high-grade AV block, severe cardiac conduction and rhythm disorders, coagulation disorders, liver and renal insufficiency, hyperthyroidism, etc.) and absolute contraindications [including cardiac decompensation, lack of compliance], particular attention must be paid to drug interactions that potentiate the effects of adrenaline, such as with digoxin, digitoxin, tricyclic antidepressants, MAO inhibitors, antiparkinsonian agents, guanethidine, and beta-blockers. However, with adrenaline concentrations of 1:100,000 or less, and when adhering to the maximum doses of local anesthetics, this potentiation is rather questionable. More important is to consider the age-related decline in metabolic function, which is why a reduction in maximum doses is recommended from the age of 60 to 65 years (Daubländer and Kämmerer 2012). Additionally, with decreasing body weight below 70 kg, the calculation of maximum doses based on body weight should be fundamentally considered.

8.7 Therapeutic Strategies in the Context of Polypharmacy and Oral Surgery

The physiological conditions in older patients are highly variable, as this is a very heterogeneous patient group (Nitschke 2012). They are characterized, among other things, by a decrease in nerve conduction velocity, muscle strength, cardiac output, vital capacity, respiratory minute volume, oxygen uptake, glomerular filtration rate, and renal plasma flow. The resulting reduced functional reserves, frailty, multimorbidity, potentially atypical symptoms, as well as diminished psychological adaptability and social isolation become key factors that must be considered when determining indications for oral surgical procedures (By the American Geriatrics Society Beers Criteria Update Expert 2015; Holt et al. 2010; Lohse 2016). Apart from the varying resilience depending on the extent of health and psychosocial limitations, further categorization of patients can be helpful for therapy planning and deciding in which setting (outpatient/inpatient) the treatment should take place. Some patients lack the ability to cooperate for an elective procedure, and in high-risk patients, there is an increased risk of a life-threatening incident during surgery due to accompanying (acute/chronic) systemic diseases. These two categories in turn present risks for physicians or dentists as well as for uninvolved third parties, but also risks for the patients themselves (Rixecker et al. 1985).

Systemic diseases affecting the oral and perioral tissues, as well as the closely related impairment of quality of life—such as hyposalivation or xerostomia (e.g., in Sjögren's syndrome or as an adverse drug reaction), restricted mouth opening and chewing function (e.g., in rheumatic diseases of the temporomandibular joint, systemic sclerosis, fibromyalgia), pain, paresthesia, inflammatory—e.g., aphthous—lesions of the oral mucosa (e.g., in systemic lupus erythematosus, Wegener's granulomatosis, fibromyalgia, giant cell arteritis), or even immune system impairments with increased risk of infection or bleeding (e.g., in systemic lupus erythematosus due to leukopenia, lymphocytopenia, or thrombocytopenia) can often negatively affect wound healing after oral surgical interventions. Conversely, adverse drug reactions associated with the treatment of these diseases (e.g., the use of immunosuppressants) can also lead to impaired wound healing. A thorough medication history in acutely and chronically ill patients is essential to identify and avoid potentially dangerous adverse drug reactions.

References

Aguiar ILS, Lins L, Falcao AFP, Sarmento VA, Santos PSS (2016) Work capacity and its relationship to oral health patients with chronic liver disease. [Portuguese]. Rev Bras Med 73:16–24

Arrieta-Blanco JJ, Bartolome-Villar B, Jimenez-Martinez E, Saavedra-Vallejo P, Arrieta-Blanco FJ (2003) Dental problems in patients with diabetes mellitus (II): gingival index and periodontal disease. Med Oral 8(4):233–247. https://www.ncbi.nlm.nih.gov/pubmed/12937385

Ausavarungnirun R, Wisetsin S, Rongkiettechakorn N, Chaichalermsak S, Udompol U, Rattanasompattikul M (2016) Association of dental and periodontal disease with chronic kidney disease in patients of a single, tertiary care centre in Thailand. BMJ Open 6(7):e011836

Bansal M, Khatri M, Taneja V (2013) Potential role of periodontal infection in respiratory diseases—a review. J Med Life 6(3):244–248. https://www.ncbi.nlm.nih.gov/pubmed/24155782

Barnett K, Mercer SW, Norbury M, Watt G, Wyke S, Guthrie B (2012) Epidemiology of multimorbidity and implications for health care, research, and medical education: a cross-sectional study. Lancet 380(9836):37–43

Bastos Jdo A, Andrade LC, Ferreira AP, Barroso Ede A, Daibert Pde C, Barreto PL, Vilela EM, Marcaccini AM, Colugnati FA, Bastos MG (2013) Serum levels of vitamin D and chronic periodontitis in patients with chronic kidney disease. J Bras Nefrol 35(1):20–26

Beers MH, Ouslander JG (1989) Risk factors in geriatric drug prescribing. A practical guide to avoiding problems. Drugs 37(1):105–112

Bergdahl M, Bergdahl J (1999) Burning mouth syndrome: prevalence and associated factors. J Oral Pathol Med 28(8):350–354

Bharateesh J, Ahmed M, Kokila G (2012) Diabetes and oral health: a case-control study. Int J Prev Med 3(11):806–809. https://www.ncbi.nlm.nih.gov/pubmed/23189233

Bianchi G, Loguercio C, Sgarbi D, Abbiati R, Chen CH, Di Pierro M, Disalvo D, Natale S, Marchesini G (2000) Reduced quality of life in patients with chronic hepatitis C: effects of interferon treatment. Dig Liver Dis 32(5):398–405

Blaizot A, Vergnes JN, Nuwwareh S, Amar J, Sixou M (2009) Periodontal diseases and cardiovascular events: meta-analysis of observational studies. Int Dent J 59(4):197–209. https://www.ncbi.nlm.nih.gov/pubmed/19774803

Brandtzaeg P (2001) Inflammatory bowel disease: clinics and pathology. Do inflammatory bowel disease and periodontal disease have similar immunopathogeneses? Acta Odontol Scand 59(4):235–243

By the American Geriatrics Society Beers Criteria Update Expert, P (2015) American Geriatrics Society 2015 updated beers criteria for potentially inappropriate medication use in older adults. J Am Geriatr Soc 63(11):2227–2246

Cekici A, Kantarci A, Hasturk H, Van Dyke TE (2014) Inflammatory and immune pathways in the pathogenesis of periodontal disease. Periodontol 2000 64(1):57–80

Chiu B (1999) Multiple infections in carotid atherosclerotic plaques. Am Heart J 138(5 Pt 2):S534–S536

Christ-Crain M, Bichet DG, Fenske WK, Goldman MB, Rittig S, Verbalis JG, Verkman AS (2019) Diabetes insipidus. Nat Rev Dis Primers 5(1):54

Clase CM, Ki V, Holden RM (2013) Water-soluble vitamins in people with low glomerular filtration rate or on dialysis: a review. Semin Dial 26(5):546–567

Clegg A, Young J, Iliffe S, Rikkert MO, Rockwood K (2013) Frailty in elderly people. Lancet 381(9868):752–762

Coffey N, O'Leary F, Burke F, Roberts A, Hayes M (2020) Periodontal and oral health status of people with Cystic Fibrosis: a systematic review. J Dent 103:103509

Cristina de Lima D, Nakata GC, Balducci I, Almeida JD (2008) Oral manifestations of diabetes mellitus in complete denture wearers. J Prosthet Dent 99(1):60–65

Dan AA, Kallman JB, Wheeler A, Younoszai Z, Collantes R, Bondini S, Gerber L, Younossi ZM (2007, Sep 15) Health-related quality of life in patients with non-alcoholic fatty liver disease. Aliment Pharmacol Ther 26(6):815–820

Daubländer M, Kämmerer PW (2012) Lokalanästhesie im Alter. Zahnärztl Mit 102:38–45

DEGAM (2017) S3-Leitlinie „Multimorbidität". Deutsche Gesellschaft für Allgemein- und Familienmedizin e.V. (DEGAM). AWMF-Register-Nr. 053-047

Deshpande RG, Khan MB, Genco CA (1998) Invasion of aortic and heart endothelial cells by Porphyromonas gingivalis. Infect Immun 66(11):5337–5343

DGMKG, DGZMK (2018) S3-Leitlinie „Antiresorptiva-assoziierte Kiefernekrosen (AR-ONJ)". Deutsche Gesellschaft für Zahn-, Mund- und Kieferheilkunde (DGZMK), Deutsche Gesellschaft für Mund-, Kiefer- und Gesichtschirurgie (DGMKG). AWMF-Registernr. 007/091

Forssell H, Teerijoki-Oksa T, Kotiranta U, Kantola R, Back M, Vuorjoki-Ranta TR, Siponen M, Leino A, Puukka P, Estlander AM (2012) Pain and pain behavior in burning mouth syndrome: a pain diary study. J Orofac Pain 26(2):117–125. https://www.ncbi.nlm.nih.gov/pubmed/22558611

Friedewald VE, Kornman KS, Beck JD, Genco R, Goldfine A, Libby P, Offenbacher S, Ridker PM, Van Dyke TE, Roberts WC, American Journal of Cardiology, Journal of Periodontology (2009) The American Journal of Cardiology and Journal of Periodontology Editors' Consensus: periodontitis and atherosclerotic cardiovascular disease. Am J Cardiol 104(1):59–68

Gani F, Caminati M, Bellavia F, Baroso A, Faccioni P, Pancera P, Batani V, Senna G (2020) Oral health in asthmatic patients: a review: asthma and its therapy may impact on oral health. Clin Mol Allergy 18(1):22

Gomes-Filho IS, Cruz SSD, Trindade SC, Passos-Soares JS, Carvalho-Filho PC, Figueiredo A, Lyrio AO, Hintz AM, Pereira MG, Scannapieco F (2020) Periodontitis and respiratory diseases: a systematic review with meta-analysis. Oral Dis 26(2):439–446

Graham DJ, Reichman ME, Wernecke M, Zhang R, Southworth MR, Levenson M, Sheu TC, Mott K, Goulding MR, Houstoun M, MaCurdy TE, Worrall C, Kelman JA (2015) Cardiovascular, bleeding, and mortality risks in elderly Medicare patients treated with dabigatran or warfarin for nonvalvular atrial fibrillation. Circulation 131(2):157–164

Granados-Principal S, El-Azem N, Quiles JL, Perez-Lopez P, Gonzalez A (2012) Relationship between cardiovascular risk factors and periodontal disease: current knowledge. In: Gasparyan AY (Eds) Cardiovascular risk factors. InTech, London, S 193–216

Gronkjaer LL (2015) Periodontal disease and liver cirrhosis: a systematic review. SAGE Open Med 3:2050312115601122

Halling F (2016) Zahnärztliche Verordnungen. In: Schwabe D, Paffrath D (Eds) Arzneimittelverordnungsreport 2016. Springer, Berlin, S 740–746

Han K, Park JB (2021) Tooth loss and risk of end-stage renal disease: a nationwide cohort study. J Periodontol 92(3):371–377

Haraszthy VI, Zambon JJ, Trevisan M, Zeid M, Genco RJ (2000) Identification of periodontal pathogens in atheromatous plaques. J Periodontol 71(10):1554–1560

Hashmi MF, Benjamin O, Lappin SL (2023) End-stage renal disease. In StatPearls. https://www.ncbi.nlm.nih.gov/pubmed/29763036

Holt S, Schmiedl S, Thurmann PA (2010) Potentially inappropriate medications in the elderly: the PRISCUS list. Dtsch Arztebl Int 107(31–32):543–551

Indriolo A, Greco S, Ravelli P, Fagiuoli S (2011) What can we learn about biofilm/host interactions from the study of inflammatory bowel disease. J Clin Periodontol 38 Suppl 11:36–43

International Classification of Orofacial Pain, 1st edition (ICOP) (2020) Cephalalgia 40(2):129–221

Ivanovski K, Naumovski V, Kostadinova M, Pesevska S, Drijanska K, Filipce V (2012) Xerostomia and salivary levels of glucose and urea in patients with diabetes. Prilozi 33(2):219–229. https://www.ncbi.nlm.nih.gov/pubmed/23425883

Iwasaki M, Borgnakke WS, Awano S, Yoshida A, Hamasaki T, Teratani G, Kataoka S, Kakuta S, Soh I, Ansai T, Nakamura H (2017) Periodontitis and health-related quality of life in hemodialysis patients. Clin Exp Dent Res 3(1):13–18

Jaaskelainen SK, Woda A (2017) Burning mouth syndrome. Cephalalgia 37(7):627–647

Jepsen S, Blanco J, Buchalla W, Carvalho JC, Dietrich T, Dorfer C, Eaton KA, Figuero E, Frencken JE, Graziani F, Higham SM, Kocher T, Maltz M, Ortiz-Vigon A, Schmoeckel J, Sculean A, Tenuta LM, van der Veen MH, Machiulskiene V (2017) Prevention and control of dental caries and periodontal diseases at individual and population level: consensus report of group 3 of joint EFP/ORCA workshop on the boundaries between caries and periodontal diseases. J Clin Periodontol 44 Suppl 18:85–S93

Kapila YL (2021) Oral health's inextricable connection to systemic health: special populations bring to bear multimodal relationships and factors connecting periodontal disease to systemic diseases and conditions. Periodontol 2000 87(1):11–16

Kaplan GG (2015) The global burden of IBD: from 2015 to 2025. Nat Rev Gastroenterol Hepatol 12(12):720–727

Kassebaum NJ, Smith AGC, Bernabe E, Fleming TD, Reynolds AE, Vos T, Murray CJL, Marcenes W, Collaborators GBDOH (2017) Global, regional, and national prevalence, incidence, and disability-adjusted life years for oral conditions for 195 countries, 1990–2015: a systematic analysis for the global burden of diseases, injuries, and risk factors. J Dent Res 96(4):380–387

Kebschull M, Demmer RT, Papapanou PN (2010) "Gum bug, leave my heart alone!"—epidemiologic and mechanistic evidence linking periodontal infections and atherosclerosis. J Dent Res 89(9):879–902

Kohorst JJ, Bruce AJ, Torgerson RR, Schenck LA, Davis MDP (2015) The prevalence of burning mouth syndrome: a population-based study. Br J Dermatol 172(6):1654–1656. https://doi.org/10.1111/bjd.13613

Larsen TB, Rasmussen LH, Skjoth F, Due KM, Callreus T, Rosenzweig M, Lip GY (2013) Efficacy and safety of dabigatran etexilate and warfarin in "real-world" patients with atrial fibrillation: a prospective nationwide cohort study. J Am Coll Cardiol 61(22):2264–2273

Lau YC, Proietti M, Guiducci E, Blann AD, Lip GYH (2016) Atrial fibrillation and thromboembolism in patients with chronic kidney disease. J Am Coll Cardiol 68(13):1452–1464

Lauritano D, Boccalari E, Di Stasio D, Della Vella F, Carinci F, Lucchese A, Petruzzi M (2019) Prevalence of oral lesions and correlation with intestinal symptoms of inflammatory bowel disease: a systematic review. Diagnostics (Basel) 9(3):77

Limdi NA, Nolin TD, Booth SL, Centi A, Marques MB, Crowley MR, Allon M, Beasley TM (2015) Influence of kidney function on risk of supratherapeutic international normalized ratio-related hemorrhage in warfarin users: a prospective cohort study. Am J Kidney Dis 65(5):701–709

Limeres J, Garcez JF, Marinho JS, Loureiro A, Diniz M, Diz P (2016) Early tooth loss in end-stage renal disease patients on haemodialysis. Oral Dis 22(6):530–535

Lins L, Bittencourt PL, Evangelista MA, Lins R, Codes L, Cavalcanti AR, Parana R, Bastos J (2011) Oral health profile of cirrhotic patients awaiting liver transplantation in the Brazilian Northeast. Transplant Proc 43(4):1319–1321

Liu YF, Kim Y, Yoo T, Han P, Inman JC (2018) Burning mouth syndrome: a systematic review of treatments. Oral Dis 24(3):325–334

Lohse MJ (2016) Psychopharmaka. In: Springer (Eds) Arzneimittelverordnungsreport 2016. Springer, Berlin, S 663–690

Lopez-Lopez J, Jane-Salas E, Estrugo-Devesa A, Velasco-Ortega E, Martin-Gonzalez J, Segura-Egea JJ (2011) Periapical and endodontic status of type 2 diabetic patients in Catalonia, Spain: a cross-sectional study. J Endod 37(5):598–601

Lutz H, Wille H (2016) Antithrombotika und Antihämorrhagika. In: Schwabe D, Paffrath D (Eds) Arzneimittelverordnungsreport 2016. Springer, Berlin, S 352

Mankia K, Cheng Z, Do T, Hunt L, Meade J, Kang J, Clerehugh V, Speirs A, Tugnait A, Hensor EMA, Nam JL, Devine DA, Emery P (2019) Prevalence of periodontal disease and periodontopathic bacteria in anti-cyclic citrullinated protein antibody-positive at-risk adults without arthritis. JAMA Netw Open 2(6):e195394

Marsh PD (2010) Microbiology of dental plaque biofilms and their role in oral health and caries. Dent Clin North Am 54(3):441–454

Mathers CD, Boerma T, Ma Fat D (2009) Global and regional causes of death. Br Med Bull 92:7–32

Mathews MJ, Liebenberg L, Mathews EH (2015) How do high glycemic load diets influence coronary heart disease? Nutr Metab (Lond) 12:6

Mauri-Obradors E, Estrugo-Devesa A, Jane-Salas E, Vinas M, Lopez-Lopez J (2017) Oral manifestations of Diabetes Mellitus. A systematic review. Med Oral Patol Oral Cir Bucal 22(5):e586–e594

McMillan R, Forssell H, Buchanan JA, Glenny AM, Weldon JC, Zakrzewska JM (2016) Interventions for treating burning mouth syndrome. Cochrane Database Syst Rev 11(11):CD002779

Mealey BL (2000) Diabetes and periodontal disease: two sides of a coin. Compend Contin Educ Dent 21(11):943–946, 948, 950, passim; quiz 956. https://www.ncbi.nlm.nih.gov/pubmed/11968145

Meurman JH, Sanz M, Janket SJ (2004) Oral health, atherosclerosis, and cardiovascular disease. Crit Rev Oral Biol Med 15(6):403–413

Moßhammer D, Haumann H, Mörike K, Joos S (2016) Polypharmazie—Tendenz steigend, Folgen schwer kalkulierbar. Dtsch Arztebl Int 113:627–633

Nam Y, Kim NH, Kho HS (2018) Geriatric oral and maxillofacial dysfunctions in the context of geriatric syndrome. Oral Dis 24(3):317–324

Neuner-Jehle S (2013) Weniger ist mehr—wie Polypharmazie vermeiden? Praxis 102:21–27

Ng KP, Edwards NC, Lip GY, Townend JN, Ferro CJ (2013) Atrial fibrillation in CKD: balancing the risks and benefits of anticoagulation. Am J Kidney Dis 62(3):615–632

Nijakowski K, Surdacka A (2020) Salivary biomarkers for diagnosis of inflammatory bowel diseases: a systematic review. Int J Mol Sci 21(20):7477

Nijakowski K, Rutkowski R, Eder P, Simon M, Korybalska K, Witowski J, Surdacka A (2021) Potential salivary markers for differential diagnosis of Crohn's disease and ulcerative colitis. Life (Basel) 11(9):943

Nitschke I (2012) Senioren—eine heterogene Patientengruppe mit vielen Unbekannten. Dtsch Zahnärztl Z 67:533–534

Noce A, Vidiri MF, Marrone G, Moriconi E, Bocedi A, Capria A, Rovella V, Ricci G, De Lorenzo A, Di Daniele N (2016) Is low-protein diet a possible risk factor of malnutrition in chronic kidney disease patients? Cell Death Discov 2:16026

Noce A, Rovella V, Marrone G, Cattani G, Zingaretti V, Limongi D, D'Agostini C, Sorge R, Casasco M, Di Daniele N, Ricci G, Bocedi A (2019) Hemodialysis biomarkers: total advanced glycation end products (AGEs) against oxidized human serum albumin (HSAox). Acta Diabetol 56(12):1323–1331

Noce A, Marrone G, Wilson Jones G, Di Lauro M, Pietroboni Zaitseva A, Ramadori L, Celotto R, Mitterhofer AP, Di Daniele N (2021) Nutritional approaches for the management of metabolic acidosis in chronic kidney disease. Nutrients 13(8):2534

Ohyama H, Nakasho K, Yamanegi K, Noiri Y, Kuhara A, Kato-Kogoe N, Yamada N, Hata M, Nishimura F, Ebisu S, Terada N (2009) An unusual autopsy case of pyogenic liver abscess caused by periodontal bacteria. Jpn J Infect Dis 62(5):381–383. https://www.ncbi.nlm.nih.gov/pubmed/19762989

Persson GR, Persson RE (2008) Cardiovascular disease and periodontitis: an update on the associations and risk. J Clin Periodontol 35(8 Suppl):362–379

Potpara TS, Ferro CJ, Lip GYH (2018) Use of oral anticoagulants in patients with atrial fibrillation and renal dysfunction. Nat Rev Nephrol 14(5):337–351

Poudel P, Griffiths R, Wong VW, Arora A, Flack JR, Khoo CL, George A (2018) Oral health knowledge, attitudes and care practices of people with diabetes: a systematic review. BMC Public Health 18(1):577

Raimann JG, Levin NW, Craig RG, Sirover W, Kotanko P, Handelman G (2013) Is vitamin C intake too low in dialysis patients? Semin Dial 26(1):1–5

Rixecker H, Kleemann PP, Tetsch P (1985) Ambulante zahnärztlich-chirurgische Behandlung bei Problempatienten. ZWR 94:900–902

Said HS, Suda W, Nakagome S, Chinen H, Oshima K, Kim S, Kimura R, Iraha A, Ishida H, Fujita J, Mano S, Morita H, Dohi T, Oota H, Hattori M (2014) Dysbiosis of salivary microbiota in inflammatory bowel disease and its association with oral immunological biomarkers. DNA Res 21(1):15–25

Sardella A, Lodi G, Demarosi F, Bez C, Cassano S, Carrassi A (2006) Burning mouth syndrome: a retrospective study investigating spontaneous remission and response to treatments. Oral Dis 12(2):152–155

Scala A, Checchi L, Montevecchi M, Marini I, Giamberardino MA (2003) Update on burning mouth syndrome: overview and patient management. Crit Rev Oral Biol Med 14(4):275–291

Schiavone V, Adamo D, Ventrella G, Morlino M, De Notaris EB, Ravel MG, Kusmann F, Piantadosi M, Pollio A, Fortuna G, Mignogna MD (2012) Anxiety, depression, and pain in burning mouth syndrome: first chicken or egg? Headache 52(6):1019–1025

Southworth MR, Reichman ME, Unger EF (2013) Dabigatran and postmarketing reports of bleeding. N Engl J Med 368(14):1272–1274

Souza IF de, Marmora BC, Rados PV, Visioli F (2018) Treatment modalities for burning mouth syndrome: a systematic review. Clin Oral Investig 22(5):1893–1905

Stolbova K, Hahn A, Benes B, Andel M, Treslova L (1999) Gustometry of diabetes mellitus patients and obese patients. Int Tinnitus J 5(2):135–140. https://www.ncbi.nlm.nih.gov/pubmed/10753433

Thomas MS, Parolia A, Kundabala M, Vikram M (2010) Asthma and oral health: a review. Aust Dent J 55(2):128–133

Van Dyke TE, Dowell VR Jr, Offenbacher S, Snyder W, Hersh T (1986) Potential role of microorganisms isolated from periodontal lesions in the pathogenesis of inflammatory bowel disease. Infect Immun 53(3):671–677

Wahl MJ (2014) Dental surgery and antiplatelet agents: bleed or die. Am J Med 127(4):260–267

Weber AA (2013) Pharmakologie der Hämostase. In: Aktories K, Förstermann U, Hofmann F, Starke K (Eds) Allgemeine und spezielle Pharmakologie und Toxikologie. Urban&Fischer, S 507–528

Wehling M (2009) Multimorbidity and polypharmacy: how to reduce the harmful drug load and yet add needed drugs in the elderly? Proposal of a new drug classification: fit for the aged. J Am Geriatr Soc 57(3):560–561

Younossi ZM, Boparai N, Price LL, Kiwi ML, McCormick M, Guyatt G (2001) Health-related quality of life in chronic liver disease: the impact of type and severity of disease. Am J Gastroenterol 96(7):2199–2205

Multimorbidity and Chronic Diseases 9

Jan-Hendrik Ortloff and Daniela Schmitz

Contents

9.1 The Phenomenon of Multimorbid and Chronic Diseases

Although patients with multiple and chronic diseases are increasingly the norm in clinical practice, multimorbidity, which is often associated with chronic diseases, is not

J.-H. Ortloff (✉)
Department of human medicine, Witten/Herdecke University, Witten, Germany
e-mail: Jan-Hendrik.Ortloff@uni-wh.de

D. Schmitz
Department of human medicine, Witten/Herdecke University, Witten, Germany
e-mail: Daniela.Schmitz@uni-wh.de

D. Schmitz et al. (eds.), *Chronic Care—Science and Practice*,
https://doi.org/10.1007/978-3-662-72298-5_9

mentioned in most guidelines and is excluded from many studies. For this reason, there is hardly any evidence-based knowledge for people with several, in some cases chronic, diseases. This means that even if guidelines for individual diseases exist and are correctly implemented in practice, the simultaneous application of multiple guidelines can lead to undesirable consequences, side effects, or contradictory treatment strategies (Deutsche Gesellschaft für Allgemeinmedizin und Familienmedizin 2017).

The treatment and care, especially for people with chronic and multimorbid conditions, are therefore not based on a single strategy and evidence base, but on different approaches, which over time also include various perspectives, fields of expertise, disciplines, and methods. In addition, care must be aligned with the priorities and goals of the patients and takes place over a longer period. The care of people with multimorbidity is therefore often fragmented, complex, challenging, and correspondingly prone to quality deficits.

On the one hand, neither multimorbidity nor the need for care are inevitable consequences of aging; on the other hand, chronic diseases in particular occur more frequently in later years of life. The term multimorbidity applies to a heterogeneous group with diverse diseases and combinations. For this reason, the treatment and care of those affected should be implemented at a high level of abstraction and should focus on dealing with multimorbidity as an independent overall situation, rather than on individual disease combinations.

Multimorbidity is a phenomenon that will continue to increase in the future due to age-related changes in society. Due to the different study populations and a lack of consensus regarding definition and operationalization, the prevalence is difficult to quantify internationally. As a result, the frequency is estimated to be between 55% and 98% (Deutsche Gesellschaft für Allgemeinmedizin und Familienmedizin 2017) or 17% to 80% (Bundesarbeitsgemeinschaft für Rehabilitation 2018) for aging societies.

9.1.1 Definition of multimorbidity

Numerous definitions and operationalizations of multimorbidity have existed for years (Marengoni et al. 2011). The required number of diseases in particular varies. The *Multimorbidity Guideline* defines the simultaneous presence of three or more chronic diseases as multimorbidity, none of which is the focus of treatment, although there may be connections (risk factors, secondary diseases, etc.). However, the literature also contains definitions that refer to two or more simultaneously occurring chronic diseases, each of which has a comparable impact on the individual disease burden (Seger and Gaertner 2020). It is also notable that these definitions refer to chronic diseases and thus exclude acute illnesses.

Furthermore, a distinction is made between multi- and comorbidity. In multimorbidity, none of the diseases can be designated as the main diagnosis, since all existing diseases have an equal influence on treatment and care. In contrast, comorbidity refers to diseases as primary when, in the presence of several diseases, a particular disease is the focus and others recede into the background. A comorbidity can, in the sense of a secondary disease, be causally related to the underlying disease or be independent of it. In this context, it can be discussed whether diseases that affect behavior (dementia, depression, neurotic-, stress-related-, and somatoform disorders) are primary or secondary diseases, or whether a multi- or comorbid condition is present.

9.1.2 Forms of multimorbidity

In the literature, multimorbidity is, among other things, divided into the statistical multimorbidity concept (frequencies), the dynamic multimorbidity concept (dynamics between problem areas), and the geriatric multimorbidity concept (Burkhardt 2019).

The statistical multimorbidity concept is based on medical diagnoses and focuses almost exclusively on quantitative aspects, such as index diseases. The dynamic multimorbidity concept additionally takes into account the respective disease phase and the interactions between disease, environment, person, activity, and participation based on the identified problem areas. To assess the situation, the process involves identifying the problem (multimorbidity pattern), determining the diagnoses and initial interventions, coordinating different measures, a re-assessment (if necessary, review/adjustment), evaluating the measures, and multiprofessional or cross-institutional documentation.

Geriatric multimorbidity, as the name suggests, refers to older and very old individuals. Geriatric patients are not clearly defined, even though the term is used in clinical practice. According to Ernst et al. (2020), immobility, tendency to fall and dizziness, cognitive deficits, incontinence, malnutrition and undernutrition, pressure ulcers, depression, anxiety disorder, chronic pain, severe visual impairment, and pronounced hearing loss are among the geriatric syndromes. In addition, the numerous interfaces, unclear responsibilities, and discipline-specific perspectives can lead to typical geriatric syndromes not being detected in time, and thus influencing factors and prevention potentials being overlooked.

9.1.3 Influencing Factors on Multimorbidity

Just as varied as the combinations of multimorbidity can be, the influencing factors are also described in the literature and are grouped into clusters, which can be found, among others, in the guideline on multimorbidity.

- Age: Numerous studies show that the prevalence of multimorbidity increases with age. One reason for this is seen in the chronicity of diseases.
- Gender: The relationship between gender and multimorbidity depends greatly on the disease spectrum studied. For this reason, there are studies in which women are more frequently affected by multimorbidity, as well as studies that demonstrate a higher prevalence in men.

- Psychological factors: Patients with chronic somatic diseases often simultaneously suffer from mental illnesses such as depression. These often exhibit complex interactions, as chronic diseases can lead to depression, while depression can also be a risk factor for the chronification of other diseases.
- Social determinants: People with low income and low educational attainment are affected by multimorbidity more frequently and at an earlier age; however, these relationships appear to depend on the respective societal structures and the specific diseases studied.
- Personal factors: Personal attitudes and intrinsic values regarding the management of chronic diseases can also influence multimorbidity, as these form the basis for compliance and coping.
- Environmental factors: Environmental influences can have a direct impact on lifestyle and thus on risk factors and behaviors. Continuous access to health-related infrastructure is also a basic prerequisite for treatment and care, which faces limitations in both urban and rural regions.
- Chronicity: The transition from a temporary to a permanent disease or symptoms can influence multimorbidity, among other things, through the resulting psychological burdens. Symptoms such as pain frequently occur in multimorbidity and increase the risk of falls, anxiety disorders, as well as cognitive or somatic dysfunctions.
- Combinations: In patients with multimorbidity, regularities in the disease spectrum occur, so that certain disease combinations are more frequent than would be expected from the prevalence of the individual diseases. These include, among others, cardiovascular, metabolic, psychological, neuropsychological, and psychosomatic diseases, as well as musculoskeletal disorders.
- Frailty: Frailty or increased vulnerability is closely interrelated with multimorbidity, as they strongly influence each other. Frailty affects people more frequently with increasing age, and various causes are assumed, such as low physiological resilience, a weak immune system, or progressive loss of skeletal and muscle mass, although only limited research findings are available so far. In addition, psychosocial factors have hardly been considered to date.

Due to the different influencing factors and the unclear distinction between multi- and comorbid disease patterns and their symptoms, it is often difficult to assign them to a specific medical specialty. The multiprofessional treatment team is therefore faced with the challenge that the interactions are less manageable and undesirable interactions become increasingly risky. In addition, as multimorbidity, vulnerability, and disease burden increase, the scope for action and resources of patients decrease.

9.2 Measuring Multimorbidity

The greatest hurdles in the treatment of patients with multimorbidity are differing approaches, contradictory recommendations, and interactions arising from the individual diseases. Initial attempts at operationalization exist, aiming to capture multimorbidity holistically. In order to assess the quality of care for people with multimorbidity, the MULTIqual (Development and Validation of Quality Indicators for Multimorbidity) was developed. The quality of care is measured using 22 indicators, which are grouped into three categories.

Under the category of *patient-centered parameters*, the indicators depression, pain, pain management, financial support needs, subjective quality of life, symptom burden, patient preferences, caregivers, as well as patient education and self-management are assessed. The category *physician-patient interaction* includes the indicators: joint agreement on treatment goals, written treatment plan, treatment-related burdens, therapy adherence (compliance with joint therapy goals), drug effects, medication review, information on potential benefits or harms of therapy options, participatory decision-making, and current medication plan. The third category, *context structures*, contains the indicators: responsibility for coordination, care documentation, and continuing education measures relevant to multimorbidity (Glassen et al. 2022). The three categories illustrate the diverse factors and their potential impact on subjective quality of life.

MULTIqual is an operationalized instrument for assessing the quality of care for people with multimorbidity, which serves as a basis for further international research. It was developed based on a systematic literature review and a two-stage consensus process with multiprofessional experts. Criticisms include the limitation of its application to the outpatient sector, the effort/benefit aspect in practice, and the reduction to the interaction between physicians and patients.

9.3 Multimorbidity as a Social Challenge

The interactions that exist at the subjective level due to multimorbidity also have societal implications, given the high number of people affected. Relevant topics in this context include research, hospitalization, quality of life, and the need for care.

9.3.1 Research

A causal relationship between multimorbidity and various variables (hospitalization, mortality, quality of life, autonomy, etc.) cannot currently be established, as the small number of studies often employ cross-sectional designs. Furthermore, research is limited by pronounced heterogeneity in the disease spectrum studied, the setting, the various data sources, and the study period (disease phase), making it difficult to draw generalizable conclusions.

A Cochrane Review investigated which interventions have an impact on relevant outcomes such as mental and physical health, economic aspects, use of services, psychosocial factors such as well-being, participation and quality of life, as well as the behaviors of those involved. Two categories could be formed. The first focuses on the organizational level of management and its coordinating activities, such as enhancing collaboration within a multiprofessional team. The second targets the behavior of patients. The results show an improvement in outcomes when interventions are aimed at risk factors or functional limitations. In addition, interventions appear to be more effective when they focus on individual risk factors or functional problems (Smith et al. 2016).

Various studies indicate a correlation between multimorbidity and mortality. Accordingly, patients with multimorbidity have, on average, a higher mortality rate than patients without multimorbidity (Marengoni et al. 2011). Mortality correlates with the number and type of chronic diseases, such as cardiovascular diseases, chronic heart failure, malignant tumors, chronic lung disease, as well as advanced liver and kidney diseases (Gijsen et al. 2001). However, there are also studies that could not demonstrate a correlation or pointed to special circumstances such as disability. Moreover, the diseases studied are conditions that, even on their own, contribute to increased mortality.

Whether mortality and multimorbidity are correlated, and whether possible associations are caused by the number of diseases or rather by the individual diseases themselves, is not clarified in the current guideline on multimorbidity (Deutsche Gesellschaft für Allgemeinmedizin und Familienmedizin 2017).

9.3.2 Hospitalization

There are also various influencing factors in hospitalization that can lead to hospital admission. The frequency of inpatient stays increases proportionally with the number of diseases, but independently of age (Glynn et al. 2011). In addition, mental illnesses such as depression, etc., tend to promote hospitalization among multimorbid patients. Another relevant indicator of hospitalization is the length of stay, as patients with multimorbidity often remain in the hospital longer and sometimes experience more postoperative complications. Furthermore, after a hospital stay, the risk of institutionalization (e.g., moving into a care facility) increases. This is especially the case if temporary immobilization occurred during the hospital stay. Moreover, permanent functional limitations may result if, for example, pre-hospital motor mobility is not regained.

9.3.3 Quality of Life

Quality of life is closely linked to subjectively perceived health. Multimorbid patients often rate their quality of life lower, experience greater psychological distress, and more frequently have depressive symptoms than the average population (Fortin et al. 2006). Here, the manifold interactions between endurance, mobility, autonomy, and quality of life become apparent, as each of these components conditions the next. In particular, chronic diseases such as visual impairments, back pain, or cardiovascular diseases can significantly reduce quality of life. Compared to hospitalization and mortality, age appears to have less impact on the assessment of quality of life. While the first chronic disease is perceived as particularly significant in certain age groups, multimorbidity with four or more diseases leads to functional and emotional impairments across all age groups (Bayliss 2014). Since the assessment of quality of life is a subjective evaluation, it should also be noted that not all influencing factors affect all domains of quality of life equally, and the adaptability and coping strategies of those affected play a central role.

9.3.4 Need for Care

A common and irreversible consequence of multimorbidity as a central health risk is the need for care, which represents a state of extreme physical, psychological, and social vulnerability. These factors, especially in combination, lead to deficient health conditions that make those affected dependent on help and care. Key factors include, for example, physical and cognitive activities as well as nutritional aspects, as these not only significantly influence the need for care but can also represent resources and potential. Even in the prevention phase (including before recurrences) of chronic diseases, appropriate measures can help reduce or prevent the need for assistance and care.

Limitations in functionality and endurance often also affect partners and caregiving relatives, as they frequently lead to loss of autonomy and institutionalization over time. The identification of pre-frailty also enables preventive measures that can positively influence the development of the need for assistance and care.

9.4 Requirements for the Multiprofessional Care Team

The World Health Organization (WHO) has published practical guidance and strategic recommendations for the appropriate care of people with multimorbidity in the *Technical Series on Safer Primary Care*, emphasizing multiprofessional care. The strategies that, according to the WHO, can be prioritized by member states are intended to focus on changes at the health policy level and can be summarized in five categories (WHO 2016).

- Implement societal changes: At the policy level, the integration of guidelines on the social determinants of health, the development of a strong primary care system within general healthcare, and research into primary care for people with multiple chronic conditions should be promoted. This requires robust workforce planning and training at the bachelor's and master's level across all areas of healthcare.
- Adopt a systemic approach: It is important to view patients holistically in terms of their physical, psychological, and social health, and to coordinate care beyond the boundaries of one's own discipline. Recommendations from individual guidelines should therefore be harmonized. To achieve this, systems must be developed that enable improved communication and coordination between organizations and across different levels of the healthcare system. In addition, physicians, nurses, therapists, and other members of the multiprofessional team should be integrated into the care of patients with multimorbidity and receive specific training in multimorbidity.
- Identify vulnerable individuals: People who require additional support due to multimorbidity should be identified as early as the primary care stage, so that targeted preventive measures and interventions can begin as soon as possible. Furthermore, the subjective interrelations between physical and mental health should be recognized so that mental illnesses are also prioritized. A combination of mental and physical multimorbidity carries the highest risk, which can negatively impact treatment outcomes.
- Improve care coordination: Assigning patients to a primary care provider should ensure that all patients with multimorbidity have care providers responsible for their care. At the system level, stratification of care provision is advisable to conserve resources for those who need them most. Furthermore, enhanced training measures, strategies for patient education and engagement, support for informal caregivers (family members), the use of shared digital medical records and information systems, as well as the promotion of self-management, are recommended.
- Simplify treatment plans: Careful management of risk factors can help reduce, for example, polypharmacy and maximize the use of non-pharmacological interventions. This includes appropriate polypharmacy, discontinuation of treatments with limited benefit, ensuring patient understanding of their treatment, the use of medication aids to promote adherence, and the introduction of technologies (such as alerts for drug interactions and reminders for timing, type, and dosage of medications).

9.5 Approaches to the Care of People with Multimorbidity

The management of multimorbid conditions focuses on cooperation between specialists, the achievement of goals, and the empowerment of self-management.

Multimorbidity leads to increased utilization of services. In the German healthcare system, these contacts are unregulated, so that examinations, diagnoses, recommendations, referrals, and treatments occur simultaneously and sequentially. The exchange of information between specialists is also unregulated, as in the case of temporary measures, the complete medical history with anamnesis, diagnostics, and treatment is rarely fully available. None of the providers has all relevant data at hand during a consultation. However, when multiple health professions are involved in the treatment of patients with multimorbidity, all parties involved (patients, relatives, specialists, etc.) should coordinate regarding diagnostics and therapy (Deutsche Gesellschaft für Allgemeinmedizin und Familienmedizin 2017).

To ensure successful treatment and care, it is necessary to raise awareness among all parties so that multimorbidity is recognized already in primary care. This requires individual needs assessment, particularly where patients are first and most continuously cared for across interfaces. This includes not only solid primary care but also needs-based management of both inpatient and outpatient rehabilitation services, as well as concrete goal setting. In addition, it is necessary to present the assessment of multimorbid conditions transparently and comprehensibly for all stakeholders and to document it throughout the entire course so that relevant impairments, contextual factors, and their interactions are apparent. Planning and implementation also require continuous review of the (partial) goals achieved and, if necessary, adjustment, taking into account professional, social, and economic resources (regional health infrastructures).

Due to its complexity and dynamics, multimorbidity requires a holistic approach, which in turn necessitates multiprofessional care. For this reason, it is essential to involve representatives of all relevant disciplines from the outset in process design and to include them participatively in the development of guidelines, so that over-, under-, or misprovision of care for patients with multimorbidity is avoided and successes in terms of *best practice* are shared. Ultimately, it is the collaboration between specialists and those affected, taking into account the different perspectives, that can lead to successful treatment of multimorbid conditions (see contribution 21).

References

Bayliss E (2014) How does multimorbidity affect patients? In: Mercer S, Salisbury C, Fortin M (Eds) ABC of multimorbidity. Wiley, S 8–11

Bundesarbeitsgemeinschaft für Rehabilitation (Eds) (2018) Multimorbidität in der medizinischen Rehabilitation. https://www.bar-frankfurt.de/fileadmin/dateiliste/_publikationen/reha_grundlagen/pdfs/Multimorbidit%C3%A4t_Final_ES.pdf. Accessed 13. Mai 2023

Burkhardt H (Eds) (2019) Umgang mit Multimorbidität und Multimedikation, 1. Aufl. Kohlhammer, Stuttgart

Deutsche Gesellschaft für Allgemeinmedizin und Familienmedizin (Eds) (2017) S3-Leitlinie Multimorbidität. Arbeitsgemeinschaft der Wissenschaftlichen Medizinischen Fachgesellschaften

Ernst F, Lübke N, Meinck M (2020) Kompendium Begutachtungswissen Geriatrie, 4. Aufl. Springer, Berlin/Heidelberg

Fortin M, Bravo G, Hudon C, Lapointe L, Almirall J, Dubois M-F, Vanasse A (2006) Relationship between multimorbidity and health-related quality of life of patients in primary care. Qual Life Res 15(1):83–91

Gijsen R, Hoeymans N, Schellevis FG, Ruwaard D, Satariano WA, van den Bos GA (2001) Causes and consequences of comorbidity: a review. J Clin Epidemiol 54(7):661–674

Glassen K, Schulze J, Breckner A, Lühmann D, Szecsenyi J, Scherer M (2022) Multimorbidität. Qualitätsindikatoren für die ambulante Versorgung von Patientinnen und Patienten mit Multimorbidität—Handbuch für die ärztliche Praxis. In: Szecsenyi J, Broge B, Stock J (Eds) QISA—Das Qualitätsindikatorensystem für die ambulante Versorgung, Bd F2. KomPart, Berlin

Glynn LG, Valderas JM, Healy P, Burke E, Newell J, Gillespie P, Murphy AW (2011) The prevalence of multimorbidity in primary care and its effect on health care utilization and cost. Family Prac 28(5):516–523

Marengoni A, Angleman S, Melis R, Mangialasche F, Karp A, Garmen A, Meinow B, Fratiglioni L (2011) Aging with multimorbidity: a systematic review of the literature. Ageing Res Rev 10(4):430–439

Seger W, Gaertner T (2020) Multimorbidität: Eine besondere Herausforderung. Dtsch Ärztebl 117(44):A-2092

Smith SM, Wallace E, O'Dowd T, Fortin M (2016) Interventions for improving outcomes in patients with multimorbidity in primary care and community settings. Cochr Database Syst Rev 3(3):12

World Health Organization (2016) Multimorbidity: technical series on safer primary care 2016. https://www.who.int/patientsaety/topics/primary-care/technical_serie/en/. Accessed 17. Feb 2023

Impacts of Chronic Diseases 10

Jan-Hendrik Ortloff

Contents

10.1 Influencing Factors on Chronic Diseases

The effects of chronic diseases are often defined using the bio-medical concepts of disease burden, health-related quality of life, and risk factors in order to achieve an objective description. However, upon closer examination, it becomes apparent that the consequences must be differentiated both at the micro level for those affected and at the macro level with regard to societal impacts, and are shaped by subjective assessments, psychosocial contextual factors, as well as the dynamics of disease progression. Consequently, the effects of chronic diseases require a perspective that calls for

J.-H. Ortloff (✉)
Department of human medicine, Witten/Herdecke University, Witten, Germany
e-mail: Jan-Hendrik.Ortloff@uni-wh.de

D. Schmitz et al. (eds.), *Chronic Care—Science and Practice*,
https://doi.org/10.1007/978-3-662-72298-5_10

multiprofessional care services in order to continuously consider the situations of those affected within an individual bio-psycho-social context.

10.1.1 Disease Burden

Disease burden describes the impact of a health problem, which is determined using quantified data and used for comparison. To this end, burden of disease studies at the global (global burden of disease) and national or regional (national burden of disease) levels capture the impact of disease burden using financial costs, mortality and morbidity rates, and other statistical parameters. Methodological cornerstones include Disability-Adjusted Life Years (DALYs), which sum the years of life lost due to mortality (relative to average life expectancy) with the years lived with health limitations or disease, in order to compare these with the average of the population under consideration. The main sources of information are health insurance routine data, survey data from studies, and mortality statistics (Robert Koch Institut 2021). From burden of disease studies, the difference between optimal health and actual health is derived and used as a comparison to assess the effects and developments of a disease.

For Germany, the results indicate age- and gender-specific as well as regional differences that highlight specific care needs. People with chronic or multimorbid conditions can influence DALY rates, as their life expectancy may deviate significantly from the average due to the combined disease burden of individual conditions. Based on DALY rates, coronary heart disease, lower back pain, and lung cancer contribute most to the disease burden. Gender differences also showed that headache disorders and dementias in women, as well as lung cancer and alcohol-related disorders in men, cause the greatest disease burden. Proportionally with age, the disease burden also increases for cardiovascular diseases, dementias, and diabetes mellitus (Porst et al. 2022). Thus, DALY rates provide an initial orientation for prevention and health measures in a region (macro level); however, even though DALY rates are determined from individual data of those affected, they offer little insight into the subjective perspective (micro level). It should also be noted that DALY rates are based on long-term surveys, and the subjectively experienced disease burden may temporarily deviate from the DALY rates of a region due to various contextual factors.

10.1.2 Health and Quality of Life

Based on the term chronic in the sense of ongoing, people with chronic diseases are affected permanently. In addition, the disease situation, even in the case of physical complaints, can be exacerbated by psychological problems and influence the assessment of quality of life. Health and quality of life are closely linked, as both concepts consist of multiple dimensions that can influence each other. Despite the pronounced interactions, it should be noted that health encompasses more than quality of life, and quality of life in turn includes more than health, as both constructs may also contain dimensions not captured by the other.

For health sciences, a coherent concept of health and a functioning transfer from theory to practice are important prerequisites for multiprofessional care. To approach such a concept, health can be subdivided multidimensionally into: health as demarcation concepts, which are closely linked to the medical interpretation and diagnosis of disease (bio-medical perspective); as functional statements for physical and social performance and work capacity or role fulfillment (sociological perspective); as homeostatic health concepts of a physical-mental balance (salutogenetic perspective); or as a flexible adaptation of body and self to changing environmental conditions (systemic demands-resources model). Thus, health encompasses physical, mental-spiritual, and social components that influence each other and also integrate potential limitations in the sense of a health-disease continuum (Franzkowiak and Hurrelmann 2018). Depending on the perspective, people with chronic diseases are therefore conditionally healthy if, despite health limitations, they achieve their life goals, lead a meaningful existence for themselves, or experience quality of life, etc.

The factors for quality of life were defined in terms of content, among others, by a European expert group and categorized into nine dimensions: material living conditions; education; main activity; health; leisure and social interaction; economic and physical security; rule of law and fundamental rights; natural environment and living environment; as well as a general sense of life. Not only indicators of general quality of life play a role here, but also indicators of individual perception (Diez 2015). In the context of chronic diseases, there is also often an attempt to objectify quality of life as health-related quality of life (Health-Related Quality of Life). A multidimensional concept is also applied here, which places the interactions of physical, psychological, and social factors in context (Robert Koch Institut 2023). Thus, the dimensions differ both between the various concepts of health and between the concepts of health and quality of life. In addition, objectively measured quality of life may decrease, while personal assessment, through the development of individual coping strategies by those affected, leads to a more positive evaluation of quality of life. An examination of quality of life in chronic diseases shows that coronary heart disease primarily affects physical functionality, while in arthritis, physical pain leads to losses in quality of life, and diabetes mellitus affects overall health status. The most pronounced impacts on quality of life are found in diseases of the cerebral vessels, gastrointestinal tract, musculoskeletal system, and kidney diseases. A particularly high overall loss of health-related quality of life is present in heart failure, chronic obstructive pulmonary disease, and arthritis. In contrast, the loss is considered low in hypertension and allergies (Güthlin 2020). People with mental illnesses may experience a higher degree of social and emotional impairment, while their physical functioning remains intact. Conversely, people with musculoskeletal diseases may have pronounced impairments in physical functioning, while their social environment remains largely unaffected. In addition to mobility restrictions, reduced resilience can lead to losses in quality of life. For example, heart failure can negatively affect physical endurance, mobility, and, in the case of dizziness symptoms triggered by heart failure, also gait. The associated limitations in mobility can, in turn, negatively impact participation and independence.

10.1.3 Risk Factors

Risk factors are of particular importance for the entire course of a disease, from etiology to prognosis and disease management, and are especially relevant for chronic illnesses, as they determine and allow assessment of the course (e.g., the occurrence of recurrences in cancer or progression in dementias). Three core factors can be identified here;

- Genetic predispositions: Biological or genetic risk factors include, among others, sex, age, as well as genetic predispositions for certain diseases, which can also lead to illnesses later in life.
- Environmental conditions: The living conditions in which people grow up and live are crucial (see Chapter 15), as they shape how individuals deal with illnesses and create access to health goods and services. This links societal provision (participation) with the utilization (involvement) of health services.
- Health behavior: Depending on intellectual, cognitive, and physiological abilities, risk factors are shaped by lifestyles. Positive and negative behaviors can be influenced by those affected and can impact both genetic predispositions and environmental conditions (Sperlich and Franzkowiak 2022).

Modern risk factor models are based on the assumption that there are connections between the development of diseases and perceived quality of life. By focusing on the emergence of diseases, risk factors represent a pathogenic perspective, which is only complemented by the protective factors of the salutogenic perspective. However, when considering the effects of chronic diseases, it should be critically noted that describing risk factors primarily allows for an assessment of medical diagnoses, which partially overlooks psycho-social aspects and thus distorts the need for necessary resources to achieve quality of life.

10.2 Impact on Primary and Secondary Diagnoses

Engaging with the burdens of disease load, reduced health-related quality of life, risk factors, and available resources can result in various interactions. Chronic illnesses can, on the one hand, represent an emotional burden because the progression of the disease is uncertain, and on the other hand, because those affected are aware of the chronic nature of their illness. Emotional imbalance, anxiety and depression, feelings of loss of autonomy and control, altered body image, as well as self-esteem and identity problems can result. It is well established that people with a chronic physical illness and a psychological comorbidity have a lower health-related quality of life and a less favorable disease course (Koch et al. 2011).

Isolated disease patterns are rare in chronic illnesses. More often, a spectrum of different diagnoses from co- or multimorbidity is observed, which can also be caused by secondary diseases. This leads to disease constellations that can be as diverse as the chronic illnesses themselves. To determine the impact of chronic diseases, it is useful, regardless of the field, to identify primary and secondary diagnoses for the current point in time.

According to a general understanding, the diseases of a *multimorbid condition* are considered to be of equal rank, as each disease in itself has comparable effects on the subjectively perceived disease burden, health-related quality of life, and risk factors. In the case of *comorbidity* (accompanying disease), diseases are instead prioritized and thus divided into primary main diagnoses and secondary diagnoses. This can be interpreted to mean that, during the current treatment period, secondary diagnoses have less impact on disease burden, health-related quality of life, and risk factors than primary diagnoses. However, such an interpretation can be misleading, especially in chronic diseases, when several illnesses are present temporarily, whose symptoms and phases may be asynchronous or alternating. Many chronic diseases have a remitting and progressive course, which includes recurring acute phases and introduces a dynamic into the burdens and treatment. The classification into primary and secondary diagnoses often focuses on disease burden, the weighting of which can change over time. In clinical practice, chronic disease patterns are assessed differently, both subjectively and temporarily, depending on the comorbid or multimorbid constellation, the type and severity of impairments, their duration and intensity. The actual chronic disease itself is then not always understood as the primary diagnosis, but often merely as a comorbidity, and is assessed in terms of its impact on the likelihood of developing other diseases (secondary diseases), the disease course, and disease management.

In addition to primary and secondary diagnoses, the ongoing need for treatment and the organization of medical, nursing, and therapeutic tasks can also pose a challenge. Prioritizing these raises the question of how and by whom, during a phase of a chronic illness, the distinction between primary and secondary diagnosis is made. An example is dementia, which is often recorded as a secondary diagnosis in the bio-medical treatment process, without giving sufficient attention to its psycho-social influence on the course of the disease. A bio-psycho-social prioritization of primary and secondary diagnoses, in contrast, calls into question the practicality of diagnosis classification and weighting, focuses on the subjective disease burden, highlights the necessity of multiprofessional care as well as the activation of resources, and emphasizes the meaningfulness of preventive measures (including prevention of recurrences), as the bio-psycho-social prioritization can sufficiently adapt to the progressive and remitting course. Fig. 10.1 illustrates that diagnoses such as phobias, depression, and (incipient) dementia without directly

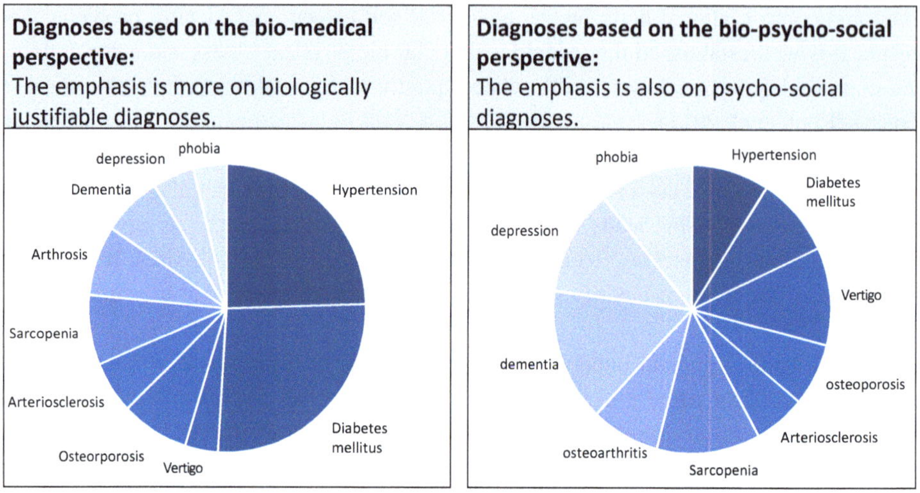

Fig. 10.1 Exemplary perspective-specific weighting of diagnoses. (Own illustration)

verifiable causes can be given less weight from the bio-medical perspective, as biologically verifiable diagnoses (hypertension, diabetes mellitus) are more obvious in acute phases. In the bio-psycho-social perspective, all (chronic) diagnoses can receive similar weighting regardless of the phase. Relevant research findings on the weighting of individual diagnoses could not be found during the research for this chapter, which is why Fig. 10.1 is intended as an allegory. The individual weighting of diagnoses represents an interesting case study for the future of chronic care.

10.3 The Relevance of Bio-Psycho-Social Perspectives

The distinction between health and illness is of central importance, as only when a condition is classified as requiring treatment is the use of resources for treatment legitimized. The bio-medical model continues to serve as the guiding principle in clinical practice, in which diseases are regarded as purely biological phenomena that can be described, explained, and treated using the methods of the natural sciences (Richter and Hurrelmann 2016). However, the assessment of a human condition is always embedded in a cultural context that cannot be captured by bio-medical instruments alone. In particular, the description and treatment of mental illnesses are considered especially susceptible to the influence of established norms, as they often lack an organic finding (Romfeld 2015). Guided by the premise that health is the norm and illness a violation of the norm, the question arises as to which cognitive, psychological, or behavioral state is defined as the norm and which standard is used to identify a violation of the norm.

To distinguish between concepts of illness, English uses the terms disease, illness, and sickness to differentiate between objectively measurable and subjectively perceived health states. Disease refers to a pathological process whose origin is sometimes indeterminate but which represents an objective deviation from a bio-medical norm. In contrast, illness is an unhealthy feeling rooted in the affected person. Illness often accompanies disease, but it can also be described even when no objective finding is possible. Sickness, in turn, refers to the duration of being ill as a status and thus also to the social consequences. Thus, disease is described as bio-medical, illness as subjectively experienced, and sickness as socially recognized illness (Von Schlippe and Schweizer 2016).

There are numerous scientific publications on many chronic diseases, such as dementias, from which, despite differentiated consideration, no consensus on diagnosis and treatment can be derived. Rather, the differences between bio-medical and bio-psycho-social perspectives become apparent, which may contradict or complement each other in content, but are experienced as coexistent in practice. In the context of dementias, a disease may be present if the illness leads to detectable protein deposits (Lewy body dementia) or to reduced brain plasticity (Vascular dementia, Alzheimer's disease). Illness can be spoken of when those affected by (incipient) dementia notice reduced cognitive performance in the form of disorientation, impaired memory, or difficulties in in the perception of executive functions, even though no bio-medical finding is yet present. This is particularly relevant in cases of mild cognitive impairment, which can be a precursor to dementia. Sickness, in turn, is present when the illness is socially recognized due to behavioral changes, reduced drive, or emotions such as anxiety and lack of motivation. In the context of the etiology of dementias, their symptoms, and the various proposed solutions for dealing with those affected, current theories and practices must take the bio-psycho-social perspective into account, as the treatment setting also has a significant impact on psychological well-being and cognitive activity. The same applies to other chronic diseases, where bio-psycho-social contextual factors can promote self-efficacy and thus influence the course of the illness. Due to the dynamic nature of chronic diseases, treatment goals are less obvious than in acute conditions and vary depending on the position of those formulating them. Considering the interactions between disease burden, health-related quality of life, and risk factors can meaningfully link the bio-medical and bio-psycho-social perspectives on health and illness, since from a bio-medical perspective, many chronic diseases represent a deviation from a state assumed to be normal (see Chap. 37). The aim of treatment is therefore not only to consider the knowledge and practices of chronic diseases in terms of their evidence or effectiveness, but also to evaluate the functionality of treatment within the given bio-psycho-social circumstances.

10.4 The Bio-Psycho-Social Model

The bio-psycho-social model of the International Classification of Functioning, Disability and Health provides an initial orientation for classifying those affected along with their contextual factors. Using the components of body functions and structures, activities, participation and involvement, as well as environmental and personal factors, health problems, available resources, and their interactions become clear. A negative example here would be a lack of infrastructure. If people with mobility impairments (body functions and structures) depend on public transportation (environmental factor), but it is not sufficiently available or accessible, this can lead to restrictions in participation. Those affected may be unable to carry out activities outside the home due to their limited mobility and, for example, may not be able to reach relatives or healthcare institutions. As a consequence of a chronic illness, social, financial, and organizational problems may develop, as well as difficulties in dealing with the complex demands of the healthcare system. However, positive developments can also arise from contextual factors if interventions are better accepted by those affected because they align with their values, beliefs, and perspectives (personal factors), are adopted in terms of compliance, and coherent goals are achieved, for example, when regained body functions allow for more activities.

By consciously considering the components, the interactions between the individual contextual factors become clear. Ultimately, health problems can be positively or negatively influenced by various contextual factors. Orientation to the bio-psycho-social model is therefore meaningful for people with chronic illnesses, as the components provide a more adequate understanding than the classic bio-medical concept with its imbalanced primary and secondary diagnoses. This also underlies a task of Chronic Care Science and Practice: to determine the contextual factors in a multiprofessional manner in order to derive equivalent goals and resources for practice.

10.5 Factors for a Bio-Psycho-Social Health Infrastructure

The comparisons of the multidimensional concepts of disease burden, health-related quality of life, and risk factors highlight the complexity of the impacts of chronic diseases (see Fig. 10.2). Effective prevention and care strategies should take into account biological, psychological (behavioral), and social contextual factors, and provide an adequate health infrastructure that can flexibly respond to the primary and secondary diagnoses of a disease phase. The starting point for this is the most detailed possible knowledge of the health or disease status, in order to analyze the need for prevention and care measures and translate this into practice.

People with chronic diseases require flexible access to care resources that must be both high-quality and low-threshold in order to meet individual and complex situations. However, it is precisely this flexible access that reaches its limits in times of staff shortages, unevenly advanced digitalization, and regionally unequal distribution of resources, etc. If access to care resources already presents challenges and barriers for those involved, this can significantly affect the individual impacts for those affected. Professionals can support those affected by promoting their active management of the situation (self-efficacy) or by facilitating access to resources. On the subjective level, coping strategies (see Chapter 18) have proven effective in managing chronic diseases and their

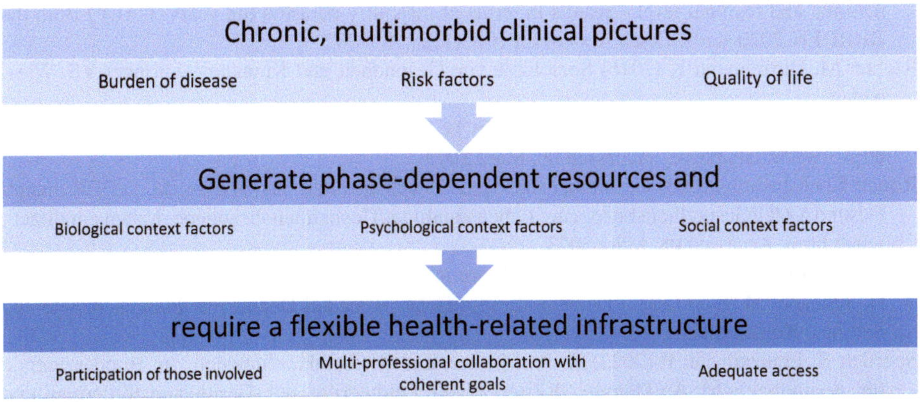

Fig. 10.2 Factors for a bio-psycho-social health infrastructure. (Own illustration)

consequences, contributing to a reduction in risk factors and disease burden as well as to the promotion of health-related quality of life.

To ensure adequate care and positively influence the impacts of chronic diseases, coordinated, multiprofessional, and cross-interface collaboration is required, which is based on successful information sharing, implemented in a participatory manner with those involved, pursues coherent goals, and provides an adaptable health infrastructure. A holistic approach in accordance with the bio-psycho-social model and its influence on disease burden, health-related quality of life, and risk factors can define primary and secondary diagnoses more accurately depending on the phase of the disease. The phase-dependent activation of available resources, in turn, closes the loop to individual contextual factors, because even the most general model can become something personal.

References

Diez SG (2015) Indikatoren zur Lebensqualität: Vorschläge der europäischen Expertengruppe und ausgewählte nationale Initiativen. Statistisches Bundesamt (Eds). WISTA, Wiesbaden, p 6

Franzkowiak P, Hurrelmann K (2018) Gesundheit. In: Bundeszentrale für gesundheitliche Aufklärung (BZgA) (Eds) Leitbegriffe der Gesundheitsförderung und Prävention. Glossar zu Konzepten, Strategien und Methoden. E-Book

Güthlin C (2020) Chronisch krank sein in Deutschland: Zahlen, Fakten und Versorgungserfahrungen. Robert Bosch Stiftung (Eds). https://www.bosch-stiftung.de/de/publikation/chronische-krankheiten-deutschland. Accessed 15. Mai 2023

Koch U, Mehnert A, Härter M (2011) Chronische körperliche Erkrankungen und psychische Komorbidität, Bundesgesundheitsblatt, Gesundheitsforschung, Gesundheitsschutz 1. https://doi.org/10.1007/s00103-010-1196-7

Porst M, von der Lippe E, Leddin J, Anton A, Wengler A, Breitkreuz J, Schüssel K, Brückner G, Schröder H, Gruhl H, Plaß D, Barnes B, Busch MA, Haller S, Hapke U, Neuhauser H, Reitzle L, Scheidt-Nave C, Schlotmann K et al (2022) The burden of disease in Germany at the

national and regional level – results in terms of disability-adjusted life years (DALY) from the BURDEN 2020 study. Dtsch Arztebl Int 2022(119):785–792
Richter M, Hurrelmann K (2016) Soziologie von Gesundheit und Krankheit. Springer VS, Wiesbaden
Robert Koch Institut (2021) Burden 2020: Was bedeutet Burden of Disease oder Krankheitslast? https://www.daly.rki.de/. Accessed 08. März 2023
Robert Koch Institut (2023) Gesundheitsbezogene Lebensqualität. https://www.rki.de/DE/Content/GesundAZ/G/Gesundheitsbezogene_Lebensqualitaet/Gesundheitsbezogene_Lebensqualitaet_inhalt.html. Accessed 08. März 2023
Romfeld E (2015) Fordert eine psychische Störung zum Heilen auf? In: Boggatz T, Brandenburg H, Schnabel M (Eds) (2022) Demenz: Ein kritischer Blick auf Deutungen. Pflegekonzepte und Settings, Kolhammer
Sperlich S, Franzkowiak P (2022) Risikofaktoren und Risikofaktorenmodell. In: Bundeszentrale für gesundheitliche Aufklärung (BZgA) (Eds) Leitbegriffe der Gesundheitsförderung und Prävention. Glossar zu Konzepten, Strategien und Methoden
Von Schlippe A, Schweizer J (2016) Lehrbuch der systemischen Therapie und Beratung I: Das Grundlagenwissen. In: Tiemann M, Mohokum M (Eds) (2021) Prävention und Gesundheitsförderung. Springer, Wiesbaden, p 234

Course Curves of Chronic Diseases as a Common Orientation Model for Multiprofessional Care Practice

11

Ulrike Höhmann

Contents

11.1 Chronic Illness as a Challenge for Coordinated Care

People with chronic illnesses require varying support from different professional groups and institutions. The physicians, nurses, therapists, counseling bodies, etc. involved must respond to both long-term and rapidly changing symptoms and care needs, ranging from acute care, nursing, rehabilitation, everyday support, prevention, to palliative care. To achieve this as seamlessly as possible, service providers must coordinate tailored intervention strategies across professions and institutions, as well as with those affected and their families. Despite the high performance of individual services, the overall situation of those affected often falls out of focus. Consequences of this fragmented care include:

U. Höhmann (✉)
Universität Witten/Herdecke, Witten, Germany
e-mail: ulrike.hoehmann@uni-wh.de

D. Schmitz et al. (eds.), *Chronic Care—Science and Practice*,
https://doi.org/10.1007/978-3-662-72298-5_11

- Patients and their families sometimes experience contradictory or incomplete intervention strategies. Potentials for recovery, rehabilitation, or quality of life remain untapped, and unnecessary suffering for those affected is preordained.
- From a societal perspective, differentiated and specialized but unconnected institutions and professions waste financial and professional resources of the healthcare system. Untapped synergies result in quality deficits.
- These problems also burden professionals:
  1. On the one hand, due to uncertainty about expectations for cooperation, therapeutic concepts, goals, ways of thinking, tasks, routines, working conditions, interests, and power claims of the respective others,
  2. on the other hand, due to the experience of discrepancy between the patients' professional care needs and their own economically triggered care routines, which reflect neither their own expertise, skills, nor understanding of quality.

  Such role stress caused by experiences of uncertainty and pressure leads to well-known consequences, such as feelings of powerlessness, loss of motivation and empathy, coldness, over-bureaucratization, and even burnout.

  The often implicit tacit agreement of lacking hope for change obscures the view of one's own professional scope for action to change one's own practice. In a resigned manner, this unintentionally stabilizes the fragmented practice and exacerbates barriers to cooperation.

Fragmented care is fostered on the one hand by institutional system design, and on the other by uncoordinated, divergent action concepts of the actors (see Contribution 20). This contribution addresses the latter point and discusses the trajectory work model as a cross-professional and cross-institutional common substantive framework for patient-centered chronic care.

11.2 A Multiprofessional Framework as Common Ground for Chronic Care

Since the 1980s, the literature on cooperation among health professions has emphasized the importance of a cross-professional framework as a necessary, though not sufficient, condition for compatible situation definitions and problem-solving to reduce profession- and institution-related care discontinuities (e.g., Brashers et al. 2001; Hornby 1993). This postulate is fundamentally based on the convictions of the theory of communicative action, according to which different actors, guided by rules, jointly strive for innovative solutions. A shared framework is intended to serve as common ground, spanning the coordination and design spaces accessible to actors for professional boundary work in care, and, through improved communication, counteracting the negative consequences of insufficient service coordination.

For chronic care, a concrete shared interpretive and communicative framework is therefore called for (e.g., Höhmann 2002), which identifies substantive and conceptual gaps in multiprofessional care practice using jointly accepted reference points, and at the same time provides substantive guidance on how care-relevant gaps can be filled with a patient-individually negotiated, needs-based, and compatible mosaic of services. In the necessary negotiation process, the involved service providers are to identify, justify, coordinate among themselves and with those affected, and arrange compatible measures within their own professional scope of action to reduce care discontinuities. In doing so, professionals simultaneously reduce role stress: they gain greater confidence in their interactions and, with shared professional definitional authority, can counter the pressure of empty, procedurally preformed action patterns. Person-centered, coordinated care strategies, in turn, strengthen substantive collaboration as well as the sense of coherence in one's own professional actions. In the long term, such trust-building learning processes can lay the foundation for multiprofessional tacit agreements and generate new everyday coordination and work routines. The prerequisite is always the professionals' willingness and ability to reflect, negotiate, and act.

A suitable common ground for this purpose must particularly meet the following substantive requirements:

- The obvious health-related care needs of people with chronic illnesses must visibly be at the center. A shared focus on the perspective of chronically ill people and their families reduces professional dominance in defining needs. Professional specializations thus serve the goal of the most effective problem-solving possible for those affected.
- The trajectory character of chronic illnesses, with the associated need for care adaptation and the resulting interactions, must be part of the concept.
- Care-relevant needs identified for people with chronic illnesses must be relatable to the everyday care tasks of direct providers, enable negotiation of professional assignments, and be able to be coordinated and integrated within the action spaces accessible to actors among professional groups and patients/families.
- Likewise, situationally significant contextual conditions of the patients/families, as well as of the providers and their institutions, must be considered in their interplay. The goal of *compatibility* of multiprofessionally delivered individual interventions requires clear professional boundaries, secured by mutual fairness norms.

11.3 The Trajectory Concept as an Exemplary Common Ground for Chronic Care

In the trajectory concept, the aforementioned model requirements for the field of chronic care are specified. It was developed between the 1960s and 1990s as the Trajectory Work Model (TWM) by the research groups around Glaser and Strauss. The starting point was to analyze, first using the example of the dying and later of people with chronic illnesses, central coping and care requirements and the related organization of medical work and its consequences for the experience of illness (Glaser and Strauss 1968; Strauss et al. 1985; Corbin and Strauss 1988). From their structural-interactive process perspective, they emphasize, similar to general social science career concepts, the interaction processes between structural conditions, the related actions of those affected and professionals, and the resulting consequences as formative opportunity structures for the course of illness:

- at the micro level, the case-specific value horizons, thinking, knowledge, feelings, and actions of those affected, families, and professionals,
- at the meso level, the case-specific institutional action patterns of care facilities, e.g., responsibilities, service priorities, work organization, routines, etc.,
- at the macro level, the case-specific economic and legal framework conditions, as well as
- feedback processes between these three levels.

The success or failure of this interplay, as well as the intended and unintended consequences, determine the course of care and illness, the changes and social disorder processes to be managed in everyday life, and thus the future prospects of those affected. This fundamental perspective, which characterizes the concept, is also followed by target group-specific specifications of the TWM (e.g., Gerhardt 1986; Höhmann 2002).

In the authors' understanding, this "model for health policy and practice" (Strauss and Corbin 1988) serves both as a conceptual guide for the work of direct care providers and for shaping the institutional level of the health system, in order to address the needs of the growing number of chronically ill individuals in the US healthcare system. Due to the high resistance to change in the German healthcare system, the first aspect is implementable in practical situations, such as in the expert standard for discharge management in nursing or in multiprofessional networking projects. The second, structural function is, at best, used as a model in a limited way. In practice, interdisciplinary analyses, reconstructions, and reflections on various chronic health phenomena in biographical, health, or (nursing science) care research predominate, provided that the subject-related management of status passages due to internal or external changes and their interactions are to be understood from a longitudinal perspective (e.g., Nittel and Seltrecht 2013).

The substantive core of the TWM was distilled from broad empirical analyses and self-descriptions of those affected and their families, not from the concepts of individual health professions. To specifically address chronicity, the concept contrasts the original medical thinking in terms of acute illness episodes with "trajectories" (trajectories as a metaphor for course curves), which are shaped by the complexity of the conditions and consequences of actions and events in the process of living with chronic illness. Thus, Strauss et al. define: "the trajectory encompasses physiological events as well as the work of every participant, the work relationships, the changing work patterns, and the arrangements that are made to carry out that work in the face of changing illness phases and life`s contingencies ..." (Strauss et al. 1985, p. 49).

From this perspective, three elements of the TWM provide concrete guidance for patient-centered, multiprofessional negotiation of functionally compatible, profession-specific interventions and task bundles:

- The attributes of chronic diseases,
- which affect key areas of life beyond the individual and require coping efforts related to them
- as well as the phases of disease progression resulting from the interactions of conditions, actions, and consequences, with typical processes of suffering and coping demands.

The common foundation is always the two basic perspectives: the subjective view of those affected and the constitutive significance of processual interactions.

The specific content focuses in detail:

11.3.1 The Attributes of Chronic Diseases

For those affected, chronic diseases mean unending demands to manage uncertainty and associated disruptions in all areas of life. The following characteristics stand out as cross-professional and cross-institutional points of orientation:

- The certainties of reliable textbook courses or conventional medical therapies are lacking. Symptoms fluctuate in the short term between highs, lows, and phases of uncertainty, shaping the *entire* life. Decisions often have to be made under uncertainty.
- Managing disease symptoms and problems requires active experimentation, making those affected experts in their own situation. There is a risk of conflicts with professional strategies as well as care disruptions, loss of control, trust, and autonomy, accompanied by confusion, accumulation of problems, etc. The order of everyday life becomes fragile.
- The disease is never *gone.* Internal and external vigilance become ingrained in one's sense of life. Thoughts and feelings often revolve around illness-related issues, care problems, role changes with depressive moods, and social isolation.
- Social networks and informal support often deliver high performance in the short term, but in the long term, there is a risk of overload and exhaustion.
- Those affected and their families primarily generate their own resources to actively normalize everyday life, combined with efforts at self-management and managing external demands, such as seeking information, selecting, coordinating, and financing support, etc.

11.3.2 Substantive Coping Tasks

Those affected themselves describe their approach to the challenges of chronic illness as work. The term *Trajectory Work Model* emphasizes this active role and effort.

Based on their research, the authors identified three areas of life that are fundamentally affected by chronic illness and require coping work: these are *everyday life, illness,* and *biography.* A fourth area is often separately grouped as invisible underlying *management requirements* (Corbin and Strauss 1988; Strauss et al. 1985; Höhmann 2002). Specifically:

- **Tasks for coping with everyday life** refer to necessary activities and routines of daily living, whose self-evidence is threatened by physical, psychological, social, or material limitations. Essentially: the entire conglomerate of personal care, household management (such as shopping, cooking, laundry, cleaning, etc.), maintaining and adapting life rhythms and spaces, social relationships, up to securing economic livelihoods, etc.
- **Tasks for coping with illness** include actions aimed at the many, sometimes changing and threatening health limitations, or at achieving the highest possible level of well-being and safety. Essentially: the spectrum of preventive, (self-)diagnostic, therapeutic, experimental, stabilizing, activating, rehabilitative, palliative, accompanying, supportive, and promoting activities with which those affected, their relatives, or professionals in their respective domains strive to prevent, control, alleviate, or cure symptoms.
- **Tasks for coping with biographical adjustment processes** encompass the internal and external actions aimed at integrating the illness, the changes to the body, its functions, and the entire life situation into one's biography. Essentially: identity adjustments, reconceptualization of the self, social role and contacts, etc., including dealing with the remaining biographical time.
- **Management tasks** underlie all coping tasks. They are necessary for **self-management** and **the coordination of various care and support services.** They are often invisible, difficult to refinance, and are frequently overlooked in professional needs assessments. Therefore, they are explicitly emphasized here. Chronic illness is akin to a high-wire act, where professional, segmented routine actions, as uncoordinated individual acts, risk missing the mark. Essentially:
  1. Self-management tasks primarily refer to efforts for emotional and behavioral self-regulation, etc.
  2. Coordination tasks, on the other hand, involve ongoing processes of organization and selection that ensure or rearrange the effectiveness of routines or support services, e.g., through information, check of the work content, or coordination.

Both the areas of life and the coping tasks are interwoven in the everyday lives of those affected in a "reciprocal impact" (Corbin and Strauss 1991, p. 165). Their separation serves an analytical function to clarify the common ground for professionals and to identify, name, and assign needs to interventions and responsibilities. The coping requirements identified within this relevance framework can serve as guidelines for negotiating profession-specific core and boundary tasks. They aim to meet the needs of those affected as fully as possible through improved cooperation and coordination among professionals, to identify and minimize gaps, and to individually tailor preventive, supportive, curative, and palliative intervention packages. The framework consists of the direct intervention priorities of the settings and professions, such as medicine, nursing, therapy professions, domestic services, etc., in the coping areas of everyday life, illness, and biographical adjustment, as well as the identification and support of management requirements, e.g., through coordinated profession-related information, coordination, counseling, or empowerment tasks to strengthen the resources of those affected.

11.3.3 Phased Nature of Progressions

The interplay of coping efforts by all parties involved, as well as the related interactions with and between subjective and objective conditions, shapes individual illness trajectories. For analytical purposes, Corbin and Strauss (1988, 1991), Corbin (1998) assign management phases to these interaction processes, each characterized by specific conditions, coping requirements, and efforts by all involved parties:

1. the pre-phase of the illness trajectory (preclinical phase)
2. the diagnostic phase/beginning of the trajectory
3. the acute phase
4. the critical phase
5. the stable phase
6. the unstable phase
7. the relapse phase
8. the deterioration phase
9. the dying phase

The guiding criterion of this common classification used by health and therapy professions is the physical progression of the disease from the professionals' perspective. No mandatory sequence is assumed; phases three to eight are considered reversible.

In contrast to this disease-inherent perspective, Schütze and Riemann, from the viewpoint of phenomenologically oriented biographical research, conceptually and theoretically oppose the subjective feelings and experiences of chronically ill individuals in the interplay of subjective and objective factors, actions, and consequences as specific processes of suffering (Schütze 1995; Riemann and Schütze 1991). They focus on the significance of phenomena that, beyond the deliberately rational action schemes of professionals and those affected, become effective for a chain of interactions and events and thus for upward or downward curves in the trajectory (potentially reversible course of illness phases), such as physical, psychological, social, and spiritual reactions to health or social changes, coincidences, gaps in care, professional mismanagement, disruption of everyday order, etc. They distinguish the following as typical phases of suffering (Höhmann et al. 1998, p. 65, modified after Riemann and Schütze 1991):

1. Accumulation of trajectory potential (subjectively interpreted threats in the preliminary stage)
2. Prominent, triggering event of the trajectory
3. Unstable equilibrium (with the illness in the background, bodily irregularities quickly create uncertainty, sometimes with over-focusing)
4. Exhaustion of (internal) action capacities (patients experience themselves as thrown, no longer as active shapers of life)
5. Development of physical or psychosocial secondary problems of the "second" order due to internal or external influences (e.g., hopelessness when therapy fails, consequences of falls with increasing mobility restrictions)
6. Unstable equilibrium begins to spiral (e.g., relapses, collapse of the support system)
7. Breakdown of the active coping orientation (external and internal transformation processes close off future perspectives)

Straightforward transitions in the multifactorial course of illness are hardly to be expected; rather, depending on the conditions, typical phases of suffering with specific coping requirements emerge. Stages three to six, and partially seven, are considered reversible.

In the sense of the Common Ground, the phases point to the individually effective constellation of conditions that influence the course of the illness. Attention is also drawn to the internal and external significance of professionally (un)coordinated actions. This provides care-relevant indications for the reconstruction, planning, and prioritization of professional interventions. In both phase models, the progression partly can be symbolized graphically as upward and downward curves with corresponding turning points.

11.4 Conclusion: The Content Orientation of Multiprofessionally Coordinated Care Practice

Two fundamental perspectives and three concrete building blocks of the TWM outline a cross-professional systematic framework for exchange, analysis, planning, coordination, evaluation, and documentation for needs-based multiprofessional design of Chronic Care practice. Systematic thinking in processual interactions of conditions and consequences of one's own decisions and actions opens up an understanding of the interconnectedness of individual Chronic Care interventions and their significance for those affected. Thus, this cross-professional, contextualizing orientation framework aims to identify and reduce actor-accessible breaking points in care that go beyond acute medical needs, with needs assessment primarily guided by the phase-specific relevant coping requirements and efforts of those affected. Chronically ill individuals and their families are understood as active negotiation partners, with their own expertise, experiences, efforts, resources, and areas of relevance—without shifting original professional responsibility onto those affected.

The concept-inherent focus of coordinated professional task bundles on the shared ratio essendi supports all professional groups in overcoming, through communicative processes of understanding, the experiences of normative pressure and normative uncertainty inherent in multiprofessional collaboration, and in grounding their multiprofessional boundary work through this coordination practice, which, even under existing regulations, can result in a tacit agreement of jointly practiced routines.

11.5 Basic Principles of Implementation

The everyday comprehensibility of the TWM enables professionals to systematically empower themselves along this framework through step-by-step cooperative self-qualification, allowing them to recognize and reflect on their professional scope of action and actively align their care practice accordingly (Höhmann et al. 1998, 2018). Personal knowledge, competence, and role requirements can largely be implemented even under structural conditions that are difficult to influence.

Concrete steps in this regard may include in particular:

- The foundation is the motivational-cognitive level. As a first step, everyday professional encounters provide opportunities for active mutual acquaintance, exchange of perspectives, and exploration of a shared understanding of care, e.g., formal case discussions, round tables, ward rounds, team or handover meetings, goal or training planning, etc., but also thematically focused informal communication situations, such as sharing a coffee in the staff room. In the course of this alignment process, the central core perspectives of the TWM can be communicated, discussed, and, if necessary, concrete temporary trials with monitoring can be designed. Due to the risk of conflicts arising from divergent interests, competition, and dominance issues, it is important to agree early on the search for fair balancing mechanisms between *winners and losers*.

- Only after this should direct care practice be operationally changed, e.g., by using guidelines based on jointly defined coping tasks—structuring, testing, reflecting on, and modifying anamneses, intervention planning, and service agreements, as well as transparently identifying, communicating, and reducing care gaps.
- For systematic cross-professional and cross-institutional sensitization, knowledge acquisition, practice of perspective alignment, and agreement on interventions, training sessions, communication training, or similar activities based on the TWM can provide qualification, ideally with the involvement of family and patient groups.
- Structural safeguards for a TWM-oriented chronic care practice are the responsibility of facility managers, in order to support staff in recognizing and utilizing their own professional scope of action for practical trials, reviews, and modifications in the work process through systematically structured development and communication processes, organizational and quality standards, etc.
  To normalize a tacit agreement on this care strategy in everyday practice, not only structural specifications but also an active communication culture, target agreements, partial role exchanges, or reciprocal job shadowing, etc., contribute.

Overall, the target perspective of the TWM described here, as a multiprofessional common ground for chronic care, challenges all actors to actively explore and shape the framework for their own intervention strategies in a needs-oriented manner.

References

Brashers V, Curry C, Harper D, McDaniel S, Pawlson G, Ball J (2001) Interprofessional health care education: recommendations of the National Academies of Practice Expert Panel on health care in the 21th century. Issues Interdiscip Care: Natl Acad Pract Forum 3(1):21–32

Corbin J (1998) The Corbin and Strauss chronic illness trajectory model: an update. Sch Inq Nurs Pract 12(1):33–41

Corbin J, Strauss A (1988) Unending work of care. Jossey-Bass, San Francisco

Corbin J, Strauss A (1991) A nursing model for chronic illness management based upon the trajectory framework. Sch Inq Nurs Pract 5(3):155–174

Gerhardt U (1986) Patientenkarrieren. Suhrkamp, Frankfurt

Glaser B, Strauss A (1968) Time for dying. Aldine, Chicago

Höhmann U (2002) Spezifische Vernetzungserfordernisse für chronisch kranke, langzeitpflegebedürftige Menschen. In: DZA (Hrsg) Expertisen zum 4. Altenbericht, Bd III. Vincentz, Hannover, S 289–428

Höhmann U, Müller-Mundt G, Schulz B (1998) Qualität durch Kooperation. Mabuse, Farnkfurt

Höhmann U, Lauxen O, Schwarz L (Hrsg) (2018) Gestaltungskompetenzen im Pflegealltag stärken. Mabuse, Frankfurt

Hornby S (1993) Collaborative care. Blackwell, London

Nittel D, Seltrecht A (Hrsg) (2013) Krankheit: Lernen im Ausnahmezustand? Springer, Heidelberg

Riemann G, Schütze F (1991) "Trajectory" as a basic theoretical concept for analyzing suffering and disorderly social processes. In: Maines D (Hrsg) Social organization and social process. Aldine, Chicago, S 333–357

Schütze F (1995) Verlaufskurven des Erleidens als Forschungsgegenstand der interpretativen Soziologie. In: Krüger HH, Marotzki W (Hrsg) Handbuch Erziehungswissenschaftliche Biographieforschung. Leske & Buderich, Opladen, S 116–157
Strauss A, Corbin J (1988) Shaping a new health care system. Jossey-Bass, San Francisco/London
Strauss A, Fagerhaugh S, Suczek B, Wiener C (1985) Social organization of medical work. University of Chicago Press, Chicago

Somatic Theories of Illness and Coping With Illness

12

Sarah Weller and Christine Thomas

Contents

12.1 Classification of Somatic Theories of Disease

The term *somatic* refers to pathophysiological processes of the body and nervous system, and thus also to mental illnesses that are to be distinguished from functional complaints. The concepts of health and disease are closely related and have undergone significant historical change. It should be highlighted that, especially in the mid-19th century, medicine increasingly established itself as a natural science and focused its attention almost exclusively on the study of diseases and their treatment. Based on this, physicians

S. Weller (✉)
Zentrum für Seelische Gesundheit, Klinikum Stuttgart, Stuttgart, Germany
e-mail: s.weller@klinikum-stuttgart.de

C. Thomas
Ärztliche Direktorin der Klinik für Psychiatrie und Psychotherapie für Ältere, Klinikum Stuttgart, Stuttgart, Germany
e-mail: c.thomas@klinikum-stuttgart.de

D. Schmitz et al. (eds.), *Chronic Care—Science and Practice*,
https://doi.org/10.1007/978-3-662-72298-5_12

asserted themselves as experts on diseases—a perspective that, along with the associated curative health care system, continues to dominate today (Faltermeier 2023). Central models for the development and management of disease at the somatic level can be classified within the tradition of this perspective.

12.2 Models of Somatic Disease Development and Management

The best-known models for the development and management of diseases are the biomedical disease model and the risk factor model, which to this day serve as essential starting points for curative and preventive medical interventions.

12.2.1 Biomedical Disease Model

Unlike the currently favored salutogenic perspective, the biomedical approach is based on a strict separation between disease and health. Disease is defined as the absence of health and, from a homeostatic perspective, as an imbalance of biochemical and physiological changes. This concept assumes a simple cause-and-effect relationship (monocausality), i.e., every illness is based on a specific cause. Causes may include infections triggered by microorganisms, endogenously arising biochemical dysfunctions (e.g., dysregulation of metabolic processes), organ defects, or functional disorders due to exogenous influences (e.g., accidents, burns). These disorders can be objectively measured (e.g., laboratory diagnostics, X-ray imaging) and subsequently assessed by comparison with population-based reference values. Based on these objective measurements, treatment is then implemented. The primary aim of this treatment is to eliminate deviations from the norm (i.e., complete cure), but in cases such as chronic diseases, it may also aim to reduce structural or functional impairment or to prevent death (Koppelin 2022). Corresponding treatment approaches include appropriate medication or surgical intervention. The physical and psychological aspects of a person are viewed separately, similar to the rationalism of Descartes, with psychological processes—such as coping with the consequences of illness—being completely disregarded in this model.

Metaphorically, the body in this model is viewed as a machine that can be broken down into its individual parts, so that treatment is approached as a technical problem-solving process. Patients are regarded as passive objects of medical treatment (Faltermeier 2023). The following example illustrates the model:

> "Ms. G. (65 years old) reports during the consultation of severe pain and burning during urination. These symptoms have persisted for about five days and are severely hindering her daily activities as well as the care of her dependent husband. Due to the severe pain and frequent urination, she can hardly sleep and even fell yesterday."

Restricted to this model approach, there would be an exclusive focus on the described somatic cardinal symptoms. The practitioners would attempt to objectify their suspicion of a urinary tract infection (etiology). In accordance with the scientific gold standard for diagnosis, a pathogen detection would be performed, in which the type and quantity of the pathogen could be determined using a midstream urine culture. If the threshold value for Ms. G. were > 105 colony-forming units (cfu)/mL urine, this would be considered proof of a urinary tract infection (Schmiemann et al. 2010) (diagnosis) and would be treated with antibiotics (cure). If a corresponding bacterium could not be detected, alternative causes would be investigated and appropriate curative measures initiated.

Although this model, and especially the causal-analytical concept, provides a fundamental basis for research, treatment, and medical prevention of infectious diseases (e.g., vaccines), it is considered inadequate for the majority of objectives in research and health care, and especially in clinical practice, due to its narrow perspective. The main points of criticism in this context are:

- No consideration of social, psychological, and behavioral aspects, nor of multiprofessional treatment approaches
- Somatic and other influencing factors (e.g., social support, stressors) are strictly separated
- The individual is regarded as passive
- Complex disease processes cannot be explained by simple causal cause-and-effect relationships
- Resources and preventive measures are disregarded
- Essential aspects such as subjective concepts of health or quality of life play no role
- Doctor-patient relationships are purely functional, focused on the detection and somatic treatment of disease, and promote a paternalistic attitude

These points of criticism, in the course of a general salutogenic paradigm shift (see Contribution 18), have led to the model being supplemented by psychological and social aspects, resulting, among other things, in the bio-psycho-social model.

12.2.2 Risk Factor Model

Especially in the 1950s, the rise in chronic and non-communicable *diseases of civilization* led to the emergence of social and preventive medicine. In the course of this development, the risk factor model was established. Unlike the biomedical model, the case-based method is largely abandoned here in favor of a statistical analysis of largely homogeneous population groups. It became clear that a disease can arise not only from a specific factor, but often several risk factors must coincide for a particular illness to occur. This model therefore also focuses on risk factors and not just on early symptoms as in the biomedical model (Franke 2012).

In the social and health sciences, risk factors are generally defined as predictors that have been empirically shown to increase the probability of a specific disease occurring in a particular population. Unlike the biomedical perspective, a risk-based approach focuses on probable associations between risk factors and diseases in population groups. Risk factors are therefore always determined statistically and do not mean that an affected individual will actually develop a particular disease. Nevertheless, especially the accumulation and interaction of several risk factors significantly increases the probability of disease (Keller and Menche 2017).

To detect risk factors, observational studies are primarily conducted, especially case-control or cohort studies. The former examine cross-sectionally and retrospectively whether individuals in the case group, who suffer from a particular disease (e.g., vascular dementia), had a certain exposure (e.g., high blood pressure) more frequently in the past than individuals without this disease (control group). Cohort studies, on the other hand, are prospective as well as longitudinal and provide data on incidence (rate of new cases), which is why they are generally considered to have greater evidential value (Ressing et al. 2010).

The WHO (2013) identifies tobacco use, harmful alcohol consumption, physical inactivity, and unhealthy diet as the most common risk factors. For Germany, studies can demonstrate the significance of the *nutrition* complex, as this can promote further risks (Plass et al. 2014).

Behavioral factors are considered the main risk factors (see Section 10) for chronic diseases, but these should always be assessed in combination with environmental factors. This concept is also reflected in the WHO's *causal chain of disease development* model (2002): Distal factors (e.g., low educational attainment) influence proximal factors (e.g., high consumption of fast food). These result in pathophysiological factors (e.g., elevated blood sugar), which in turn lead to specific diseases (e.g., diabetes) and result in corresponding disease consequences (e.g., impaired functioning). Based on the risk factor model, preventive medical implementation focuses on strategies for individual behavior change (e.g., dietary modification, promotion of physical activity), whereas a setting-based approach targeting living environments plays a significantly lesser role (Franke 2012). This approach can be illustrated using the example of dementia:

> "The most common cause of dementia is Alzheimer's pathology, which underlies about 75% of all dementia cases (Thyrian et al. 2020). There is still no promising therapy available that can prevent the disease or delay its progression. However, 30% of all Alzheimer's dementia cases are attributable to modifiable risk factors such as high blood pressure or overweight in midlife, late-life depression, diabetes mellitus, physical inactivity, smoking, and low educational attainment (Livingston et al. 2020), which specifically target high-risk individuals."

The risk factor model continues to be of great importance for targeted prevention and treatment:

- The further development into a multifactorial disease process addresses the increasing prevalence of chronic diseases
- The identification of risk factors is based on scientific evidence
- Patients are regarded as active participants and psychological factors are recognized

Nevertheless, the risk factor model is also associated with three points of criticism:

- Increasing medicalization
- Neglect of protective factors
- Diseases occur despite avoidance of risk factors

12.3 Summary

Although disease models with a somatic orientation, also in light of their historical development, are of great importance for selected curative or preventive treatment approaches for individual diseases, from today's perspective they are largely unsuitable for broad application in clinical practice. Instead, somatic causes should be embedded in a holistic therapeutic approach. Especially in view of the rising prevalence of chronic diseases and age-related multimorbid disease patterns, health and illness should be considered from a salutogenic perspective, and the often complex interactions of biological, social, and psychological aspects should be assessed, taking into account environmental and individual factors. Finally, the definition and the question of the need for treatment of a disease, in addition to a scientifically based somatic approach, should always be aligned with subjective parameters such as health-related quality of life, thus enabling joint assessment and planning of therapy. Medical-scientific guidelines are also addressing this challenge by directly involving patients in guideline development, as participatory decision-making is particularly essential in chronic diseases. Over time, diseases interact with physiological and pathological aging processes and can reinforce their impetus. Therefore, consideration of psychosocial concerns, individual interpretations of illness, and proven coping mechanisms is crucial for treatment management, treatment success, and individually experienced quality of life.

References

Faltermeier T (2023) Gesundheitspsychologie, 3. akt. Aufl. Kohlhammer, Stuttgart

Franke A (2012) Modelle von Gesundheit und Krankheit, 3. Aufl. HUBER, Bern

Keller C, Menche N (2017) PFLEGEN. Gesundheits- und Krankheitslehre. Elsevier, München

Koppelin F (2022) Public Health: Ansätze, Theorien und Strukturen. UTB, München

Livingston G, Huntley J, Sommerlad A, Ames D, Ballard C, Banerjee S (2020) Dementia prevention, intervention, and care: 2020 report of the Lancet Commission. Lancet 396(10248):413–446

Plass D, Vos T, Hornberg C (2014) Trends in disease burden in Germany: results, implications and limitations of the Global Burden of Disease study. Dtsch Arztebl Int 111(38):629–638

Ressing M, Blettner M, Klug SJ (2010) Auswertung epidemiologischer Studien. Dtsch Arztebl International 107(11):187–192

Schmiemann G, Kniehl E, Gebhardt K (2010) Diagnose des Harnwegsinfekts: Eine systematische Übersicht. Dtsch Arztebl Int 107(21):361–367

Thyrian JR, Boekholt M, Hoffmann W (2020) Die Prävalenz an Demenz erkrankter Menschen in Deutschland – eine bundesweite Analyse auf Kreisebene. Nervenarzt 91:1058–1061

World Health Organisation (2002) The World Health Report: reducing risks, promotinghealthy life. www.who.int/publications/i/item/9241562072. Zugegriffen: 01. März 2023

World Health Organisation (2013) Global action plan for the prevention and control of noncommunicable diseases (2013–2020). www.who.int/nmh/events/ncd_action_plan/en/. Zugegriffen: 01. März 2023

Sociological Perspectives on the Social Construction of Illness and the Implications for the Experience and Treatment of Illness

13

Werner Vogd

Contents

13.1 Sociological Perspectives on Illness

Whether scientifically grounded or not, ultimately all concepts of health and illness are of cultural origin. They are based on *socially supplied meaning*, which communicatively and performatively creates its own plausibility. Not too long ago, homosexuality was considered an illness. In the Middle Ages, it was not uncommon to interpret behavioral abnormalities as expressions of possession by demonic forces.

The sociological perspective on illness and health focuses attention on the relationship between body, consciousness, and communication. For analytical reasons, it is helpful to initially consider these three spheres separately, following Luhmann (1995):

W. Vogd (✉)
Fakultät für Gesundheit (Department für Humanmedizin), Lehrstuhl für Soziologie, Universiät Witten/Herdecke, Witten, Germany
e-mail: Werner.Vogd@uni-wh.de

D. Schmitz et al. (eds.), *Chronic Care—Science and Practice*,
https://doi.org/10.1007/978-3-662-72298-5_13

- The *body* represents the trillions of processes that occur simultaneously in a living organism (activities of the organs, metabolic processes in every cell, the chemical reactions of the involved molecules). However, organs, cells, and molecules do not think or understand. They do not know what meaning is. They are based solely on the fact that countless processes occur simultaneously and, from moment to moment, link together into a complex event that cannot be fully comprehended by outsiders.
- *Consciousness* stands for the psychological processes by which sensory perceptions—such as visual impressions and sensations—are linked with thoughts. Thoughts are accompanied by meaning, which means that perceptions acquire a specific significance within the horizon of other possible interpretations (for example, when a patient has felt exhausted for weeks, but does not interpret the fatigue as a sign of overwork and lack of sleep, but rather as an indication of illness).
- The term *communication* refers to social systems, that is, all those processes in which meaning is conveyed through linguistic and symbolic actions (for example, when a doctor tells a patient that he is *depressed* and prescribes fluoxetine).

Neither the psyche nor communication can ever fully address, let alone comprehend, everything that happens with the body. Only a highly selective construction of meaning is ever created. It is only in this way that a particular perspective on the situation can be generated. This perspective does not have to be correct. With regard to meaning, it is generally less about whether the suggested causal relationship is true, and more about whether it is socially and psychologically plausible. Let us first consider some relations between body, psyche, and communication that are relevant to our topic.

Relation between Consciousness and Body

Consciousness cannot directly control or observe the internal processes of the body to which it owes its existence (no body, no consciousness). Only in the case of pain so severe that it comes into focus, or in the case of organ impairment, does the body become a subject of consciousness.

A multitude of pathological bodily processes (consider the onset of cancer or high blood pressure) do not necessarily involve perceptible symptoms, and even when there is some discomfort or pain, consciousness still does not know what these bodily sensations mean. Ultimately, consciousness can interpret these sensations less through *self-knowledge* and only through socially supplied meaning. This, of course, also applies to health-damaging or health-promoting influences: Whether cholesterol in butter, hormone replacement therapy during menopause, workplace stress, etc., are harmful to health (or not) is not self-evident, but only appears plausible (or not) in the context of a socioculturally established framework of communication. Therefore, on the one hand, even extremely life-threatening working conditions, as Hien (1994) demonstrates using the example of the chemical industry workforce, can be reinterpreted in a counterintuitive way within certain milieus (e.g., "That only makes me stronger"). On the other hand, health-promoting measures (such as a vaccination) can be perceived as harmful and excessively risky. Causal assumptions regarding health and illness are social constructions and are thus the result of social and cultural relationships that convey the associated meaning.

Relation between Communication and Body

From placebo research, we know that the mere act of communication can influence bodily processes toward healing, and conversely, negative prognoses can have effects up to and including psychogenic death (Kächele 1970). In ethnomedicine, these processes are known as *white or black magic* (Rösing 2006), and in medical sociology as threat through stereotypes (Vogd and Feißt 2022). What is meant here is that diagnoses can have a stigmatizing effect and—especially in the case of mental illnesses, as a self-fulfilling prophecy—can themselves create the conditions for further chronicity of the illness process.

This raises the fundamental question of the consequences of medicalization (Illich 1976), especially since therapeutic interventions carried out as a result of a diagnosis often perpetuate the need for treatment. It is often difficult to distinguish whether the chronicity of the illness is due to the treatment or the original condition.

Relation between Psyche and Communication

First, it is important to understand that the process of meaning in communication is different from what happens in the consciousness of those affected as interpretation. A patient may be admitted to psychiatry as schizophrenic. However, this does not mean that they themselves see themselves as mentally ill. General practitioners may point out to patients that they have a poor diet and drink too much alcohol, but this does not mean that this perspective is adopted and behaviors are changed (compliance). From the medical or nursing side, a lack of insight into illness or even denial may be criticized. This does not prevent patients from superficially agreeing in order not to jeopardize the role structure of the doctor-patient relationship.

Conversely, patients may be very well aware of the problems of their physical condition, while in the doctor-patient interaction or in contact with relatives, they act as if things are not so bad (Glaser and Strauss 1979).

Such decouplings are primarily an expression of the fact that the sphere of meaning that creates and maintains a social identity is different from the one that builds and stabilizes psychological identity. In this sense, it is not unusual for people to express themselves in a role-appropriate manner within certain contexts, even though they may see things quite differently a little later. From a social-psychological perspective, this is less about lying or self-deception. Rather, it is an expression of continuing to comply with the familiar conventions of different social contexts.

13.2 Medical Treatment is Always Also Symbolic Healing

From the proposed sociological perspective, it should be emphasized once again that every operation of meaning selectively highlights certain relationships from the sea of possible causal connections, thematizes them, and marks them as relevant for its own practice. For a homeopath, a spiritual healer, or a rheumatologist, the respective postulated connections are *real*, and accordingly, he or she will assert these in doctor-patient communication. Since patients' consciousness has no direct access to the processes of their bodies, they have no choice but to rely on the socially provided meanings that appeal to them and to interpret events according to the scripts that come with them (for example, that chronic back pain can be cured by spinal surgery or by taking up a yoga practice).

With regard to the two spheres of consciousness and communication, these scripts are both subjective (they can appear in consciousness and become relevant) and objective (they appear as components of discourses that, according to the prevailing cultural standards, regard the connection as true). This does not preclude the possibility that the postulated connections can be scientifically investigated (in the previous example, for instance, with a control group receiving a sham spinal surgery).

In light of the preceding discussion, the old ethnomedical insight holds true that it is above all a matter of coordinating the only selective access of psyche and communication to the body in such a way that the process appears convincing to all involved. Dow (1986) therefore speaks of symbolic healing.

13.3 Specific Relations in Chronic Illnesses

In all of this, it must be considered that illnesses and disabilities challenge psychological and social identity (threat of stereotypes). To avoid the resulting crises, it may be attractive for those affected to pretend that everything is fine. For example, many people with dementia try to cleverly cover up their memory gaps to show visitors that everything is normal with them. From the perspective of psychological integrity, as Goffman (1963) shows in dealing with stigma, it can be helpful to see oneself as normal and healthy and to act accordingly in interactions as if everything were fine (see Contribution 37). Anyone who questions another person's integrity (which easily happens when weaknesses are addressed) must expect resistance—because it is always also about continuing to be seen as a person (and not just as disabled or ill).

It should also be noted that physical, psychological, and social processes each have their own rhythms, which brings its own set of problems. The consequences of health-damaging behavior are rarely felt immediately, but often only become apparent years later. Only in the case of severe pain—such as in an acute heart attack—is the causal nexus between physical complaints and conscious suffering immediately present on the psychological level.

With other clinical pictures, however, the temporal horizons diverge. For example, cancer is now often detected at a point when the patient is not yet clinically or sensually aware of suffering from it. This leads to a situation in which often dramatic bodily interventions are required that radically change the patients' lifeworld, without them experiencing any urgency as a self-evident implication of the immediate present. The threat of death and a future marked by severe suffering initially appears to patients in such cases only as a communicatively constructed facticity, which, however, is not psychologically experienced in relation to their own bodily processes. Medical communication conveys that one has no choice but to submit to the prescribed therapy protocols. Yet, in consciousness, considerable doubts arise as to whether all this is right (Vogd 2013).

13.4 Concluding Remarks

The sociological perspective on health and illness draws attention to the role of social relationships and the role of communication expressed therein. Discrepancies in the understanding of illness can arise on the factual, temporal, and social levels. It also becomes clear how the attribution of illness can shape and thus threaten the social and psychological identity of those affected (see Contribution 18). Especially in the case of stigmatized chronic diseases, the question of the cultural embedding of the treatment process arises.

References

Dow J (1986) Universal aspects of symbolic healing: a theoretical synthesis. Am Anthropol 88:56–69

Glaser BG, Strauss AL (1979) Awareness of dying. Chicago, Aldine

Goffman E (1963) Stigma: Notes on the management of spoiled identity, Englewood Cliffs, NJ, Prentice-Hall

Hien W (1994) Chemische Industrie und der Krebs: Zur Soziologie des wissenschaftlichen und sozialen Umgangs mit arbeitsbedingten Krebserkrankungen in Deutschland. Verlag für Neue Wissensschaft, Bremerhaven

Illich I (1976) Limits to medicine: Medical nemesis: The expropriation of health. Boyars. London

Kächele H (1970) Der Begriff „psychogener Tod" in der medizinischen Literatur. Z Psychosom Med Psychoanal 16:105–129

Luhmann N (1995) Social Systems. Stanford (California), Stanford University Press

Rösing I (2006) Die Schließung des Kreises: Von der Schwarzen Heilung über Grau zum Weiß: Nächtliche Heilungsrituale in den Hochanden Boliviens. Zweitausendeins, Kronig

Vogd W (2013) Arzt-Patient-Interaktion aus medizinsoziologischer Perspektive. In: Nittel D, Seltrecht A (Hrsg) Krankheit: Lernen im Ausnahmezustand. Springer Verlag, S 456–468, Wiesbaden

Vogd W, Feißt M (2022) Therapeutische Arrangements im Maßregelvollzug. Studien zur Leerstellengrammatik und den Bezugsproblemen in der forensischen Psychiatrie. Velbrück Wissenschaft, Weilerswist

Psychological and Psychosomatic Approaches to Illness

14

Michaela Stratmann

Contents

14.1 Subjective Well-Being and Experience of Illness

The definition of illness as a deviation from the norm must take into account not only somatic symptoms but also functional, statistical, diagnostic, and therapeutic norms (Kessler 2021). How people assess their own well-being depends not only on their physical condition but is also influenced by psychosocial factors. The assessment of well-being and capacity to act as diminished initially occurs through interoception, whereby symptom perception and interpretation do not necessarily have to correspond with external observation. A divergence between subjective well-being and medical and/or

M. Stratmann (✉)
Junior Professorship of Interprofessional and Collaborative Didactics in Medical and Health Study Programmes, Faculty of Health, Witten/Herdecke University, Witten, Germany
e-mail: michaela.stratmann@uni-wh.de

D. Schmitz et al. (eds.), *Chronic Care—Science and Practice*,
https://doi.org/10.1007/978-3-662-72298-5_14

psychological findings can be based on misperception, such as in anorexia with differing internal and external norms, in hypochondria with excessive self-perception and overvaluation of bodily sensations, or in individuals with a lack of self-perception, resulting in delayed diagnosis and treatment opportunities.

14.2 Psychological Models of Illness

14.2.1 Behavioral Models

In learning theories, observable behavior, which manifests on the physiological and motor levels as well as the verbal-cognitive level, plays a central role. The development of problematic, unhealthy behavior is determined by physical dispositions, environmental conditions, and the consequences of the behavior exhibited. Behavioral changes are acquired through various learning processes, which can also interact, particularly in the cognitive components of internal prediction and self-description (Faller and Lang 2019). Classical and operant conditioning are based on associative learning through the linking of stimuli or events. The likelihood of classical conditioning increases the more frequently a conditioned and an unconditioned stimulus occur together (contingency), the greater their temporal and spatial proximity (contiguity), the more salient the conditioned stimulus is and thus stands out from the environment, and the better we are biologically prepared for the pairing (so-called preparedness). Classical conditioning is confirmed in clinical studies, for example, in the occurrence of nausea during chemotherapy. In operant conditioning, the change in behavioral probability is controlled by its consequences. The frequency of a behavior increases if a pleasant consequence follows and decreases if an unpleasant consequence follows. Operant conditioning is clearly evident in clinical practice, for example, in avoidance behavior maintained by negative reinforcement in phobias.

Behavioral changes associated with illness that have been acquired or maintained through learning processes are to be unlearned through behavioral modification within the framework of (cognitive) behavioral therapy, and health-promoting behaviors are to be developed. Initially, a behavioral analysis is conducted using the so-called SORKC model by Kanfer, which considers the five conditional factors for explaining human behavior. In the first step, the problem behavior (**R**) is described as precisely as possible on three levels: observable behavior, internal experience (emotions/cognitions), and physiological accompaniments. The subsequent analysis links the behavior to the preceding situation (**S**), organismic variables (**O**), such as an innate disposition, the subsequent consequences (**C**), and the associated contingencies (**K**) (Deinzer and von Knesebeck 2018). Once the conditions of illness behavior, for example in phobic anxiety, have been precisely diagnosed, behavioral modification can begin by changing negative thought patterns and learning new behaviors to unlearn the anxiety.

14.2.2 Psychobiological Models

Psychobiology examines the effects of psychological processes (e.g., stress) on biological processes as well as the consequences of physical changes on experience and behavior, since mutual influence is assumed (Kessler 2021). Stress represents an adaptive response of the organism to stimuli (stressors) that can affect the organism externally, such as noise or organic pathogens, but also intrapsychically. In Selye's stress model, the physiological responses to stressors are described as a general adaptation syndrome, which aims to restore internal balance, or homeostasis. In the initial alarm phase, the body responds by releasing catecholamines. If the stress persists, the body enters the resistance phase and responds with cortisol release. The duration of stress exposure is pathogenetically significant, as the increased hormone release cannot be maintained indefinitely. In the subsequent exhaustion stage, the body can no longer respond to the stressor, and the conditions for functional dysregulation and disease development are present. For example, prolonged sympathetic activation can lead to an increased cardiovascular risk. Prolonged, especially uncontrollable stress has an immunosuppressive effect and promotes physical, psychosomatic, and psychological disorders.

The neural basis of pain experience is the pain network, in which the primary sensory cells (nociceptors) detect tissue damage caused by intense mechanical, thermal, and/or chemical stimuli (Deinzer and von Knesebeck 2018). This warning and protective function of acute pain no longer applies in chronic pain, which can persist for months or years, as tissue damage can often no longer be demonstrated. On a psychological level, there are clear differences between acute pain, with short-term changes such as anxiety, insight into the pain event, and activation, and chronic pain, with depression, attentional shifts, and withdrawal. Especially for chronic pain, the concept of a pain memory is used. Memories of pain experiences leave traces at the cortical and subcortical levels and result in increased sensitivity to pain stimuli. Harmless, normally non-painful stimuli then trigger pain through the underlying mechanism of long-term potentiation. Neuronal plasticity is considered the likely basis of pain memory. In cases of severe persistent pain, such as chronic back pain, headaches (migraine, tension headache), or persistent somatoform pain disorder, a multimodal therapy is indicated, including medication and psychological interventions such as biofeedback, through which patients learn that physical processes can be influenced by psychological factors.

14.2.3 Psychodynamic Models

According to Freud, personality consists of three agencies, which, in his structural model, exist in a dynamic equilibrium (Faller and Lang 2019). The *id* is the source of primary drives and is always unconscious. The *superego* represents values, norms, and moral concepts and develops at the end of the Oedipal phase. The *ego* is the representative of the reality principle and mediates in the conflict between the impulses of the id and the demands of the superego. This fundamental opposition between bodily needs (id) and the socially sanctioned means of satisfying those needs through norms and rules (superego) can lead to intrapsychic conflicts, which are experienced as psychological arousal or anxiety. The ego attempts to mediate by integrating the contradictory needs or by defending against instinctual impulses. If this fails, and the conflict cannot be resolved or only through poor compromises, symptoms and thus psychosomatic illnesses develop as a pseudo-solution. This results in two advantages: primary gain, when the conflict tension or psychological arousal is alleviated by the defense mechanism, and secondary gain, which refers to the external benefits of the sick role and all subsequent reliefs or gratifications, such as exemption from work obligations or disability pension.

Defense mechanisms thus represent a good psychological protective reaction for coping with psychological stress, which, however, can become problematic if patients do not face reality over the long term. In life-threatening illnesses, for example, patients may initially deny the severity of their illness, behave in a demonstratively cheerful manner (reaction formation), or discuss their diagnosis in a completely matter-of-fact and detached way (isolation). Defense mechanisms manifest in varying degrees of maturity. With mature defense mechanisms, such as rationalization or turning into the opposite, psychological conflicts are regulated intrapsychically, so that social relationships are only secondarily burdened. In contrast, with immature defense mechanisms, such as splitting or projective identification, other people are involved in an attempt to stabilize one's own psychological equilibrium, which can lead to a significant strain on relationships. In psychoanalytic therapy, unconscious conflicts are made conscious through specific techniques, such as free association, dream analysis, or the revival of earlier conflicts within the therapeutic relationship (transference). Through this therapeutic process and the realization of appropriate conflict resolution, psychosomatic symptoms ultimately become unnecessary.

14.2.4 Social Psychological Models

The social psychological models of health and illness behavior focus on the influence of the psychosocial environment, social roles, norms, and personal attitudes. Based on the assumption of a continuum between health and illness (Binneböse et al. 2022), health is not seen as a static state, but as a constantly changing position. This is determined by the interplay of risk and protective factors, which include physical-material, psychological, as well as familial and social aspects. Psychological risk factors include, for example, stressful life events, especially experiences of loss, lack of social integration, learned helplessness, and depression. Psychological protective factors that counteract the development of illness are internal locus of control, self-efficacy expectation, dispositional optimism, and hardiness (resilience).

Resistance resources are considered the core of salutogenesis and are regarded as an essential potential for coping with stressors. People with many and pronounced resources can cope better with stress and thus move in a positive direction on the health-illness continuum. The sense of coherence has been postulated as an outstanding protective factor for health promotion, understood as a comprehensive, enduring, and dynamic confidence (see contribution 18). A strong sense of coherence is associated with better subjective health, fewer complaints, and a significantly lower degree of somatoform disorders. In contrast, the lowest values for sense of coherence are found in psychosomatic and mentally ill patients.

14.3 Coping With Illness

People's illness behavior is also shaped by subjective theories of illness, especially in severe and chronic diseases, where the treatment goal is usually not a cure, but rather that those affected must learn to live with the illness (Faller and Lang 2019). The cognitive explanatory patterns regarding the causes and course of the illness include rationalizations or spiritual thinking, such as viewing the illness as a test from a higher power. Subjective theories of illness are often not expressed unprompted and are not always conscious, but they have a clear impact on compliance and coping with illness. Problem-focused coping strategies aim to eliminate or improve the stressful situation. They include seeking information and actively participating in treatment. Emotion-focused strategies are used to reduce the unpleasant emotions caused by the situation, without directly addressing their cause. These include avoidance, distancing, and passivity in treatment. Another important factor in coping with illness is social support, which is largely determined by the size, stability, and quality of a person's social network and has a positive impact on physical, psychosomatic, and mental health.

References

Binneböse M, Frommer J, Franzkowiak P, Junne F (2022) Psychosomatische Perspektive. In: Bundeszentrale für gesundheitliche Aufklärung (BZgA) (Hrsg) Leitbegriffe der Gesundheitsförderung und Prävention. Glossar zu Konzepten, Strategien und Methoden. https://doi.org/10.17623/BZGA:Q4-i098-3.0. Zugegriffen am 28.10.2025

Deinzer R, von dem Knesebeck O (Hrsg) (2018) Online Lehrbuch der Medizinischen Psychologie und Medizinischen Soziologie. German Medical Science GMS Publishing House. https://books.publisso.de/de/publisso_gold/publishing/books/overview/46. Zugegriffen am 28.10.2025

Faller H, Lang H (Hrsg) (2019) Medizinische Psychologie und Soziologie, 5., überarb. Aufl. Springer, Berlin/Heidelberg

Kessler H (2021) Kurzlehrbuch Medizinische Psychologie und Soziologie, 4., überarb. Aufl. Georg Thieme, Stuttgart/New York

Human-Environment Relationships in the Context of Illness

15

Julia Kirch

Contents

15.1 Humans and Environment in Interaction

The discipline of environmental psychology examines the relationship between humans and the environment. As a subfield of psychology, it deals with the interactions between people and their physical as well as sociocultural environment. Architectural psychology in particular focuses on human behavior and experience in built environments. The task of this research field is to investigate and analyze human behavior in and requirements for their built environment, and to translate these findings in such a way that they lead to architecture oriented toward human needs.

J. Kirch (✉)
Frankfurt University of Applied Sciences, Frankfurt, Deutschland
e-mail: julia.kirch@a-sh.de

J. Kirch
alsh Sander Hofrichter Architekten, Ludwigshafen, Deutschland

D. Schmitz et al. (eds.), *Chronic Care—Science and Practice*,
https://doi.org/10.1007/978-3-662-72298-5_15

Environmental psychological concepts assume that humans and the environment are in constant exchange; the relationship is considered transactional, and this exchange is referred to as the human-environment dialectic: humans shape the environment around them, which in turn influences human behavior and well-being. The connecting element between humans and the environment is the activity between space and person, through which people relate to their environment.

The special feature of the relationship to the built environment is that this exchange process takes place permanently, is unavoidable, and affects everyone. In Western societies, people spend almost all their time in built environments. The built environment should therefore be the answer to human needs, so that built space serves people as well as possible. Spaces and objects that are the result of a user-oriented process are also referred to as *Human-Centered Design* (see Contribution 26). A central criterion for successful architecture is often the extent to which it contributes to enabling independence. Independence is made possible when the fit between individual abilities and the opportunities offered by the environment is as high as possible. The challenge here is that people and their abilities differ, but there is only one environment that must provide an answer to various abilities.

15.2 The Human as the Measure of Planning

Designing the environment is a negotiation process between various—sometimes opposing—requirements. The result is often a compromise based on the cross-section of the population. The idea of the "human as the measure of planning" is challenged by the fact that society is so diverse that a single solution cannot fit all users equally. In everyday life, this is evident, for example, in ATMs that are difficult to reach for people in wheelchairs, or in children who use stair steps as seating. The design philosophy of Universal Design pursues precisely this goal: that the environment should be usable by as many people as possible equally. In doing so, the Universal Design standard fulfills the requirement of the current planning norm DIN 18040 (p. 3) for barrier-free construction, which states in the foreword: "The aim of the standard DIN 18040-1 is to design the built living environment so that it is accessible and enables as many people as possible to use it in a conventional way, without particular impediments and basically without help from others."

The special feature of environmental design in the context of illness is that for people with physical and/or cognitive impairments, dependence on the environment increases. This is illustrated by the *Competence Press Model*, formulated by Lawton and Nahemow in the 1970s (Lawton and Nahemow 1973). The model shows that socially appropriate behavior and well-being are the result of a balance between environmental demands and individual competencies to cope with these demands. When coping competencies are reduced, dependence on the environment increases because a lower level of environmental demands can be managed. If individual competencies are diminished, environmental demands should also be adjusted accordingly so that the range of well-being and socially appropriate behavior can be achieved.

Disability, therefore, is not a personal characteristic, but the discrepancy between personal abilities and the demands of the environment. This is demonstrated by researchers Verbrugge and Jette in their model of the *Disablement Process* (roughly: process of becoming disabled) (Verbrugge and Jette 1994). In this concept, disability is not seen solely as a question of individual abilities, but is placed in the context of environmental demands. When assessing and designing environments, the focus should therefore not only be on the personal abilities of people with impairments, but also on the environmental demands, which, through their characteristics, contribute to either restricting or enabling independence.

15.3 The Fit Between People and Space

Architecture is significant because it is omnipresent and almost inescapable—people in Western countries spend almost 90% of their time indoors. Architecture directs gazes and movements—it is the concrete, material space in which social interactions take place. Because it is perceived not only visually but also physically, it is also referred to as the *Second Body* (Koppen and Vollmer 2021) or *Third Skin*, alongside the skin and clothing. In contrast to clothing, which usually offers a selection of different sizes and fits for various body shapes (it should be noted that even with clothing, many people who do not conform to the norm have difficulty finding suitable garments), architecture as the third body is even more challenging. Since built space is static and long-lasting, there is a greater reliance on average values than is the case with clothing, so that a building can serve different users for many years. In this case, architecture is a compromise. Here, the environment often has only one—unchangeable—form. And that is supposed to fit as many people as possible. How can this succeed, and what can serve as orientation standards?

People seek environments that match their orientations. Whether the environment meets individual needs can be assessed. The so-called "person-environment congruence" can be examined on four evaluation levels (Fuhrer 1996):

1. **Ergonomic congruence:** *Does the space fit my body shape, size, and anatomy?*
2. **Cognitive congruence:** *Can I easily find my way around, and does the space match my cognitive abilities?* The brain creates a "cognitive map" of the environment, which helps with orientation. For people with cognitive impairments, a clear spatial structure is important so that relevant places can be recognized directly.
3. **Emotional congruence:** *Do I find the space pleasant?* The evaluation of material, color, and form is subjective and depends on experience and culture. Control over the space, for example through clarity, contributes to a sense of well-being and safety.

4. **Motivational congruence**: *Can I design and use the space according to my wishes?* This aspect concerns the need for territoriality, self-determination, and personal expression. In private spaces, appropriation enables people to identify with their space and form a close connection.

15.4 Architecture as Medicine?

These basic needs apply initially to all people, regardless of physical or cognitive limitations. The differences lie in the degree of dependence on the environment and the spatial response. The Disablement Process theory posits that people are not *limited* but are *made limited* by unsuitable environments, as the space does not meet their needs. If the environment were appropriately designed, even people with limitations could live largely independently and the concept of *disability* would become obsolete.

Individual constitution, illnesses, and care needs determine the objectives of the space and the environmental radius. Independence in terms of mobility is not always the primary goal. In certain situations, such as being bedridden, the focus should be on safety, privacy, and control in the immediate vicinity of the bed.

The term Healing Environment has received much attention in recent years, especially in the field of healthcare buildings. It refers to the potential of the environment to contribute to recovery or illness. Studies show that the built and social environment can have both positive and negative effects on well-being and health. Environmental medicine deals with the prevention, diagnosis, and treatment of health problems related to environmental factors. Here, harmful chemical substances in building materials and indoor air, as well as physical influences such as noise, are significant.

Considering environmental medical aspects is an important part of health promotion, as harmful influences have been proven. However, in the case of serious illnesses, the term *Healing Environment* must be viewed in the context of medical treatment. Architecture cannot completely cure illness, but it can support independence and well-being by creating a good fit between people and their environment. The potential of the environment should be understood as supportive, as Koppen and Vollmer have formulated with the term *Supportive Environment*.

15.5 Vulnerability as Opportunity

People with limitations are particularly dependent on their environment. Observing this dependence can help to reveal weaknesses in design (Kirch and Marquardt 2021). For a human-centered environment, the standard should not be the most independent or fittest person, but rather people with limitations. This leads to the realization of an inclusive environment. An environment that works for people with limitations is often also suitable for people without limitations, as they are generally more adaptable and less dependent on their environment. Limitations can also be temporary, for example, with a broken limb or when using a stroller. In such situations, an accessible environment is highly valued. Limitations can therefore be seen as an opportunity when they are used as a *seismographic sensitivity* and serve as a starting point for planning good environments.

In design, it is important that objects and buildings possess aesthetic qualities in order to be widely accepted. If products are obviously designed for specific limitations, their adoption can be difficult. A successful example is accessible bathrooms, whose aesthetic design can now be found in many new and renovated bathrooms. Minimalist design, high comfort, and neutral labels contribute to increased acceptance.

15.6 Current Needs

Physical condition, cognitive and social abilities are not static characteristics, but are influenced by the environment. Health is promoted when the environment enables the greatest possible freedom of action and individual abilities are preserved for longer. This should be considered from neighborhood planning down to the door handle. Barrier-free planning is associated with additional costs of about 5–10% and requires early planning. The more advanced the planning or construction, the more expensive it becomes to create accessible environments. In terms of public infrastructure, much has been achieved in recent years through the implementation of DIN 18040, but much remains to be done.

There is currently a lack of innovation in the development of housing concepts and care facilities, especially regarding the social aspects of architecture and the promotion of social encounters and social diversity. The built environment is more than craftsmanship and ticking off accessibility checklists: architecture is the framework for social interactions and individual expression. The role of architecture in enhancing quality of life and well-being is always part of the system. It seems that the potential inherent in the built environment is still far from fully realized. Here, the societal level intersects with the personal level—framework conditions set the parameters within which projects are implemented. If more structural and social innovations are to be pursued, the framework conditions for this must also be created in legal and financial terms.

References

Fuhrer U (1996) Person-Umwelt-Kongruenz. In: Kruse L, Graumann C, Lantermann E-D (Hrsg) Ökologische Psychologie: Ein Handbuch in Schlüsselbegriffen. Beltz, München, S 143–153

Kirch J, Marquardt G (2021) Towards human-centred general hospitals: the potential of dementia-friendly design. Arch Sci Rev 0(0):1–9

Koppen G, Vollmer TC (2021) Architektur als zweiter Körper: Eine Entwurfslehre für den evidenzbasierten Gesundheitsbau. Gebr. Mann, Berlin

Lawton MP, Nahemow L (1973) Ecology and the aging process. In: Eisdorfer C, Lawton MP (Hrsg) The psychology of adult development and aging. American Psychological Association, Washington, S 619–674

Verbrugge LM, Jette AM (1994) The disablement process. Soc Sci Med 38(1):1–14

Social Determinants of Health and Chronic Diseases

16

Manfred Fiedler

Contents

16.1 Social Backgrounds of Illness

As early as 1848, Rudolf Virchow described medicine as a social science and pointed to the connection between poverty and illness. At that time, this connection could easily be traced back to the objective living conditions of the large number of agricultural and industrial workers: income insecurity, and consequently food insecurity, cramped and unhygienic living conditions, lack of occupational safety in physically demanding jobs, and inadequate or nonexistent care in the event of illness or accidents. Improvements in income, working, and living conditions, as well as the now widespread protection against health risks in much of Europe, have made the social question appear largely resolved. Today, the relationship between poverty, social inequality, and health is more inconspicuous and subtle. Education, social status, general living conditions, or capabilities for self-realization have expanded the understanding of social disadvantage beyond income

M. Fiedler (✉)
Department of human medicine, Witten/Herdecke University, Witten, Germany
e-mail: manfred.fiedler@uni-wh.de

D. Schmitz et al. (eds.), *Chronic Care—Science and Practice*,
https://doi.org/10.1007/978-3-662-72298-5_16

and wealth inequality. The scientific foundation for this is social epidemiology, which measures the distribution of diseases among population groups based on social criteria or characteristics.

16.2 The Conceptual Understanding of Social Determinants of Health (SDH)

A quarter of a century ago, the British epidemiologists Marmot and Wilkinson published their overview study on SDH for the WHO, subtitling it "The solid facts" (Wilkinson and Marmot 2003). In it, they summarized and systematized the results of numerous studies. Unlike the German concept of social indicators, which records the distribution of social factors in the population and derives more or less well-founded statements about social conditions, SDH starts from the social determinants of diseases. The focus is thus on an empirically valid understanding of the social determinants of illness and health. Conceptually, SDH is embedded in a comprehensive understanding of pathogenic and health-promoting factors. While there is a formal similarity to concepts of social distribution, SDH is a practical care concept rather than a distributional policy concept, even though social interventions can certainly be derived from a public health perspective. For example, Wilkinson and the British epidemiologist Kate Pickett, based on the comparison of social and epidemiological data, have identified social inequality as a determinant of a country's health status, affecting all population groups and only solvable through distributional policy (Wilkinson and Pickett 2009).

Such analyses remain only a supplementary understanding for the topic of SDH, as they cannot be directly implemented in care practice.

In contrast, the field of social medicine, which has been established in Germany for a long time, has interfaces with SDH, as it also deals with the determinants of health, taking into account its paramedical reference disciplines. There is also a substantive connection to salutogenesis, particularly when it comes to abilities to cope with stressors and factors that promote health (Antonovsky 1997).

16.3 Domains of Social Determinants

This section briefly explicates the domains of the concept by Wilkenson and Marmot:

1. Income—Education

Income poverty is one of the *oldest* determinants of disease. Nevertheless, its substantive scope has been relativized, as personal factors, such as physical disabilities or addiction disorders, lead to higher expenses. However, it is undisputed that education is a decisive factor, as education as a personal resource both secures access to higher income and strengthens the ability to develop health literacy. At the same time, there is a direct link between income and education, since parental income and parental education increase educational opportunities at a very early stage. Studies show that children from educationally disadvantaged families acquire chronic diseases at an early age. Early education can also have positive effects on the development of dementia-related changes over the life course.

2. Social Distress

Distress refers to stress factors that cannot be managed by the individual. These can be found in the immediate living environment of people, i.e., in the family, with and among relatives, in the neighborhood, and in school and work contexts. The Healthy Worker Effect has long been known, meaning that people in employment are, on average, healthier than those who are unemployed, which is partly due to the frequent loss of employment because of illness, and partly due to the strain that unemployment entails. At the same time, working conditions in the context of physical, psychological, and mental stress are relevant factors for health and disease. Conflicts in the home environment, (chronic) illness, but also the loss of family ties, such as in separated families, require coping actions.

3. Social Support—Social Cohesion

Social support is a health-promoting factor. Studies show that people with no or few social contacts are more likely to experience dementia-related changes. Loneliness has become an overarching psychopathological factor due to non-medical measures during the coronavirus pandemic. In addition, for people with chronic illnesses, social support is beneficial for coping with everyday life affected by the chronic condition.

4. Nutrition—Food Security

In health science discussions, nutrition is often associated with questions of lifestyle. At the same time, a number of diseases, such as obesity, cardiological and angiological diseases, e.g., in type II diabetes mellitus, are linked to malnutrition. However, nutrition is not just a behavioral problem; eating disorders are themselves a disease. Moreover, eating behavior is socialized—by family, social reference groups, and society, for example, in the form of food traditions. Severe overweight is more prevalent in low-income social groups, also because access to balanced, high-quality foods is unequally distributed. Conversely, food insecurity is also a growing problem in high-wage countries. Children who are undernourished or malnourished experience developmental disadvantages and are often less able to learn adequately, thus also facing educational disadvantages.

5. Social Status

Social status is predominantly a characteristic for the distribution of diseases, less an explicit social determinant. However, certain manifestations of social status or stratification can be captured as SDH, which is why a brief overview follows.

i. Social Minorities—Subculturality
   Social minorities represent a special social group with self-defined or socially acquired characteristics. These subcultural groups include, for example, communities shaped by religious beliefs. Studies show that such social communities often have different interpretations of illness and symptoms, a different understanding of corporeality and body-related shame, and thus of touch, especially in the context of nursing, medical, and therapeutic care. This can lead to professional services being rejected, not sought at all, or only when suffering is severe.
ii. Migration—Foreign Language
   For a large proportion of people with a migration background, the official language is often a foreign language in everyday home life. This means that access to health services is significantly more difficult, therapeutic instructions are not or insufficiently followed (non-compliance), entitlements and services are not known, or their significance is not recognized (see contribution 28).
iii. Stigmatization
   Stigmatization is the devaluation or discrimination of people based on personal characteristics and traits. This includes, not least, certain chronic diseases, especially mental illnesses. Old age and frailty are also often perceived as a stigma. The result can be a feeling of worthlessness, self-stigmatization, and ultimately social withdrawal. For people with chronic illness, experienced stigmatization can lead to an intensification of the disease and its symptoms.
iv. Environmental Conditions—Housing
   Living conditions and immediate environmental conditions are distributed unequally across social groups. People with low social status often live in smaller residents with more people, which are less well insulated against cold and heat, and are less often accessible or barrier-free. Residential areas are more often characterized by higher levels of harmful environmental emissions, such as noise or environmental gases. Dense housing, few green spaces, and difficult social milieus with anxiety-inducing spaces are also health-damaging conditions, which also have a higher potential for social and family conflicts.

16.4 Fields of Action

In conclusion, we would like to highlight scientific and practical fields of action, which can only serve as spotlights and, from our perspective, should gain increasing importance.

1. Life Phase Analysis
   The importance of life phase analyses (Robert Koch Institute 2017) arises from several factors. On the one hand, it is evident that lifestyles, such as those shaping health behaviors, are learned early and are thus transmitted within families and social environments. For example, the relationship between obesity and the social status of families is well researched. The opportunity for education as a resource for health-competent behavior is also distributed unequally across social groups. This is clearly demonstrated by the various in-depth evaluations within the KIGGS study on the health of children and adolescents in Germany (Kuntz et al. 2018) or the GEDA studies on the health of adults in Germany (Saß et al. 2017). The Lancet Dementia Study also points to the importance of age-specific interventions to prevent, delay, or influence the course of dementia, for example through targeted educational support in childhood and adolescence (GBD 2019 Dementia Forecasting Collaborators 2022).
2. Disease Prevention—Health Protection
   The numerous studies on social determinants of health demonstrate the necessity of prevention strategies oriented toward social groups. In fact, we now know a great deal about these relationships, but less about effective solutions to address them. Studies show, for example, that families with low parental educational status, at risk of poverty, and/or with a migration background have less knowledge of health promotion measures and make less use of them (Ehlen et al. 2021; Epstein and Street 2011). From this, it can be concluded that prevention and health promotion measures targeting socially vulnerable groups must be outreach-based, oriented toward real-life settings, neighborhood-based, and appropriately participatory for the milieu.
3. Coping with Illness
   In healthcare practice, the importance of patient-centered care (PCC) has been discussed for several years. The nursing expert standard *Relationship Building in the Care of People with Dementia* clearly emphasizes the strong focus on the relationship between professionals and those affected. Eppstein and Street (Epstein and Street 2011) go even further, speaking of personal, professional, and organizational relationships. In the understanding of Rawann and Moretz (Rawson and Moretz 2016), particular focus is placed on the family in relation to the eight principles (see Fig. 16.1) of Harvey Picker, while also referencing a biopsychosocial model.
   What is special here is the focus on the family, the living environment, and the social context. Such an approach to person-centeredness can be linked to the issue of social determinants, as the professional relationship requires knowledge of specific, person-related, real-life information.
   In particular, in youth social work, the social history (see Fig. 16.2) is a well-known tool, for example in assessing the need for early interventions. It also plays an important role in assessing family predispositions, especially with regard to addiction disorders or obesity.
   The systematic further development of instruments for assessing social risks, disease conditions, the ability to adhere to therapy, and also health resources that can be activated by those affected would be helpful and necessary with reference to SDH.

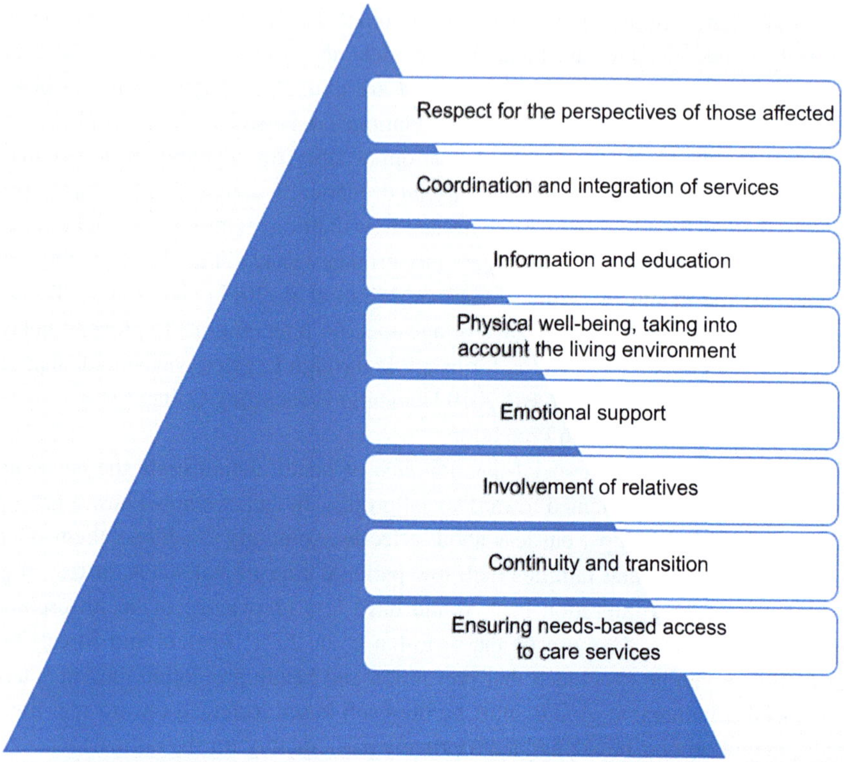

Fig. 16.1 Eight Principles of PCC. (Own illustration based on (Rawson and Moretz 2016))

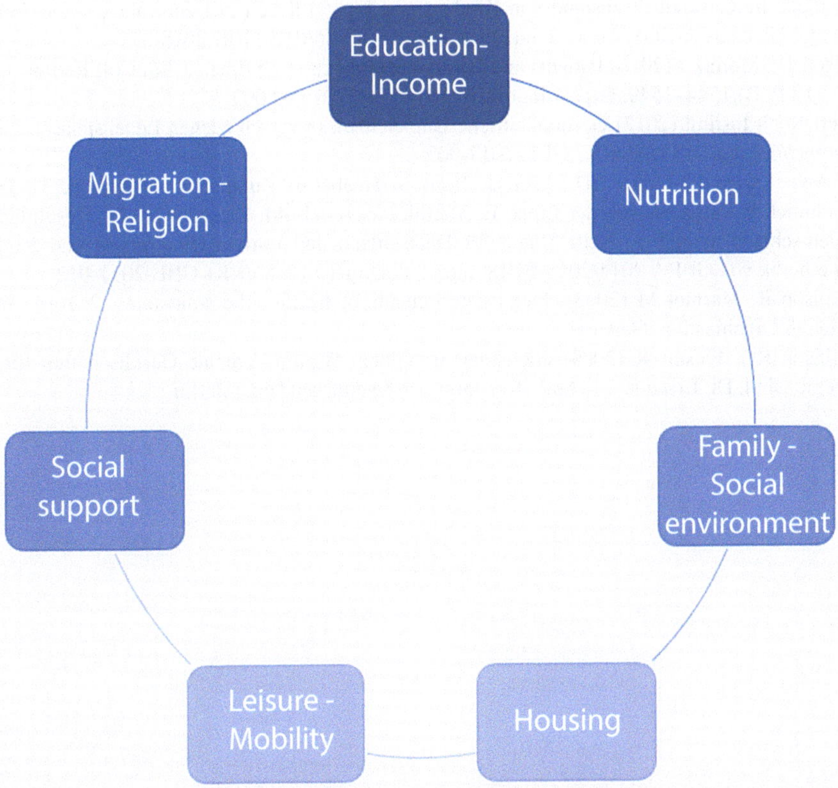

Fig. 16.2 Subject areas of a social history. (Own illustration)

References

Antonovsky A (1997) Forum für Verhaltenstherapie und psychosoziale Praxis: Band 36. Salutogenese: Zur Entmystifizierung der Gesundheit (Schulte N, Übers) (Franke A, Hg). dgvt Verlag, Tübingen

Ehlen S, Henning L, Rehaag R, Dreiskämper D (2021) Soziale Determinanten der Kenntnis und Inanspruchnahme kommunaler Gesundheitsförderung und Prävention für Kinder. In: Forum Kinder- und Jugendsport 2(1):27–40. https://doi.org/10.1007/s43594-021-00037-6

Epstein RM, Street RL (2011) The values and value of patient-centered care. Ann Family Med 9(2):100–103. https://doi.org/10.1370/afm.1239

GBD 2019 Dementia Forecasting Collaborators (2022) Estimation of the global prevalence of dementia in 2019 and forecasted prevalence in 2050: an analysis for the Global Burden of Disease Study 2019. Lancet Pub Health 7(2):e105–e125. https://doi.org/10.1016/S2468-2667(21)00249-8

Kuntz B, Rattay P, Poethko-Müller C, Thamm R, Hölling H, Lampert T (2018) Soziale Unterschiede im Gesundheitszustand von Kindern und Jugend lichen in Deutschland – Querschnittergebnisse aus KiGGS Welle. 2. https://doi.org/10.17886/RKI-GBE-2018-076

Rawson JV, Moretz J (2016) Patient- and family-centered care: a primer. J Am Coll Radiol: JACR 13(12 Pt B):1544–1549. https://doi.org/10.1016/j.jacr.2016.09.003

Robert Koch-Institut (2017) Gesundheitliche Ungleichheit in verschiedenen Lebensphasen.Berlin. https://doi.org/10.17886/RKI-GBE-2017-003

Saß A-C, Lange C, Finger JD, Allen J, Born S, Hoebel J, Kuhnert R, Müters S, Thelen J, Schmich P, Varga M, von der Lippe E, Matthias Wetzstein M, Ziese T (2017) „Gesundheit in Deutschland aktuell" – Neue Daten für Deutschland und Europa Hintergrund und Studienmethodik von GEDA 2014/2015-EHIS. https://doi.org/10.17886/RKI-GBE-2017-012

Wilkinson R, Marmot M (2003) Social determinants of health—the solid facts, 2. Aufl. World Health Organization, Geneva

Wilkinson RG, Pickett K (2009) Gleichheit ist Glück: Warum gerechte Gesellschaften für alle besser sind, Dt. Erstausg., 1. Aufl. Tolkemitt bei Zweitausendeins, Berlin

Professional Approaches to Dealing with Subjective Illness Experience

17

Heike Becker

Contents

17.1 Subjective Experience of Illness in Relation to Life Context

Depending on the life context, with its prevailing systems of thought and socially constructed processes regarding health and illness, the conception and experience for affected individuals varies individually (Faltermaier 2017). Consequently, the subjective experience of illness is closely intertwined with the respective biography and identity of those affected (see Contribution 29).

How subjectivity, and thus personal experience, can be taken into account in the context of experiencing illness with and without cognitive impairments is presented below, based on the theoretical backgrounds and profession-specific perspectives of Tom

H. Becker (✉)
Faculty of Health, Witten/Herdecke University, Witten, Germany
e-mail: heike.becker@uni-wh.de

D. Schmitz et al. (eds.), *Chronic Care—Science and Practice*,
https://doi.org/10.1007/978-3-662-72298-5_17

Kitwood's person-centered approach, Christoph Held's three worlds principle, and Naomi Feil's validation.

17.2 Person-Centered Approach According to Kitwood

With regard to people with dementia, a shift in perspective occurred between 1987 and 1995. This approach considers and understands the concept of the person from an ethical-philosophical perspective.

The person-centered approach of social psychologist and gerontologist Tom Kitwood is based on Carl Rogers' client-centered psychotherapy (see Contribution 21).

The focus is no longer on the person *with dementia,* but on the*person with* dementia. According to Kitwood, personhood is "[...] a standing or status that is bestowed upon an individual by others in the context of relationship and social being. It implies recognition, respect, and trust" (translation from German) (Kitwood 2022, p. 35).

This perspective also includes the understanding that every person, regardless of their cognitive abilities and competencies, is unique and differs, for example, in culture, gender, temperament, social class, lifestyle, appearance, taste, interests, and personal history (Kitwood et al. 2022).

17.2.1 Ways of Accessing the Subjective World of a Person with Dementia

Kitwood et al. (2022) describe seven ways to gain access to the person. These are:

- Accounts written by affected individuals in the early stages of the illness.
- Attentive listening during interviews or group work. Perceiving expressions such as fear of losing control, feelings of being lost, and worries about becoming a burden.
- Imaginative interpretation of what people say in everyday life and translating metaphorical descriptions, for example, when a person describes their changed memory as a picket fence with sturdy slats (lasting memories from long-term memory) and rotten slats or gaps (new memories from short-term memory).
- Learning from people's behavior in their actions and attempts to continue former everyday activities, which increasingly fail, and their interpration of the causes. Observing the development of challenging behavior as an attempt to counteract the fear of losing meaning.
- Interviewing people who have experienced an illness with dementia-like features, such as meningitis or depression.
- Interpreting poetic language, for example, "You are standing in the fog."
- Role play to switch into the perspective of a person with dementia.

17.2.2 Kitwood Flower

Kitwood presents the most important psychological needs of people with dementia in the form of a stylized flower, whose center is *love*. This is surrounded by the five petals *comfort, attachment, inclusion, occupation* and *identity*. There is no hierarchical order among the needs. In dementia, depending on personality, an individual pattern of needs develops, in which love stands as the all-encompassing need (Kitwood et al. 2022).

- *Love* stands for unconditional acceptance and emotional giving without an expectation of direct reward.
- *Comfort* means giving a person warmth and strength so that they remain intact when they are at risk of falling apart due to illness.
- *Attachment* refers to the need for a kind of safety net similar to primary attachments in the first years of life.
- *Inclusion* describes the feeling of belonging to a group. This is especially important in the relatively closed world of an institutional living environment.
- *Occupation* involves people in the process of life and is important for maintaining self-esteem.
- *Identity* means knowing who you are and what your past is. It is formed through doing things with others.

The person-centered approach offers a shift in perspective beyond deficit-oriented medical classifications of diseases and enables those affected and those involved to meet as equals within a dialogical I-Thou relationship, regardless of cognitive abilities and competencies (see Contribution 21).

17.3 Three Worlds Concept According to Held

The concept developed by Swiss gerontopsychiatrist Christian Held is based on the stages of dementia and their adaptation to changing needs and requirements, as well as the corresponding adaptation of the environment to create a designed experiential world. The three experiential worlds are the world of lack of success, the world of aimlessness, and the world of defenselessness. It is essential that the living spaces of the three worlds are separated from each other (Held and Ermini-Fünfschilling 2006).

In the world of *cognitive lack of success*, those affected have mild dementia. Here, individuals are included according to their abilities. Discreet assistance is provided to avoid *helpless* or *embarrassing* situations, with the aim of psychological relief.

People with moderate to severe dementia live in the world of cognitive *aimlessness*. This is characterized, among other things, by a diminished sense of ownership, declining language and social skills, childlike rediscovery of the environment, restless wandering, and uncontrolled relief even in public spaces.

To allow the urge for restless wandering to be expressed, the environment in this world is adapted through the design of outdoor areas and corridors, which also allow meals to be taken outside of fixed time structures (Held and Ermini-Fünfschilling 2006).

People in the final stage of dementia live in the world of *cognitive defenselessness*. This is characterized by the loss of language and gestures, as well as the need for protection from external influences and sensory overload. People in this stage of dementia are completely dependent on help, and their center of life is limited to their immediate surroundings. To provide them with a protected space and at the same time protect them from loneliness, Held developed the care oasis living arrangement. These are inhabited simultaneously by several people with dementia and are characterized by the fact that the individual living and sleeping areas merge seamlessly into one another. The interiors of a care oasis are designed in a restrained manner and with muted colors to prevent sensory overload. Stimuli such as scents, sounds, visual stimuli, and movements are experienced by the residents according to their individuality. In addition, the open design facilitates the participation of residents in the everyday life of other co-residents (Held and Ermini-Fünfschilling 2006).

The Three Worlds Concept demonstrates how an individual adaptation of the living environment to the changing needs of people with dementia can be achieved over the course of the illness. The goal is to improve the quality of life of those affected and those involved through a successful daily structure and adapted environment. This includes, among other things, a significant reduction in challenging behavior and a decrease in the use of sedative medications.

17.4 Validation According to Feil

The founder of Validation is the social worker Naomi Feil, whose person-centered approach is also based on Carl Rogers' client-centered counseling. In addition, Erikson's theory of life stages (Erikson 2015) and Maslow's hierarchy of needs are incorporated. The fundamental principle of Validation is an appreciative attitude. In the early 1970s, Feil described four stages of disorientation and their specific manifestations.

1. Stage (impaired/unhappy orientation): significant recognition of deficits with attempts to compensate for them.
2. Stage (time confusion): withdrawal of the affected person into their past life with their own sense of time and place.
3. Stage (repetitive movements): loss of cognitive and language abilities. Nonverbal expression through, for example, rhythmic tapping or restless wandering.
4. Stage (vegetating): complete apathy, staring blankly into space (Feil and Klerk-Rubin de 2017).

Although gestures, facial expressions, and language are lost over the course of a dementing illness, communication and closeness are still possible through Validation. Validation means that people with dementia and their behavior, even in the most confused state (challenging behavior, see contribution 21), are recognized as valid (validated) by caregivers who appreciatively accept that those affected are in their own world and experience it as real. Furthermore, Validation is a form of communication that seeks to understand and reflect the needs and feelings of those affected, who can hardly express themselves.

Validation is based, among other things, on the following principles:

- Every person is unique and valuable
- Disoriented people are accepted as they are
- Empathetic listening restores dignity, builds trust, and reduces anxiety
- Validation accompanies people, but does not lead them
- People are supported in expressing their emotions to satisfy their basic needs
- Challenging behavior has reasons, often unresolved tasks or processed traumas from the past (Feil and Klerk-Rubin de 2017).

The goals of the method include, among others, restoring self-esteem, reducing stress, improving verbal and nonverbal communication, and increasing well-being. In addition, Feil assumed that people with dementia have the need to complete unresolved tasks or resolve conflicts from their past. Specially trained staff therefore have the task of supporting those affected in this process. The foundation of Validation techniques is the building of trust and closeness, as well as verbal and nonverbal communication (Feil and Klerk-Rubin de 2017).

Validation, with its principles, demonstrates that in the subjective experience of illness, the individual life experience of those affected is a factor to be taken seriously in the care setting, and that communication is also possible on a nonverbal level.

17.5 Conclusion

The approaches presented place the person and their subjective experience of illness, rather than the dementia diseases or chronic illness itself, at the center. They thus focus on identifying competencies and meeting (basic) needs through verbal and nonverbal communication, as well as appropriate adaptations of living environments. These are promoted by the concepts mentioned, but are based on behavioral (e.g., non/verbal communication, simple language), local (e.g., dementia-sensitive wards), and structural (e.g., disease management programs) separation in specific areas created for those affected.

Separation versus inclusion of people with dementia or chronic illness is a subject of controversial debate, as the social paradigms of our time are inclusion, participation, and involvement.

This raises the question of whether and to what extent the approaches presented contribute to inclusion, since inclusion, alongside Validation, can lead to cognitive activation, self-efficacy, and participation. Even though the approaches presented mainly refer to people with dementia, they can also be applied to people with other chronic illnesses, such as schizophrenia. Here, the symptoms of those with mental illness (auditory hallucinations) are also accepted as real for them.

There are different approaches regarding the causes of challenging behavior. On the one hand, various factors are discussed, such as the brain's limited adaptability due to pre-existing damage, to changing (self-)perceptions, as well as changes in neurotransmitters at nerve connections. In contrast, Feil assumes that challenging behavior is based on an unresolved past with unfinished tasks and experienced traumas that have not yet been processed intrapsychically. Maslow's hierarchy of needs and Erikson's model of psychosocial development, for example, support this assumption. Nevertheless, Validation in particular shows that in the subjective experience of illness, the individual life experience of the affected person is an important and serious factor in the care setting.

References

Erikson HE (2015) Identität und Lebenszyklus, 27. Aufl. Suhrkamp, Frankfurt am Main

Faltermaier T (2017) Gesundheitspsychologie, 2., überarb. u. erw. Aufl. Kohlhammer, Stuttgart

Feil N, Klerk-Rubin de V (2017) Validation. Ein Weg zum Verständnis verwirrter alter Menschen, 11., überarb. Aufl. Ernst Reinhardt, München

Held C, Ermini-Fünfschilling D (2006) Das demenzgerechte Heim: Lebensraumgestaltung, Betreuung und Pflege für Menschen mit Alzheimerkrankheit: 9 Tabellen, 2., vollst. erneuerte u. erw. Aufl. Karger, Basel

Kitwood T (2022) Was heißt es eine Person zu sein. In: Kitwood T, Brooker D, Müller-Hergl C, Güther H (Hrsg) Demenz: Der person-zentrierte Ansatz im Umgang mit verwirrten, kognitiv beeinträchtigten Menschen, 9., vollst. überarb. u. erw. Aufl. Hogrefe, Bern, S 34–56

Kitwood T, Brooker D, Müller-Hergl C, Güther H (Hrsg) (2022) Demenz: Der person-zentrierte Ansatz im Umgang mit verwirrten, kognitiv beeinträchtigten Menschen, 9., vollst. überarb. u. erw. Aufl. Hogrefe, Bern

Salutogenesis, Resilience, Coping 18

Heike Becker and Jan-Hendrik Ortloff

Contents

18.1 Salutogenesis, Resilience, and Coping

People with chronic illnesses, as a vulnerable group, are exposed to increased levels of both physical and psychological stressors as well as risk factors. If those affected exhibit less flexibility in adapting to new situations, stressors and risk factors may be further heightened. For this reason, especially in the context of chronic illnesses, it is important not only to consider the contextual factors that lead to a health problem, but also the beneficial factors that contribute to recovery. Against the backdrop that progress in health can only be made if, in addition to researching pathogenesis, attention is also paid to health-promoting factors, the health scientist Antonovsky (1997) developed the model of salutogenesis.

H. Becker (✉)
Faculty of Health, Witten/Herdecke University, Witten, Germany
e-mail: heike.becker@uni-wh.de

J.-H Ortloff
Department of human medicine, Witten/Herdecke University, Witten, Germany
e-mail: jan-hendrik.ortloff@uni-wh.de

D. Schmitz et al. (eds.), *Chronic Care—Science and Practice*,
https://doi.org/10.1007/978-3-662-72298-5_18

18.1.1 Salutogenesis

Salutogenesis does not view health as the opposite of illness, but rather as a continuum between illness and health. Accordingly, health is a dynamic interaction of stressful risk factors (stressors) and relieving protective factors for coping with stress (coping). Three fundamental risk factors are distinguished, which may arise from relatively persistent negative life conditions, the experience of a traumatic event, or combinations of both (Patterson 2002). It is important to note that a risk factor such as a chronic illness does not necessarily lead to a stressful situation per se, but can serve as an indicator for psychological processes that may result in either resilient coping or a stressful situation. The decisive factor here is the individual's coping mechanisms during the confrontation with the new situation. The individual health status thus also results from the interactions between risk and protective factors, their relationship to each other, and socialization with regard to dealing with risk factors.

According to Antonovsky, a balanced relationship between risk factors and coping mechanisms contributes to the maintenance of health or provides the basis for it (see Fig. 18.1). The key concept of salutogenesis is the sense of coherence. This is formed from the feelings of comprehensibility, manageability, and meaningfulness.

Comprehensibility refers to the knowledge and structured processing of one's own actions as well as the engagement with the actions of others through anticipation and interpretation. Manageability refers to the extent to which individuals are able to meet demands and stressors with the resources available to them, and thus perceive these as manageable. Resources are defined as available if they can be controlled by the

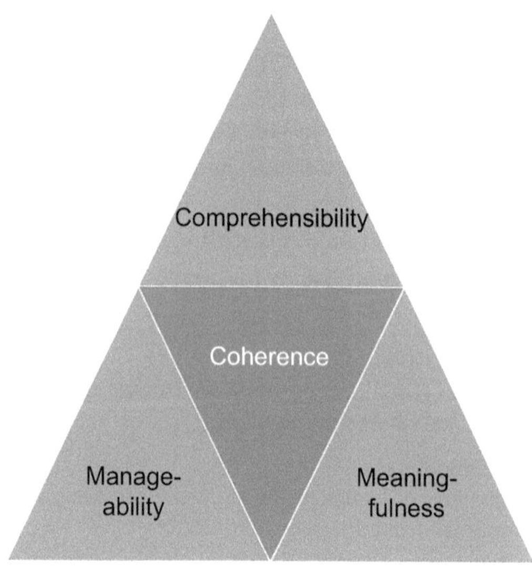

Fig. 18.1 Coherence pyramid. (Own illustration)

individuals themselves or by close helpers. Meaningfulness connects the resources invested with the goals pursued (Antonovsky 1997; Faltermaier 2017). Critics of Antonovsky's health model point to the lack of subjective experience and the absence of socioeconomic aspects. As a result, Faltermaier developed the integrative model of salutogenesis based on the original model. In addition to the component of health concepts, Faltermaier adds the action-oriented component of health *action* to the model. This reflects the subject-oriented perspective with reference to the lay health system in real life. In contrast stands the professionally oriented concept of health *behavior* (Faltermaier 2017).

18.1.2 Resilience

Resilience is an ambiguous term without a universally accepted definition. There are a multitude of different definitions from various disciplinary perspectives (Felten 2000). These relate, among other things, to terminology, basic mechanisms, specific boundaries, and their operationalizations (Haase 2004). In the social and health sciences, the term resilience is often used to describe the strength of a person to overcome adverse life circumstances without sustaining lasting physical, psychological, or social impairments, and to restore a subjective state of normalcy (Obrist and van Eeuwijk 2006). Resilience also describes the ability to face or adapt to existentially difficult situations and at the same time to derive a learning value from them (Sotzko 2013). Furthermore, although the foundations of resilience are laid in early childhood, they can be (further) developed over the course of life.

Until now, two levels of resilience have been distinguished, which differ in their conceptual perspectives and research foci. The first level focuses on psychological and physical characteristics of individuals that can have a protective effect in the face of adverse life circumstances. This perspective viewed resilience as a relatively fixed subjective trait. The second level expands this perspective to include external determinants that lie outside the person, such as social components of everyday life (Davis et al. 2009).

Recent research has expanded the concept of resilience to include risk factors such as chronic life difficulties, and thus understands it as a developmental process that unfolds within the framework of a complex person-environment interaction. Additionally, a third level is being discussed in research, which primarily focuses on the implementation of prevention and intervention measures. These imply health behavior and health action. Most concepts of resilience thus share a common perspective with the model of salutogenesis (Mergenthaler 2012). Resilience is both a process and a phenomenon that involves positive adaptation. This refers to two aspects: on the one hand, the maintenance of normal development despite existing negative influences, and on the other, the restoration of psychological functioning after it has been reduced by negative influences (Reimann and Hammelstein 2006).

18.1.3 Coping

Coping is based on the stress model by Lazarus. According to this model, stress arises from an imbalance between demands from stimuli (stressors) and a person's coping resources within a dynamic person-environment relationship. The model is founded on a transactional coping concept, in which a subjective evaluation process takes place. Consequently, the subjective assessment of stressors—which can be psychosocial, physical, or biochemical in nature—and the subjective coping competence (coping) are decisive for the health effects.

A core element of this theory is cognitive appraisal, which explains why people respond differently to objectively equivalent stressful situations. Therefore, the subjective evaluation of a situation determines whether it is perceived as stressful or not. Lazarus distinguishes three types of appraisal: primary appraisal, secondary appraisal, and reappraisal. The primary appraisal assesses the extent to which the stressor affects one's own well-being. The evaluation occurs in three qualities: first, that the stimulus is irrelevant; second, that the stimulus is positive; and third, that the stimulus requires immediate action and is therefore stressful. The degree of stressfulness is then assessed by determining whether harm or loss has already occurred (harm or loss), whether harm or loss is expected (threat), or whether it is a (challenge), which is associated with positive expectations (Mittelmark et al. 2022).

After the primary appraisal is completed, the secondary appraisal follows. Here, it is weighed whether the situation can be managed with the available resources. If the person identifies their resources as insufficient, this triggers a stress reaction that initiates an individual coping strategy. The orientation of the strategy depends, among other things, on the quality of the event, the cognition, and the socialization of the evaluating person. Lazarus describes the secondary appraisal as a three-part process. First, the available coping strategies are evaluated to make a selection. The selected coping strategies are then combined, subsequently applied, and finally evaluated. Based on a summary of the coping strategies used so far, as well as new insights and information, the situation is reappraised. Depending on whether the outcome is evaluated as a success or failure, the use of coping strategies can be fine-tuned, discarded, or continued. Lazarus distinguishes;

- problem-focused coping, which is situated at the level of the stressors or the situation. After gathering information in advance, the person pursues a coping strategy characterized by immediate action or omission in order to adapt to or overcome the stressful situation.
- emotion-focused coping, which focuses on reducing stress-induced arousal to regain emotional balance.
- cognitive-focused coping, which, after combining different coping strategies, involves a reappraisal of the personal circumstances. Here, the focus is on a shift in perspective, away from the burden and toward the accepted challenge (Monat and Lazarus 1991).

18.2 Summary

The discussion makes it clear how closely intertwined socialization, identity, life experience, and subjective experience of illness are in coping with disease. Guided by the question: *which factors and risks contribute to resilience in people with chronic illnesses, and under what conditions?* it becomes evident that, in addition to pathological factors, the resources available to people with chronic illnesses are also essential for the recovery process. A key task of the multiprofessional treatment team is therefore to secure and restore the postulated protective factors, as well as to derive implications for action and forecasts for further necessary competencies. These can already be identified during the medical history in order to promote a sense of coherence through individual goal setting. For people with chronic illnesses, coherence can also arise from the implementation of health-promoting measures, provided these are based on personal knowledge, individual goals, and active engagement with (im)material resources as well as the illness and its treatment options. In order to restore a balance between stressors and coping resources, as well as a level of functioning typical for the individual, those affected need mental flexibility. Ultimately, it may be precisely this mental flexibility that enables the development of resilience and adaptation to adverse situations. A multiprofessional treatment team can provide supportive guidance by considering different perspectives, developing individual coping strategies, fostering self-efficacy, and encouraging an optimistic outlook.

References

Antonovsky A (1997) Salutogenese: Zur Entmystifizierung der Gesundheit. Deutsche Gesellschaft für Verhaltenstherapie (dgvt) Verlag, Tübingen

Davis M-C, Luecken L, Lemery-Chalfant K (2009) Resilience in common life: introduction to a special issue. J Personal 77(6):1637–1644

Faltermaier T (2017) Gesundheitspsychologie: Grundriss der Psychologie, Bd 21, 2., überarb. u. erw. Aufl. Kohlhammer, Stuttgart

Felten B-S (2000) Resilience in a multicultural sample of community-dwelling women older than age 85. Clin Nurs Res 9(2):102–123

Haase J-E (2004) Resilience. In: Petersen S-J, Bredow T-S (Hrsg) Middle range theories: application to nursing research. Williams & Wilkins co., Philadelphia, S 341–367

Mergenthaler A (2012) Gesundheitliche Resilienz, Konzept und Empirie zur Reduzierung gesundheitlicher Ungleichheit im Alter. Springer VS, Wiesbaden

Mittelmark M-B, Bauer G-F, Vaandrager L, Pelikan J-M, Shifra S, Eriksson M, Lindström B, Meier Magistretti C (2022) The handbook of salutogenesis, 2. Aufl. Springer Open, Cham

Monat A, Lazarus RS (1991) Stress and coping: an anthology, 3. Aufl. Columbia University Press, New York, S 189–206

Obrist B, van Eeuwijk P (2006) Einleitung. In: van Eeuwijk P, Obrist B (Hrsg) Vulnerabilität, Migration und Altern: Medizinethnologische Ansätze im Spannungsfeld von Theorie und Praxis. Seismo, Zürich, S 10–24

Patterson J-M (2002) Understanding family resilience. J Clin Psychol 58(3):233–246

Reimann S, Hammelstein P (2006) Ressourcenorientierte Ansätze. In: Renneberg B, Hammelstein P (Hrsg) Gesundheitspsychologie. Springer Medizin, Berlin/Heidelberg, S 13–28

Sotzko V (2013) Resilienz-Coaching oder von der Kunst, die zweite Geige zu spielen. In: S. Degenkolb-Weyers (2016) (Hrsg) Resilienz in therapeutischen Gesundheitsfachberufen Entwicklung eines Konzeptes zur Resilienzförderung. Springer Fachmedien, Wiebaden

Health Literacy

19

Simone Hatebur, Jan-Hendrik Ortloff and Heike Becker

Contents

19.1 Health Literacy

The term health literacy (HL) originates from the Anglo-American language area. HL refers to the extent to which those affected are able to engage with their illness and make appropriate decisions.

To date, there has been no systematic development or substantive engagement regarding the translation and the resulting consequences for practice. Therefore, both terms are often used synonymously in reference to individuals and collectives (Abel et al. 2018;

S. Hatebur (✉)
Faculty of Health, Witten/Herdecke University, Witten, Germany
e-mail: simone.hatebur@uni-wh.de

J.-H Ortloff · H. Becker
Department of human medicine, Witten/Herdecke University, Witten, Germany
e-mail: jan-hendrik.ortloff@uni-wh.de

H. Becker
e-mail: heike.becker@uni-wh.de

D. Schmitz et al. (eds.), *Chronic Care—Science and Practice*,
https://doi.org/10.1007/978-3-662-72298-5_19

Dierks and Schaeffer 2023). In the 1970s, the use of the term HL was still limited to the field of school health education (education on health issues). Subsequently, further development and differentiation into two areas of work took place. In the context of development cooperation, HL is a significant element in adult education and in the area of empowerment in community development. In the medical care system, HL is found in connection with subjective approaches to patient leadership and health promotion, focusing on understanding health information as well as corresponding actions and compliance.

Health promotion expands this focus to include the perspectives of everyday practical knowledge from individual life worlds, the handling of health and illness against the background of socialization, the communication of specialist knowledge regarding health risks, and the implementation of health-promoting framework conditions. By enabling individuals to access health-relevant information, HL promotes the management of one's own health through participation, co-determination (autonomy), as well as through participation and inclusion. Specifically, this ability means finding, understanding, and evaluating health information in order to make health-related decisions (Abel et al. 2018).

19.2 National Health Literacy

Regardless of the health-related topic (prevention, therapy, prognosis, etc.), understandable and accurate information is necessary in order to make meaningful decisions. This means applying knowledge in a motivated and targeted manner and being able to make decisions based on one's own opinion.

The *National Action Plan for Health Literacy* (Schaeffer et al. 2020) contains four areas of action, which include the promotion of health literacy in all living environments, an individualized and health-literate design of the health system, the exercise of health literacy with chronic illness, and the systematic research of health literacy. The overall goal is to engage all organizations and stakeholders in the health sector to adopt, implement, and anchor the recommendations of the action plan as comprehensively as possible in practice. Three of the recommendations relate directly to people with chronic illnesses: integrating health literacy into the care of people with chronic illness, strengthening self-management skills of people with chronic illness and their families, and promoting health literacy for coping with everyday life with chronic illness. The quality and extent of health literacy in the population depend not only on individual prerequisites but also on the professional quality and availability of the information provided, as well as on a health-related infrastructure.

A study on the health literacy of the population in Germany found that more than half of the population (58.8%) have low health literacy. In the process of information processing *(finding, understanding, evaluating, applying)*, it is the step of evaluation that is most difficult for the population. In addition, health literacy is distributed unequally across social groups, and the majority of respondents have low competence in navigating the health system. In particular, people of older age, with chronic illnesses, migration experience, as well as those with low social status or low educational attainment, have on average lower health literacy. The study also shows that people with multiple chronic illnesses have lower health literacy than those with only one chronic illness (Schaeffer et al. 2020).

It is well known that low health literacy leads to further negative consequences and unhealthy behaviors such as poor nutrition, less mobility, and lack of compliance. In the further course, a subjectively perceived low quality of life, frequent sick days, and increased use of the health system may also result. Consequently, people with chronic illnesses are often disproportionately affected when they also have low health literacy. Nevertheless, people with chronic illnesses can be supported through health literacy.

19.3 Practical Transfer

Since the Ottawa Charter for Health Promotion (1986), empowerment has become a normative guiding principle in the context of the World Health Organization, understood as a structural or behavioral health resource. Accordingly, empowerment refers to a psychological, social, cultural, or political process through which individuals and social groups are enabled to express their needs and concerns, develop strategies for participation in decision-making, and take appropriate action.

Empowerment is a continuous process aimed at enabling people to utilize their personal and social resources and to shape their social environment (Brandes and Stark 2021). The literature does not provide a uniform definition, but there are challenges in operationalizing the empowerment concept. It is used in the sense of enabling and empowering disadvantaged population groups to reduce social inequality and to support vulnerable groups such as people with chronic illnesses.

The empowerment process promotes participation and community building, taking into account and incorporating the given conditions and structures. The goal is to develop and enhance e the skills that enable individuals to take control of their lives and their social environment acting independently and responsibly.

Psychoeducation involves structured interventions for specific clinical conditions such as dementia or schizophrenia. These interventions are designed to inform patients and their relatives about the illness and its treatment, thereby fostering understanding. The professional content is adapted to the respective target group and translated in such a way that it is comprehensible to participants. The aim is to enable individuals to manage their illness independently and responsibly, and to support them in coping with the illness. For chronic conditions in particular, understanding the illness and its treatment is a fundamental prerequisite to self-determined management and successful everyday coping.

Psychoeducation programs are offered as individual or group sessions by various healthcare professionals and may include variable modules (German Society for Psychiatry and Psychotherapy, Psychosomatics and Neurology 2019). Frequently, the individual modules (including illness definition, symptoms and early warning signs, medication, therapy, dealing with affected individuals, stressors, crisis plans) are offered weekly so that participants can gradually acquire the content. In addition to promoting understanding of the illness and autonomy of those affected, professional support and exchange with other affected individuals also contribute to empowerment.

The method of social network intervention, as a systematic support tool, focuses for example on identifying individuals' social connections, stabilizing or expanding insufficient networks, and identifying potentials (Galuske and Bock 2013). Thus, networks and network interventions enable people with chronic illnesses to participate and be included. Participation means that networks are accessible without barriers for people with chronic illnesses, and inclusion means that those affected are aware of and can use the available networks.

Network research distinguishes between primary, secondary, and tertiary network types. Primary or microsocial networks refer to direct personal contacts in the areas of family, kinship, friendships, and neighborhood. Secondary or macrosocial networks develop, for example, through the workplace, leisure facilities, and the education system. Tertiary or mesosocial networks are situated between the private and public sectors. These include, for example, self-help groups and non-governmental organizations (Galuske and Bock 2013).

Networks and their quality can be illustrated both quantitatively and qualitatively. The distance between individual connection points visualizes the spatial and, if applicable, emotional distance. The characteristics of the individual connection points can also indicate the frequency and quality of the respective contacts.

According to von Kardorff (1995), important parameters of analysis are:

- *Interaction criteria*, which refer, for example, to the frequency, reciprocity, and directness or indirectness of a connection
- *Interaction content,* which includes, for example, emotional support, instrumental help, and value orientation
- *Quality of interaction*, for example, focusing on intensity, accessibility, duration, resilience, dependency, and control.
- *Role of participants*, for example, regarding centrality, gatekeeper, excluded individuals, or bridge-building function
- *Structural characteristics* such as size, density, and clustering
- *Functions* such as emotional support and cognitive orientation

The resources and competencies resulting from social relationships often enable individuals to cope with stressful situations and to gain new perspectives. Older adults often report fewer social contacts than younger adults; however, the number does not differ with regard to emotionally significant social contacts, but rather to peripheral social contacts that have been deliberately discontinued (Wrzus et al. 2013). Applied to people with multimorbid and chronic illnesses, this means that they consciously maintain their social contacts, assume interpersonal roles in later life stages, and benefit from long-lasting relationships.

19.4 Conclusion

In the field of multiprofessional care for chronic illnesses, HL, empowerment, psychoeducation programs, and social network interventions involve creating structures that enable and realize a self-determined and responsible life.

Knowledge, motivation, and competencies initially enable individuals to find, understand, assess, and apply health information. In combination with situational and individual factors during the course of illness, they also facilitate coping with illness, prevention (e.g., of relapses), and health promotion. These are implemented through societal and environmental components, which also include health-related infrastructure.

References

Abel T, Bruhin E, Sommerhalder K, Jordan S (2018) Health Literacy/Gesundheitskompetenz. In: Bundeszentrale für gesundheitliche Aufklärung (Hrsg) Leitbegriffe der Gesundheitsförderung und Prävention: Glossar zu Konzepten, Strategien und Methoden. https://leitbegriffe.bzga.de. Zugegriffen am 25.05.2023

Brandes S, Stark W (2021) Empowerment/Befähigung. In: Bundeszentrale für gesundheitliche Aufklärung (Hrsg) Leitbegriffe der Gesundheitsförderung und Prävention: Glossar zu Konzepten, Strategien und Methoden. https://leitbegriffe.bzga.de. Zugegriffen am 25.05.2023

Deutsche Gesellschaft für Psychiatrie und Psychotherapie, Psychosomatik und Nervenheilkunde (Hrsg) (2019) S3-Leitlinie Psychosoziale Therapien bei schweren psychischen Erkrankungen: S3-Praxisleitlinien in Psychiatrie und Psychotherapie, 2. Aufl. Springer, Berlin

Dierks M-L, Schaeffer D (2023) Gesundheitskompetenz in Deutschland. In: Schwartz FW, Walter U, Siegrist J, Kolip U, Leidl R, Busse R, Amelung V, Dierks M-L (Hrsg) Public Health: Gesundheit und Gesundheitswesen, 4. Aufl. Elsevier, Berlin, S 490–500

Galuske M, Bock K (2013) Methoden der Sozialen Arbeit: Eine Einführung, 10. Aufl. Beltz Juventa, Berlin

Kardorff E v (1995) Soziale Netzwerke. In: Flick U, Kardorff E v, Keupp H, Rosenstiel L v, Wolff S (Hrsg) Handbuch qualitativer Sozialforschung, 2. Aufl. Beltz Psychologie-Verlags Union, Berlin, S 402–405

Schaeffer D, Hurrelmann K, Bauer U, Kolpatzik K (Hrsg) (2020) Nationaler Aktionsplan Gesundheitskompetenz: Die Gesundheitskompetenz in Deutschland stärken. KomPart, Berlin

Wrzus C, Hänel M, Wagner J, Neyer FJ (2013) Social Network changes and life events across the life span: a meta-analyses. In: Staats M, Steinhaußen J (Hrsg) (2021) Resilienz im Alter. Beltz Juventa, Berlin, S 93–95

Setting-Specific Care: Connectivity as a Challenge

20

Ulrike Höhmann

Contents

20.1 Setting-Specific Care

The healthcare provision and support for people with chronic illnesses should ensure health, social participation, independence, well-being, and dignity for those affected and their relatives at all stages of illness, individually and at a high professional level. To achieve this, the individual services provided by the participating institutions and professional groups across all settings must be compatible and interconnected. It has long been lamented that this is rarely achieved (e.g., SVR 1987, 2007). In particular, four mutually reinforcing characteristics of the healthcare system systematically fuel this failure:

U. Höhmann (✉)
Universität Witten/Herdecke, Witten, Germany
e-mail: ulrike.hoehmann@uni-wh.de

D. Schmitz et al. (eds.), *Chronic Care—Science and Practice*,
https://doi.org/10.1007/978-3-662-72298-5_20

1. the dominant biomedical and acute care paradigm,
2. the programmatic nature of service delivery,
3. the rigidity of conditional regulatory mechanisms, and
4. the overarching profit orientation of the health care system.

It is especially the latter, the profit orientated logic of competition, that permeates all service processes, as has often been criticized. In doing so, it amplifies the dysfunctions of the other three characteristics, which are outlined individually below:

20.2 The Reductionism of the Overarching Biomedical and Acute Care Paradigm

Health policy analyses (e.g., Badura 1996; Rosenbrock and Gerlinger 2014) have long described the pervasive influence of the biomedical and acute care emergency paradigm, which reduces and inadequately addresses the needs of people with chronic illnesses in particular. Based on business management calculations, it structures an overly simplistic orientation of both care offerings and service delivery, creating blind spots and gaps in care. This almost unquestioned logic of action especially promotes and consolidates the political-strategic, scientific, and economic dominance of biomedical services, which are often dubiously justified as evidence-based. With often high individual quality, specialized repair agents in autonomous settings work to eliminate classified individual symptoms, such as in high-performance diagnostic and surgical clinics, specialized specialty or rehabilitation centers, etc. This perspective also permeates the financial support of research, industrial development, and education.

Conversely, this systemic prioritization leads to the conceptual and economic subordination of communicative, non-apparatus-based medicine and those settings that provide complex health, prevention, rehabilitation, or palliative care services delivered by less influential health and social professions.

Despite differences in financing models in detail, all settings struggle with competitive, often short-term profit orientation. The focus on lucrative core assignments and low standby costs secures their own resources and becomes the bottleneck of their operational capacity. Supported by the financial preference for repair medicine, the paradigmatic dominance of the biomedical perspective thus shapes a technicist understanding of health, reduced primarily to physical needs and oriented mainly toward apparatus-based medicine focused on objectively measurable data. Dysfunctional health and even macroeconomic consequences of ignoring complex, and thus unmeasurable, functional interrelationships are particularly evident in the care of people with chronic illnesses, such as dementia, or when treatment after hospital discharge lacks continuity.

The appeals of scientific analyses that challenge biomedical and acute care thought structures in light of the needs of people with chronic illnesses (e.g., Höhmann 2002; SVR reports 1987, 2007) and call for systemic management of complexity have hardly any structural impact. Cross-setting service integration is systematically lacking, with few exceptions, such as treatments under § 39 and § 115 d SGB V.

Beyond this reductionist understanding of disease, the other system characteristics mentioned above also reinforce connectivity problems between settings.

20.3 Siloed Services Due to the Programmatic Nature of Care

Referring to Luhmann's (1972) analysis of the increasing differentiation and specialization of all systems in modern societies sheds further light on structural problems of autonomy, connectivity, and fit. With the programmatic nature of modern support systems, Luhmann explains the self-referentially isolated and sluggishly adaptable modes of operation of social subsystems, including the various care settings, their organizations, and professions. Each program is specialized in addressing a defined segment of life's problems. The legal entitlement of those affected to program services arises from previously defined legal and financial rules for problem assignment and design.

In the first step, a person's problems are assigned to the responsible program. This involves breaking down the complex support and care needs of an individual according to the legally and financially codified rules of responsibility and assigning them to the available program services of a setting, for example, determining care needs according to the regulations of the Social Long-Term Care Insurance (SGB XI) within the framework of outpatient or inpatient care settings. A setting can serve several programs, such as outpatient care providing services under both SGB XI and SGB V (Statutory Health Insurance) (see Article 41).

Needs and services rarely coincide.

In the second step, professionals decide, based on applicable legal and funding rules, on the specific design of their services with which they address the identified and programmatically assigned needs in their setting.

They then determine which of the support needs they will address, with which services, to what extent, and with which personnel, in accordance with the rules.

This program logic entails three main problems:

First, cross-boundary, person-centered coordination between programs, such as outpatient care with home-based orthopedic physiotherapy, is not considered. Nor, secondly, is the systematic question of whether a program offers sufficiently broad and differentiated solutions for the individual's complex problem constellations. Gaps in care due to unmet additional needs are often accepted with regret or completely ignored by professionals. The latter occurs especially when, thirdly, needs that systematically transcend program boundaries are not even identified in business-driven needs analyses of the programs. As a system-compliant way of dealing with unmet needs, those affected are often helplessly shunted to the patchwork of other programs, which, following the same logic, creates new problems of fit and further points of discontinuity.

20.4 Increased Difficulty for Needs-Based Justice Due to a Conditional Understanding of Rules

Opportunities to flexibly adapt program boundaries to better address problems struggle with a system-inherent conditional understanding of rules, according to which benefit decisions can only be made on the basis of previously formulated rules. Any expansion of program boundaries first requires new rules that legally assign problem categories and intervention options to systemic areas of responsibility and funding. Only then are new conditional because-justifications for new benefits available. This lengthy mechanism is often lamented as a fundamental barrier to change, even as a form of existential aftercare (Luhmann 1972, p. 365).

However, blanket criticism risks overlooking the other side of this mechanism. The aim of justifying benefits through because-rules is to ensure equal treatment and neutrality of professional assistance, to exclude arbitrariness, and to guarantee the predictability of legal entitlements to certain benefits, for example, within the insurance principle. Even if this limits the substantive scope of professional care actions appropriate to the situation.

It is especially chronically ill individuals with fluctuating symptoms and complex needs who suffer from the restrictions of conditionally justified, de-individualized benefit offerings, which are usually governed by business management calculations and a biomedical care paradigm. As a result, professional providers also risk losing the sense of coherence in their work, particularly when their interventions fall short of their professional competencies.

Systematic flexibilization and changes to conditional rules are therefore slow and fall to non-health professions, who, in turn, must change existing rules and/or define new ones.

Attempts by direct providers to expand their professional capacity to act through more problem-appropriate in order to-justifications—such as by identifying gaps in program regulations or by networking services—often remain unstable, partial, or model-based. In individual cases, they can improve needs-based justice and stimulate innovation. However, secure, norm-compliant foundations arise only through legislative and executive safeguards of new because-rules.

In conclusion, it is particularly the everyday practical autonomy of this rule principle in service provision that is considered worthy of criticism. Especially in cases of procedurally inflated rigidity, implicit biomedical reductionism, or the excessive prioritization of business objectives, direct providers and non-health professions have active opportunities for change. Below the level of structural conditions, their professional behavior can meaningfully break through obstructive routines.

20.5 Shared Challenges for Health and Non-Health Professions

Actors in all care settings are structurally embedded in the autonomous, legal-economic, and conceptually organizational logics of their silos. This relationship limits their capacity for change, but does not prevent it (Höhmann et al. 2018), as long as they are actively aware of their professional and conceptual scope for action. Non-health professions can then systematically question and break through the autonomous conditional rules in their decision-making and interpretive practices. Direct providers—especially in teams—can identify, modify, and counteract procedurally inflated processes, strangling pseudo-justifications due to professional-conceptual gaps, and dysfunctional routines, and instead define, claim, and test requirements for professional-content fit. This not only positively influences the needs-based justice of care, but also the professional sense of coherence. In summary, three actor-accessible starting points can be identified along the system characteristics:

1. The conceptual limitations of the bio- and acute medical paradigm must be professionally reviewed in each individual case, and substantive professional scope for action should be used to identify patient-specific needs and align one's own treatment strategies with them as much as possible. Networking activities that seek a cross-setting common ground can smooth connections to further programs (see Contribution 11).
2. Assignment and design rules of programs should be recognized as changeable. One's own substantive and professional interpretive and action scope can be conceptually expanded in a more needs-based way within the team and tested in practice (e.g., through anamnesis categories, case discussions, etc.). A shared conceptual common ground (see Contribution 11) can help to relate autonomous limitations of practice processes to each other in a more case-appropriate and flexible manner. Systematic program gaps should be purposefully brought into the political system, for example, at regional round tables.
3. The practice of conditional rule justifications must be specifically reviewed in light of the care needs of people with complex requirements. Their protective function against arbitrariness and unequal treatment only holds as long as rules are not legitimized solely formally or mechanically inflated to become unchangeable, routine-forming mechanisms. Those responsible for institutions and direct providers should seek out their own practice-guiding rule interpretations, instructions, and routines. They will discover that they themselves can influence a more needs-based chronic care practice. The prerequisites are motivation and an appropriate professional attitude.

References

Badura B (1996) Patientenorientierte Systemgestaltung im Gesundheitswesen. In: Badura B, Feuerstein G (Hrsg) Systemgestaltung im Gesundheitswesen. Juventa, S 225–310

Höhmann U (2002) Spezifische Vernetzungserfordernisse für chronisch kranke, langzeitpflegebedürftige Menschen. In: DZA (Hrsg) Expertisen zum 4. Altenbericht. Band III. Vincentz, S 289–428

Höhmann U, Lauxen O, Schwarz L (Hrsg) (2018) Gestaltungskompetenzen im Pflegealltag stärken. Mabuse

Luhmann N (1972) Formen des Helfens im Wandel gesellschaftlicher Bedingungen. In: Otto HU, Schneider S (Hrsg) Gesellschaftliche Perspektiven der Sozialarbeit I. Luchterhand, S 21–43

Rosenbrock R, Gerlinger T (2014) Gesundheitspolitik. Hans Huber
SVR (Sachverständigenrat für die Begutachtung und Entwicklung des Gesundheitswesens) (2007) Kooperation und Verantwortung. Nomos
SVR (Sachverständigenrat für die konzertierte Aktion im Gesundheitswesen) (1987) Jahresgutachten. Nomos

Person- and Patient-Centeredness as Care Concepts

21

Helen Güther and Heike Baranzke

Contents

21.1 Personhood

The concept of the person is ambiguous and is not always used as a technical term. In everyday language, it refers, among other things, to individual, concretely countable human beings. In ethics and law, person is a term for humans as bearers of inalienable human and fundamental rights, who must be treated as equal *subjects* and, in contrast

H. Güther (✉)
Fakultät für Gesundheit, Department für Humanmedizin, Universität Witten/Herdecke, Witten, Germany
e-mail: helen.guether@uni-wh.de

H. Baranzke
Fakultät für Geistes- und Kulturwissenschaften, Bergische Universität Wuppertal, Wuppertal, Germany
e-mail: baranzke@uni-wuppertal.de

D. Schmitz et al. (eds.), *Chronic Care—Science and Practice*,
https://doi.org/10.1007/978-3-662-72298-5_21

to objects, must not be subject to the control of others. Personalist philosophers such as Martin Buber and social philosophers like Axel Honneth emphasize the ethical necessity of mutual interpersonal or societal recognition of personhood. Empirical psychological approaches, in this context, point to the factual necessity of dialogical communication and interaction for the development and maintenance of an individual's personal sense of self. However, this also means that personhood can be disregarded or even denied in social interaction (depersonalization), thereby ultimately calling into question the community of persons based on human rights. The social practice of recognizing personhood thus proves to be fragile.

21.1.1 The Problem of Depersonalization

Worldwide, people with chronic mental (e.g., schizophrenia and depression) or cognitive-degenerative impairments (dementias) are particularly exposed to depersonalizing practices. They are perceived as people with conspicuous behaviors that do not meet society's expectations of normality. As a result, they are at risk of having their human and fundamental rights—especially those to self-determination and social participation—relativized or restricted, and of suffering exclusion and discrimination (see contribution 37). With regard to the situation of people with dementia, reference can be made to the work of social psychologist and theologian Tom Kitwood, who, at the end of the 20th century, revealed how care professionals and relatives, despite well-meaning intentions, demean, shame, label, infantilize, or simply ignore people with dementia. Such a discriminatory practice, which does not treat people as equal subjects of the social community, he termed "malignant social psychology" (Kitwood et al. 2022). This is accompanied by a deficit-oriented, medicalized perspective (Foucault), which focuses on the medical diagnosis of a chronic cognitive illness in perception and professional action, and derives the personal status from it. This increases the risk of pathologizing the person as a whole. That is, those affected are involuntarily reduced to an existence as patients, i.e., as bearers of disease symptoms, and degraded to a passive *object* of medical treatment. The exercise of human rights to self-determination and participation by patients is not supported in such a treatment process. For people with chronic cognitive impairments, such a depersonalizing practice is particularly risky, as a deeply rooted hypercognitivist paradigm in Western culture ties the recognition of legal personhood to the cognitive abilities of human individuals (Wetzstein 2010), thereby fostering a discriminatory basic attitude. This is often legitimized in medical-ethical discourse by an interest-based ethical concept of person.

21.1.2 Human Rights-Based vs. Interest-Based Concepts of Personhood

Since the 1970s, the human rights-based concept of personhood—according to which the rule of law is demonstrated by the fact that state organs respect and guarantee the inalienable human rights of all people—has faced opposition in the *medical-ethical* debate on personhood. Here, the discussion centers on whether all humans are equally persons (human rights-based concept of personhood) or whether moral personhood is tied to empirical performance criteria that a human individual must first fulfill in order to claim rights adapted to their abilities (interest-based, objectifying concept of personhood).

The human rights-based concept of personhood expresses the *pre-state (pre-positive), natural legal personality*, i.e., the equality of all people regardless of their individual characteristics and abilities. All humans are regarded as equal subjects with inalienable human rights such as the right to physical integrity, the protection of life, the free development of personality, social participation, and more. Since the UN Universal Declaration of Human Rights (1948), inalienable human rights are founded on the ethical idea of universal human dignity, which is inherent to every human being by virtue of being human. This forms the human rights-political equivalent of moral personhood and has been enshrined in constitutional law since 1949 in Article 1 of the Basic Law of the Federal Republic of Germany, as in many other constitutional democracies.

In contrast, within the framework of the analytic-philosophical discourse on rights, which does not distinguish between pre-positive and positive (politically enacted) rights, an *interest-based, objectifying concept of personhood* has been developed. This ties personal legal claims to specific interests of individual rights holders, which must be demonstrated by empirically measurable abilities. The trigger was the fiercely debated sociopolitical discussion in the USA since the 1960s about the liberalization of abortion and end-of-life measures for the terminally ill, which was linked to the question of the value of the life of an unborn or terminally ill person. With Dworkin (1993), the debate about an interest-based ethical concept of person was extended to the situation of people with dementia and thus potentially to the value of life of all chronically cognitively impaired people, by tying the right to life or the interest in continued living to the presence of cognitive self-determination abilities. A natural will to live, expressed in affective enjoyment of life, does not meet this cognitive standard. Accordingly, Dworkin distinguishes between critical interests (*critical interests*), which he sees as present in people of average intelligence and which are valid across time, and currently experience-related interests (*experiental interests*), which he bases on the individually given abilities for emotional and sensory experience such as joy or pain. He grants only critical interests the possibility of grounding the right to self-determined action. Experience-related interests, on the other hand, he considers only as a basis for a right to care. The obvious medical-ethical explosiveness of the interest-based ethical concept of person for chronically (cognitively) impaired people results from the denial of natural legal personhood and ability-independent human rights due to limited, especially cognitive, abilities. Instead, the identification of limitations in abilities should be used empirically to determine the type and extent of support needs, in order to assist people with chronic impairments in exercising their inalienable human right to self-determination (advocacy support). In the logic of an interest-based ethical concept of person, however, the most vulnerable and most in need of protection are left without protection.

21.2 The Care Concepts of Person- and Patient-Centeredness

Differently connoted understandings of the term *person* are also subject to the various care concepts of person- and patient-centeredness, even though they may initially appear related. Upon closer examination, their different roots and consequences for practice become apparent.

Person-Centeredness

Congruence, empathy, and acceptance form the central elements of the non-directive psychotherapy developed by Carl R. Rogers, which—initially aimed at the professional group of psychotherapists—serves to reflect the professional *attitude* of practitioners. The co-founder of humanistic psychology initiated a programmatic shift in perspective from psychoanalysis by regarding clients seeking advice as experts in their own lives, while professional therapists should see themselves as advocates accompanying them. Under the influence of Martin Buber's I-Thou philosophy, Rogers increasingly complemented the initially chosen term client-centered therapy (Client-Centeredness) with the concept of person-centered therapy, which reflects the helper relationship in a dialogical manner. Person-centeredness thus does not describe an outcome-oriented therapeutic *technique*, but rather an understanding, learning, and assisting *attitude* in shaping the therapeutic relationship, in which the person in need of help is actively involved in the treatment process as the expert of their own life (subjectivation). The focus on individualized relationship-building makes person-centeredness particularly relevant for (medical, nursing, educational, etc.) care concepts in the training of professionals who accompany people in need of assistance over a longer period or permanently.

In contrast, the notion of *persons*-centeredness arises from the discourse on social policy reform initiatives within rehabilitation care and calls for the structural and organizational differentiation and identification of specific needs of groups of people requiring different treatment. Unlike person-centeredness, it does not focus on reflecting the professional attitude of practitioners, but rather on specifying rehabilitation services for specific groups (people with dementia, depression, schizophrenia, etc.), combined with efficiency-oriented organizational development (Baranzke and Güther 2023).

Patient-Centeredness

In the context of (clinical) healthcare, the term *patient orientation* has become the most common German translation of patient-centeredness. Its roots also lie in the psychotherapeutic context. Unlike Rogers' humanistic-psychological concept of person-centeredness, patient-centeredness originates from the more medically oriented psychoanalytic school, which maintains the classic expert-oriented therapist-patient hierarchy. The starting point is marked by the writings of Enid Balint, who, at the end of the 1960s, emphasized the uniqueness of every patient. Numerous further publications have led to an increasingly prominent, but also increasingly ambiguous, concept of patient-centeredness, which is broadly defined and variously interpreted in research and practice—possibly facilitated by semantic imprecision in translation. Moreover, the conceptual definition is primarily based on scientific and clinical expertise, not on the experiences of those affected. According to the empirically derived conceptualization, a high degree of contextuality is revealed. For example, in the US literature review by Mead and Bower (2000), patient-centeredness is characterized by five core dimensions: 1) recognition of patients as individuals; 2) the associated psychosocial understanding of illness that goes beyond biomedical diagnostics; 3) sharing of power and responsibility; 4) a therapeutic alliance; and 5) the consideration of professionals as persons as well. The German variant of patient orientation, in an expert survey, additionally includes organizational and social policy dimensions: patient empowerment; individualized services; patient outcomes such as satisfaction and quality of life measurements; health policy participation; coordination and teamwork. Accordingly, the conceptual understanding also varies with respect to the associated care practices. For example, in the care of multimorbidity, the Delphi study by Kivelitz et al. (2021) finds that, in addition to the individuality of patients, patient orientation focuses especially on doctor-patient communication; the involvement of patients in nursing processes; the physical, cognitive, and emotional support of patients; as well as the inclusion of family members and friends.

In particular, the German-language discourse on patient orientation—similar in some respects to the economic concept of customer orientation—features not only individualistic and social policy, but also organizational connotations, thus creating tension with the aim of an equitable relationship as envisioned by the concept of person-centeredness. Consequently, Zill et al. (2021) note that the care concept of patient-centeredness, on the one hand, has high *outcome relevance*, reflected in improved health behavior and status of patients, associated cost reductions in the healthcare system, and higher job satisfaction among physicians. They also point to the 2013 introduction of the *Patient Rights Act* to strengthen patient safety, information, and participation, which can be traced back to the discourse on patient orientation. However, in its implementation in practice, patient-centeredness often proves to be little more than "lip service for marketing purposes" (Zill et al. 2021, p. 53).

21.3 Person-Centered Care (PCC) in Challenging Behavior

The following reflects on Kitwood's concept of PCC in the context of the two care concepts of person- and patient-centeredness. This is done, firstly, because Kitwood made it his central task to counteract the depersonalization of people with dementia by providing a practical action framework, and secondly, because it is a fundamental, basic concept that can be transferred to the situation of people with chronic cognitive impairments.

Drawing on Rogers, Kitwood called for Person-Centered Care (PCC) as protection against depersonalization, i.e., the willingness to accept those affected, with their psychological and cognitive changes, as persons and experts on themselves (acceptance), to recognize their competencies, to empathize with their situation (empathy), and to be guided by their will (non-directivity). Like Rogers, Kitwood also emphasized the necessity of genuineness (congruence/authenticity) on the part of the caregiver for successful interpersonal, dialogical relationship-building, which gives (self-)reflection on one's *attitude* central importance. The person-centered impulses inspired a new perception of and approach to so-called challenging behavior. The term originated in the field of special education, with the aim of averting the dangers of self-harm, harm to others, and social exclusion for people whose behavior is perceived as conspicuous from a cultural perspective, particularly those with intellectual disabilities (Baranzke and Güther 2023), and to enable professionals to provide positive behavioral support. The expression is intended to encourage empathetic understanding of disruptive behaviors such as wandering, vocalizing, aggression, or depression from the perspective of those affected, in order to examine possible underlying causes such as unrecognized pain, discomfort, anxiety, or boredom. Conspicuous behaviors can thus be reinterpreted as meaningful nonverbal communication and understood and valued as legitimate forms of expression. They are then no longer viewed primarily as symptoms of organic brain impairment, but are examined to determine whether they are expressions of unmet needs. What is crucial here is the recognition not only of physical but especially of psychosocial needs, such as social inclusion, meaningful activities, and self-actualization (need-driven-behavior model according to Kolanowski). The assurance of a psychosocial relationship as a foundation precedes the provision of physical needs. In this way, Kitwood expands the biomedical perspective to include psychosocial dimensions, creating a bio-psycho-social model of dementia that enables him to consider exogenous causes for challenging behavior that lie in the social environment—though he had not yet incorporated the emancipatory impetus of the disability movement into his concept of PCC.

21.3.1 Critique of Person-Centered Care

While Kitwood shares with the early disability movement the criticism of the medicalization and medical depersonalization of people with chronic impairments, just as people with disabilities do not want to be reduced to their functional deficits and made passive objects of medical treatment by the medical-scientific perspective, Kitwood also rejects the reduction of people to their organic brain impairments and their degradation to objects of treatment. Whereas Rogers' person-centeredness, influenced by Buber's concept of personhood, conceives the psychotherapeutic relationship as a dialogical relationship between (two) equal *subjects*, Kitwood operates with a bio-psycho-social preconception of personhood and thus with a primarily *empirically objectifying attribution concept* that converges with the concept of patient-centeredness. This leads to a conceptual ambiguity, which means that PCC, despite its claim to subjectivization, can be subtly misunderstood as a therapeutic, outcome-oriented concept with which challenging behavior can be measurably reduced or prevented. The PCC concept, with its bio-psycho-social orientation and without explicit reference to human rights, thus risks exacerbating the problem of depersonalization. There is a danger that people with behavioral challenges will continue to be discriminated against. The empirically oriented bio-psycho-social approach remains tied to an outcome-oriented expectation that focuses on measurable effects rather than on a change in perspective and attitude among professionals. This *hinders* an unbiased encounter with people exhibiting challenging behaviors. They continue to be labeled, for example, as (dementia) patients (labeling). In the context of challenging behavior, there remains a risk that subjectively justified behavior will continue to be devalued, for example, as a disruption to organizational processes and subject to control (normalization). In this context, the study by Doyle and Rubinstein (2014) is noteworthy, as it documents the persistence of a cultural matrix of *othering* despite PCC training for professionals. In an ethnographically studied, PCC-oriented nursing home, challenging behavior continued to be interpreted and sanctioned as pathological. Professionals distanced themselves from those affected instead of addressing their concerns. Against this background, it is not surprising—though all the more alarming—that many studies also document the mis- and overuse of psychopharmacological treatment to control symptoms in people with challenging behavior, despite the increased mortality risk for those affected (Güther et al. 2021). The body of research thus shows that, without a foundation in human rights ethics, PCC often fails in practice to overcome the medically objectifying care framework through subjectivization of those affected, and instead all too often remains stuck in a behaviorist, objectifying interventionism. Thus, contrary to Kitwood's intentions and in contrast to the emancipatory disability movement—which, according to the principle: *We are not disabled. We are being disabled!*—the subject status for people with chronic cognitive impairments and dementia remains diffuse in the PCC concept. Consistent person-centered care therefore requires a clear positioning that is unequivocally oriented toward a human rights-based person-centeredness and goes beyond previous approaches such as the one discussed here by Kitwood. This should not be measured by the quantity of its influence, but should be qualitatively defined, taught, and cultivated as an advocatory, solidaristic, and respectful practice through casework.

21.4 Case Work

In everyday practice, understanding cases should occupy a central role in person-centered approaches to managing challenging behavior. A *case* refers to situations, circumstances, or individual phenomena to which different actors (e.g., members of various professions) attribute different meanings. For example, in the context of caring for a person with chronic psychological or cognitive-degenerative impairments, a behavior perceived as challenging by professional staff may constitute a case requiring the development of solution strategies. However, it is always necessary to examine and sensitize oneself to the perspective of those affected. Methodologically, case work is a hermeneutic process of interpretation that focuses on understanding the lived experiences of individuals. Methodically, this requires the process of case reconstruction in the form of case discussions. Documents such as care records, situation descriptions, and reported subjective impressions related to a case must be compiled. These serve as an information base and foundation for interpretive work. To correctly interpret behavior and uncover *blind spots* in one's own interpretive habits, it is necessary to open up different perspectives. For instance, increased restlessness may be diagnosed from a medical-psychiatric perspective as symptomatic misbehavior. From the perspective of caregivers, the behavior may appear disruptive and overwhelming, as organizational processes can no longer be smoothly maintained in the face of chronic staff shortages. Physical therapists may value wandering as beneficial training in the service of fall prevention. From the perspective of those affected, however, the same behavior may be an expression of, for example, habit (biography), boredom (neglect), inner tension, or unrecognized pain (Schrems 2019).

The following core elements of case work in the sense of person-centeredness should be highlighted:

1. *Understanding attitude and willingness to engage in dialogue:* On the part of professionals, an attitude oriented toward understanding and a willingness and competence for dialogical conversation are required. This means openness to problem definitions and solutions, as well as a willingness to actively listen, learn, and explore. Familiar solutions and ways of thinking must be continually reviewed, reconsidered, or further developed.
2. *Perspective and expertise of those affected:* Personal viewpoints and experiences must be specifically elicited. At the very beginning of case work, it should be clarified for whom the *case* is actually considered relevant—and for whom it is not! This may require skilled communication and individuals who can advocate for the perspective of those affected, especially in the case of people with chronic cognitive impairments such as dementia. Furthermore, the expertise of chronically ill individuals in assessing their own situation must be taken into account (empowerment).
3. *Multiprofessionalism:* Case work is shaped by professional perceptions. Therefore, as many perspectives as possible should be incorporated into the case work in order to capture and represent the complexity of the case as fully as possible. To this end, case discussions should be conducted with all professions involved in the case, as well as with those affected and/or their advocates, in order to open up differentiated approaches to the case.
4. *Documentation and self-evaluation:* To do justice to the hermeneutic learning process of case work, it is necessary to document assumptions, problem definitions, and agreed-upon solutions in writing and in a way that is comprehensible to all, in order to secure information and to be able to evaluate and, if necessary, correct the process.

5. *Organizational development:* The implementation of case work also requires the organization to provide the willingness, time, space, and professionals to guide the dialogical learning process of case work. In addition, established procedures and familiar hierarchies may need to be reconsidered and abandoned in favor of an inclusive organizational culture (cultural change). This promotes democratic organizational development, which enables greater diversity competence beyond individual cases.
6. *Professional language:* Since our language shapes our perception and thus our professional actions, a person-centered professional language must be developed. The technical term *challenging behavior* illustrates the importance of a reflective use of terminology and the need to develop a professional language of one's own in order to realize the paradigm and attitude shift, and thus person-centeredness as a care concept.

References

Baranzke H, Güther H (2023) Die Entdeckung der PERSON mit Demenz in der stationären Langzeitpflege. In: Brandenburg H (Hrsg) Pflegehabitus in der stationären Langzeitpflege von Menschen mit Demenz. Personzentrierte Pflegebeziehungen nachhaltig gestalten. Kohlhammer, Stuttgart, S 39–99

Doyle PJ, Rubinstein RL (2014) Person-centred dementia care and the cultural matrix of othering. Gerontologist 54(6):952–963

Dworkin R (1993) Life's dominion. An argument about abortion, euthanasia, and individual freedom. Alfred A. Knopf, New York

Güther H, Baranzke H, Höhmann U (2021) Herausforderndes Verhalten bei Personen mit Demenz. MMW Fortschritte der Medizin 2021 163(S3):52–60

Kitwood T, Brooker D, Müller-Hergl C, Güther H (Hrsg) (2022) Demenz: Der person-zentrierte Ansatz im Umgang mit verwirrten, kognitiv beeinträchtigten Menschen, 9., vollst. überarb. u. erw. Aufl. Hogrefe, Bern

Kivelitz L, Schäfer J, Kanat M, Mohr J, Glattacker M, Voigt-Radloff S, Dirmaier J (2021) Patient-centeredness in older adults with multimorbidity: results of an online expert delphie study. Gerontologist 61(7):1008–1018. https://doi.org/10.1093/geront/gnaa223

Mead N, Bower P (2000) Patient-centredness: a conceptual framework and review of the empirical literature. Soc Sci Med 51(7):1087–1110

Schrems B (2019) Fallarbeit in der Pflege. Grundlagen, Formen und Anwendungsbereiche, 3., überarb. u. erg. Aufl. facultas, Wien

Wetzstein V (2010) Kognition und Personalität: Perspektiven einer Ethik der Demenz. In: Kruse A (Hrsg) Lebensqualität bei Demenz? Zum gesellschaftlichen und individuellen Umgang mit einer Grenzsituation im Alter. Akademische Verlagsgesellschaft, Heidelberg, S 51–70

Zill J, Zeh S, Scholl I (2021) Patientenzentrierte Versorgung. In: Brinkhaus B, Esch T (Hrsg) Integrative Medizin und Gesundheit. Medizinisch Wissenschaftliche Verlagsgesellschaft, Berlin, S 47–58

Palliative and End of Life Care as Care Concepts

22

Christine Dunger

Contents

22.1 Basic Concepts of Palliative Care

The founder of the hospice movement was Dame Cicely Saunders, who, as a nurse, social worker, and physician in London in the 1960s, witnessed how inadequate the care was, especially for cancer patients at the end of life. In 1967, she established the first modern hospice, which still exists today (Oechsle and Scherg 2019).

C. Dunger (✉)
Lehrstuhl für Sozialphilosophie und Ethik im Gesundheitswesen,
Universität Witten/Herdecke, Witten, Germany
e-mail: Christine.Dunger@uni-wh.de; christine.dunger@pmu.ac.at

C. Dunger
Institut für Pflegewissenschaft und -praxis,
Paracelsus Medizinische Universität, Salzburg, Austria

D. Schmitz et al. (eds.), *Chronic Care—Science and Practice*,
https://doi.org/10.1007/978-3-662-72298-5_22

In the course of her work at St. Christopher's Hospice in London, she defined the principles of palliative care. Over time, these have been modified (Oechsle and Scherg 2019; May 2016), but have essentially been maintained:

- Treatment takes place in the setting of choice; inpatient, e.g., in a hospice, hospital, nursing home, or at home with the support of outpatient services such as nursing services, hospice associations, etc.
- The physical, psychological, social, and spiritual needs of patients and their families, as well as those of the care team, should be taken into account.
- The human aspect should take precedence, while what is medically and technically possible should recede into the background.
- The goal of therapy is to improve the quality of life for patients.
- Individualized treatment is the priority.
- An interprofessional, trained team is required.
- Openness and honesty are the foundation of the trust relationship among all involved.
- The integration of volunteers into care is necessary.
- There is central coordination of the care team.
- Continuous support is provided to those affected and their families, even beyond the death of the patient.
- Central to this is the acceptance of dying and death as part of life, which also means that death is neither hastened nor delayed.

The currently valid definition of palliative care describes it as an approach to care "to improve the quality of life of patients and their families who are facing problems associated with life-threatening illness. This is achieved by preventing and alleviating suffering through early identification, careful assessment, and treatment of pain and other physical, psychosocial, and spiritual problems" (WHO 2020).

The focus of palliative and end-of-life care is therefore on the relief of pain and other distressing symptoms. Psychological and spiritual aspects are integrated into the care provided. This is intended to ensure support that helps patients live as actively as possible until death and takes into account the needs of family members both during the patient's illness and in the period of bereavement. (WHO 2020)

22.2 General and Specialized Palliative Care

Thus, even in the face of serious illness associated with the need for assistance and care, people should be enabled to live with dignity until the end and to die with dignity. To achieve this, care services must be adapted to the life situation of those affected. Not only specialized palliative care is needed, but also general palliative care, i.e., end-of-life care that is low-threshold and integrated into routine care. These services are available in both outpatient and inpatient settings (see Fig. 22.1).

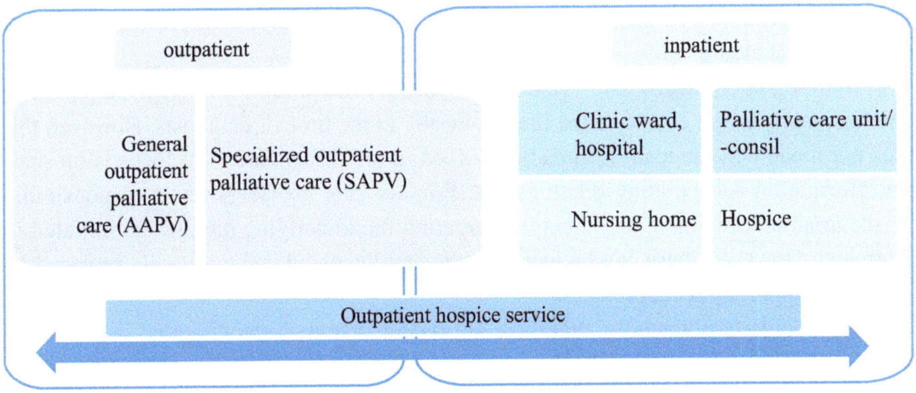

Fig. 22.1 Care services. (Own illustration, oriented towards the German Health Care System)

Outpatient palliative care services are part of the **general outpatient palliative care (AAPV)** and are responsible for people with severe illnesses in their familiar environment: Specially trained nursing staff care for and support palliative patients in close cooperation with hospice services and other local providers. Physicians with the **additional qualification in palliative medicine** alleviate distressing symptoms with the aim of achieving the best possible quality of life for seriously ill people and their families. In **outpatient hospice services,** volunteers are involved in supporting seriously ill people and their families. They provide advice on outpatient care, work with physicians and nursing services, and support the family during the dying process and the period of mourning.

The **specialized outpatient palliative care (SAPV)** aims to maintain quality of life and self-determination as much as possible. SAPV teams visit seriously ill patients wherever they are needed, whether at home or, for example, in care or integration facilities.

Palliative care units are specialized hospital departments where people with advanced, life-limiting illnesses are cared for. The goal is to relieve symptoms as much as possible and improve quality of life, so that seriously ill people can spend their remaining time in their usual environment whenever possible. If discharge is no longer possible, the multiprofessional team of the palliative care unit supports the dying and their families. In inpatient **hospices,** full-time and volunteer staff care for and support seriously ill people and their families in a homelike environment according to their personal needs. A palliative care service in the sense of a **consultation service** offers palliative care for patients in all hospital wards as a specialized team with various professional backgrounds. This care includes both continuous and early palliative medical consultation as well as supplementary co-management in the case of complex symptoms and needs.

There are thus many ways to integrate palliative care at an early stage, without the primary focus being on the last days or weeks of life. The goals of palliative care should therefore not only come to the fore when previous therapies aimed at cure or life extension are replaced. Rather, palliative care should begin as early as possible in the sense of *early integration.* For this, the structures of general palliative care presented here are important in standard care.

Early integration means that seriously ill patients come into contact with the palliative care team early in the course of the illness, ideally at the time of diagnosis. However, this does not mean that the team is already involved in providing care. The focus is on sharing information and building relationships. Primary care providers retain responsibility for the treatment regimen, and therapies targeting the underlying disease are initiated or continued. However, these can be increasingly supplemented and eventually replaced by palliative support as needed.

It is particularly noteworthy that there are repeated studies showing that good quality of care, which incorporates palliative services and specifically promotes quality of life, also has a positive impact on the course of the illness. Thus, a combination of curative and palliative elements within a therapy ensures that overall quality of life is improved and can even lead to an extension of life expectancy.

22.3 Course of Illness and Therapy

These concepts and established care structures correspond to the more recent approaches and ideas of palliative care. In the past, the so-called *surprise question* was often used as an initial screening for a palliative situation: "Would I be surprised if this person were to die within the next six months?" The time frame outlined by this question describes the final phase of life for people for whom specialized palliative care may become relevant in the coming weeks and months. Like all predictions, this prognosis is not always accurate. However, it is not only an indication of the remaining time, but also of the expected burdens, functional limitations, and needs of those affected as well as their relatives and loved ones.

In a certain sense, the question also implies that palliative care begins when a cure is no longer achievable. This reflected the focus at the beginning of the development of hospice and palliative care structures. At that time, patients with tumor diseases were the main focus. In the meantime, especially in recent years, the target group has been expanded to include patients with severe organic, chronic diseases, such as cardiovascular diseases (May 2016).

Today, it is therefore generally advocated that curative and palliative care should complement each other over the course of illness, with the palliative focus gaining increasing importance in chronic, incurable, and progressive diseases (Finn and Malhotra 2019). Fig. 22.2 illustrates the difference between the two approaches.

The courses of chronic, progressive diseases are, of course, highly variable (see Sect. 11). Thus, the trajectory models for diseases such as cancer, organ failure, and frailty in old age as well as dementia-related changes are highly individual and indicate that the respective care needs also differ (Lynn and Adamson 2003). They also show that, within the general decline, there can be phases of improvement and regeneration.

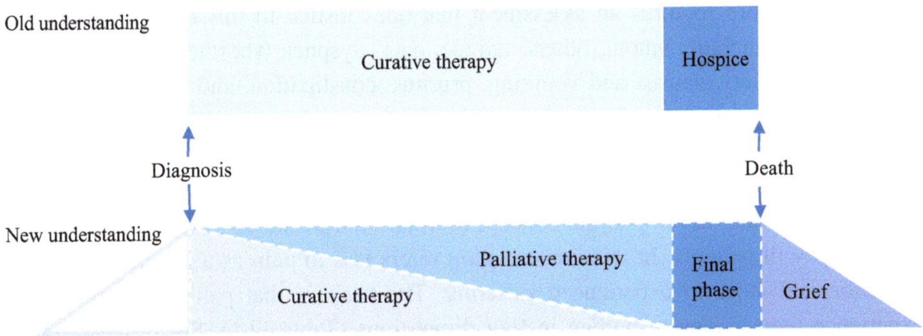

Fig. 22.2 Course of illness and therapy. (Own illustration, adapted from Lynn and Adamson 2003)

The corresponding care services should therefore be oriented to these trajectories. This requires good communication and appropriate assessments regarding current needs, as well as the ability to respond adequately.

For general palliative care, this perspective on the course of illness appears particularly relevant. After all, it is not exclusively about the last days, weeks, or months. The people affected require support that is appropriate to their current situation. This may look completely different in the case of acute care for a worsening COPD than during a pain episode of a resident in a nursing home or the increasing spatial fixation of a person with dementia in an outpatient setting.

22.4 Support Between Mandated Care and Existential Challenges

Good, safe, and patient-centered care ultimately takes place in the direct interaction between those affected and both professional and volunteer helpers. Against this background, two aspects are given special consideration, which highlight the particularities and approach of palliative care and end-of-life care. The starting point for both approaches is that seriously ill and dying people must come to terms with the fact that their abilities are declining and fading, their private and professional roles are changing significantly, and their autonomous will is being pushed into the background (Wasner and Pankofer 2014).

22.4.1 Symptom Relief

Distress manifests on various levels and can be mutually reinforcing. For example, psychosocial symptoms may occasionally present as physical symptoms. Comprehensive care therefore requires an assessment that does justice to this complexity. Palliative symptoms include, among others, fatigue, pain, dyspnea (shortness of breath), loss of appetite, anxiety, nausea and vomiting, pruritus, constipation, and delirium. There is varying quality of evidence for the treatment of these symptoms, as described in the S3 guideline "Palliative Medicine for Patients with Incurable Cancer" from the Oncology Guideline Program (2019).

Cicely Saunders developed the concept of Total Pain in the context of care planning for seriously ill patients. In this context, *pain* refers less to pain as a physiological phenomenon and more to experienced suffering. The basis is that palliative patients can experience their symptom burden in four dimensions (Table 22.1). Since these dimensions are interrelated and influence each other, all should be included in care planning, alleviation of suffering, and the promotion/maintenance of quality of life (Oechsle and Scherg 2019).

Symptom relief can thus become a complex process that cannot be standardized across all patients.

22.4.2 Individual Aspects of Experience and Diversity at the End of Life

Despite all individuality, it is clear that the experience of loss in particular reflects the psychosocial situation of those affected and triggers deep sadness (Wasner and Pankofer

Table 22.1 Symptoms in the four dimensions of the Total Pain concept. (Oechsle and Scherg 2019)

Dimension	Methods of Assessment
Physical	Pain or other physical symptoms are perceived and expressed individually by those affected. Assessment tools such as the visual analog scale can be used, which can also serve to evaluate the effectiveness of interventions.
Psychological	Distress at this level often interacts with physical complaints. Concerns and ruminating thoughts, for example about family or dying, should be acknowledged and, if necessary, discussed or expressed in other ways.
Social	People have various roles that, in their perception, they can no longer fulfill during the dying process and as illness progresses. This often leads to internal conflicts that can cause or influence symptoms. Involving the relatives of those affected and being aware of their burdens, as well as facilitating open communication, can provide support here.
Spiritual	Religious beliefs, questions of meaning and existence become relevant as people confront the end of their existence. Questions may arise about "why" or "what comes after." Here, too, it should be possible to speak openly about one's own thoughts.

2014). Confronting one's own mortality means reflecting on and experiencing the loss of one's own future, as well as social roles and security. Added to this is the loss of autonomy and the question of how to shape the final phase of life and the place of dying in light of this diminishing autonomy. Finally, it is also significant how the farewell from relatives and loved ones can be arranged.

The particular challenge that palliative care and end-of-life care must now address is a specific diversity at the end of life (Schnell 2023). This refers to an irreducible asymmetry between dying and continuing to live, which exists only at the end of life and in no other area of life or healthcare. "No one can take dying away from another. Death is always one's own death. Communication between doctor and patient takes place at the boundary of silence, because at the end of life the shared world of meaning necessary for dialogue between I and You fades away" (Schnell 2023, p. 108).

In addition to all professional and organizational challenges, there is thus a particular ethical challenge. This means responding to dying people who are not simply patients, and that symptom control alone is not sufficient.

The contribution of palliative care and end-of-life care can only be considered a healthcare service in the narrow sense. More broadly, it is a societal task, dedicated to the social regulation and interpretation of dying as well as the shaping of human life.

In summary, it should be noted that palliative care and end-of-life care are team efforts that place humanity and existential experience at the center, but cannot be viewed separately from the course of illness and require high professional standards.

References

Finn L, Malhotra S (2019) The development of pathways in palliative medicine: definition, models, cost and quality impact. Healthcare 7(22):1–10. https://doi.org/10.3390/healthcare7010022

Lynn J, Adamson DM (2003) Living well at the end of life adapting health care to serious chronic illness in old age. RAND white papers: Santa Monica, Pittsburgh

May A (Hrsg) (2016) Patientenverfügungen. Handbuch für Berater, Ärzte und Betreuer. Springer, Berlin

Oechsle K, Scherg A (Hrsg) (2019) FAQ Palliativmedizin. Antworten – prägnant und praxisnah, 1. Aufl. Elsevier, München

Schnell MW (2023) Der Tod als Andersheit. In: Schönefeld D, von Gahlen-Hoops W (Hrsg) Soziale Ordnungen des Sterbens. Theorie, Methodik und Einblicke in die Vergänglichkeit. Transcript, Bielefeld, S 103–14

Wasner M, Pankofer S (Hrsg) (2014) Soziale Arbeit in Palliative Care. Kohlhammer, Stuttgart

WHO (2020) Palliative Care. Online im Internet: Palliative care (who.int). Zugegriffen: 25. Sept. 2023

Emergency and Critical Care as Care Concepts

23

Hans Lemke

Contents

23.1 Introduction

The terms Intensive Care and Critical Carc are often used interchangeably to refer to the care of individuals in a medically critical condition in an intensive care unit. Severe acute injuries or illnesses often result in emergency medical and thus time-critical care (Emergency Care), so that intensive and emergency care must be considered as a continuous care process. The increasing number of elderly people adds complexity, as with advancing age, additional chronic comorbidities must be identified more frequently alongside the acute illness or injury.

Emergency medical initial treatment with stabilization and, if necessary, emergency intervention is usually followed by monitoring, further treatment, and care of the acutely

H. Lemke (✉)
Klinik für Unfall-, Hand- und Wiederherstellungschirurgie, Klinikum Dortmund gGmbH, Dortmund, Germany
dr.h.lemke@t-online.de

D. Schmitz et al. (eds.), *Chronic Care—Science and Practice*,
https://doi.org/10.1007/978-3-662-72298-5_23

seriously ill or injured person in the intensive care unit. Here, too, the early identification of all comorbidities plays an essential role in the success of therapeutic measures and survival.

23.2 The Development of Emergency Medicine in Recent Decades

Emergency medicine as a whole has changed significantly in recent decades. It was recognized very early on that patient survival depends crucially on the optimal coordination and linkage of the individual interfaces within the rescue chain. The outcome for patients thus depends on the quality of care at each individual link in the chain (First Aid 2004).

The rescue chain (see Fig. 23.1) refers to the individual phases that the patient passes through from the emergency event, through first aid by laypersons, to admission to the intensive care unit.

Thirty years ago, emergency medical transports were primarily conducted according to the *load and run* principle, usually without preclinical stabilization measures. This preclinical strategy changed with the nationwide introduction of the Medical Director of Emergency Services *(ÄLRD)* for every emergency service. After many years without emergency medical experience and the corresponding additional qualifications in emergency medical services, the introduction of the Medical Director of Emergency Services shifted the focus to better training and qualification of active emergency physicians. Now, all physicians involved in emergency rescue must provide proof of emergency medical expertise, and the ÄLRD must ensure that only physicians who have regularly acquired at least 20 continuing education points in recognized emergency medical training within a two-year period are deployed in public emergency services. The introduction of additional qualifications and the obligation for regular continuing education has led to a significant improvement in the quality of preclinical care.

23.3 Structured Care Processes Using the Example of Trauma Care

Based on the ATLS® measures (Advanced Trauma Life Support) in the trauma surgery shock room, the preclinically initiated, time-critical emergency medical initial care was developed in the form of Prehospital Trauma Life Surgery *(PHTLS®)* and adapted to the

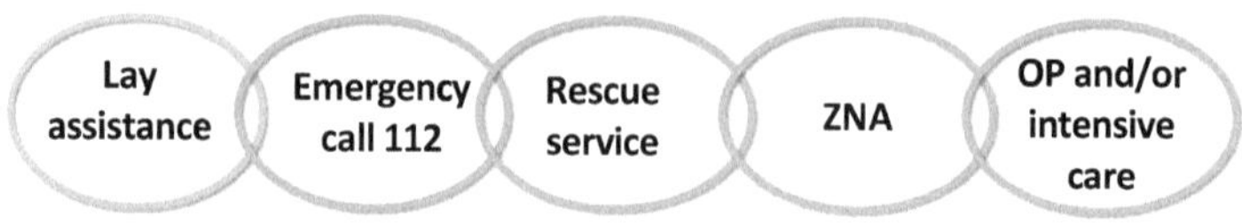
Lay assistance
Emergency call 112
Rescue service
ZNA
OP and/or intensive care

Fig. 23.1 Rescue chain. (Own illustration)

ATLS® standard. Due to its high effectiveness, the structured approach was also included as a recommendation in the S3 Polytrauma Guideline of the German Society for Trauma Surgery (DGU).

The standardized, priority-oriented, preclinical approach (Wölfl et al. 2008) aims to

- quickly and accurately assess the patient's condition
- rapidly identify the critical patient
- facilitate the decision between on-site treatment or immediate transport.

The goal of the standardized approach is to:

- avoid secondary injuries
- keep track of time
- ensure consistent quality of care.

With the introduction of the function of the Medical Director of Emergency Services (ÄLRD), the equipment technology on emergency vehicles has also been significantly further developed. In addition to monitoring modules for patients' vital parameters, more diagnostic options such as 12-lead ECG, sonography, and telemetry are now being used.

Until just a few years ago, the handover of patients from the emergency services to the hospital team was the greatest weakness in the entire rescue chain. Due to noise and incompletely staffed teams in the shock room, as well as a lack of standards and minimum requirements, many important pieces of information were lost during this critical phase. With the establishment of local, regional, and supraregional trauma centers initiated by the DGU (German Society for Trauma Surgery [DGU] 2019) and the associated requirements, there has been a significant improvement in patient handover in the shock room. In cases of life-threatening injuries or illnesses, a time-critical and concise handover from emergency physicians now takes place in a calm atmosphere in the presence of all relevant specialties (shock room team) and the shock room leader, following a standardized handover protocol based on the ABCDE rule (Hodgetts et al. 2006):

This is supported by mandatory procedures for all shock room members according to *ATLS®* (Advanced Trauma Life Support), which are made available to all shock room staff in the form of shock room guidelines. This is a training concept with standardized diagnostic and therapeutic procedures for the early in-hospital initial care of severely injured (polytraumatized) patients in the shock room. The main goal is to recognize and treat life-threatening conditions through regular application of the ABCDE scheme (see Fig. 23.2). Each letter stands for a specific point that must be addressed before moving on to the next. These procedures must be regularly reviewed by the responsible physicians and continually adapted in the local shock room guidelines. Every trauma center has such a statute for the treatment of severely injured patients (interdisciplinary and interprofessional Standard Operating Procedures—shock room), which is agreed upon by all specialties and professional groups and outlines the responsibilities for the initial treatment of severely injured patients. The current version of the statute must be

Care according to the ABCDE scheme	
Airway	Securing the airway
Breathing	Advice on and treatment of respiratory functions and their disorders
Circulation	Advice and treatment of circulatory functions and their disorders
Disability	Determination of (newly occurring) neurological deficits
Exposure	Complete physical examination for signs of injury

Fig. 23.2 Care according to the ABCDE scheme. (Own illustration)

accessible to staff. Staff must be familiar with its contents. The qualifications of individual shock room members, as well as the size and equipment of the shock room, are clearly defined (DGU 2019) and are recertified every three years by independent auditors.

After the shock room handover of the severely injured/ill patient, standardized diagnostic cycles are carried out, strictly following the ATLS® scheme (Advanced Trauma Life Support) (DGU 2019). After FAST sonography, trauma CT scan and/or ECG and laboratory tests, a rapid decision is made as to whether an emergency operation, cardiac catheterization, placement of a chest drain, or other life-saving interventions are required, or whether patients should be transferred directly from the shock room to the intensive care unit.

For patients with minor or moderate injuries or illnesses who are not in acute life-threatening condition, immediate triage is performed in the Central Emergency Department (ZNA) after handover by the emergency services, usually by specially trained nursing staff, many of whom now have the additional qualification of *specialist emergency nursing*. For the initial assessment (triage), most hospitals in Germany use either the Emergency Severity Index *(ESI)* (Grossmann et al. 2009) or the Manchester Triage Scale *(MTS)* (Mackway-Jones 2011). While the ESI may only be applied by specially trained specialist emergency nursing staff in a *ZNA* (German Hospital Association [DKGeV] 2019) and is based on the urgency of the illness/injury and the expected resource consumption of the patient (see Fig. 23.3), the MTS may also be used by non-physician ZNA staff without specialist emergency nursing training.

The MTS refers to the initial categorization of patients newly arriving in the ZNA. The goal is to quickly establish safe and transparent treatment priorities. Depending on vital parameters and symptoms, patients are assessed according to the severity of their illness or injury and assigned to one of five different levels of treatment urgency, each marked by a specific color (see Fig. 23.4). The color coding allows the urgency of treatment to be quickly identified visually. Depending on the color category, the first

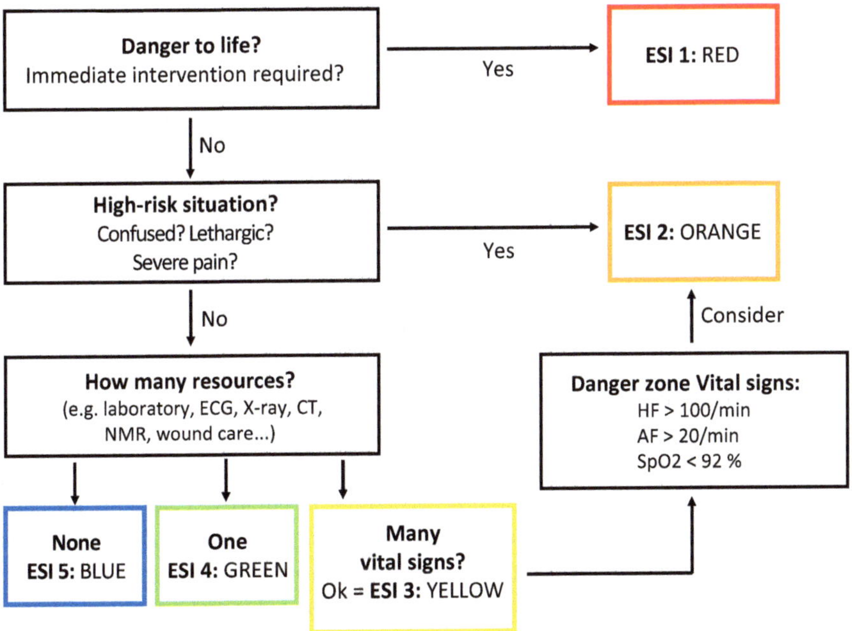

Fig. 23.3 Emergency Severity Index. (Created by ZNA Klinikzentrum Nord, Klinikum Dortmund gGmbH based on: Gilboy et al. 2005)

Priority levels in the MTS

Digit	Name	Color	Max. Time	Control assessment at the latest after
1	Immediately	Red	0 minutes	
2	Very urgent	Orange	10 minutes	10 minutes
3	Urgent	Yellow	30 minutes	30 minutes
4	Normal	Green	90 minutes	90 minutes
5	Not urgent	Blue	120 minutes	120 minutes

Fig. 23.4 Manchester Triage System (MTS). (Created by ZNA Trauma Clinic, Klinikzentrum Nord, Klinikum Dortmund gGmbH based on: Mackway-Jones et al. 2011)

physician contact must be guaranteed within a defined time window. This ensures that more seriously ill/injured patients are prioritized for necessary diagnostics and medical treatment over less seriously ill/injured patients (Mackway-Jones 2011).

23.4 The Geriatric Patient

In particular, patients aged 70 years and older must receive special consideration in light of physical and cognitive decline and age-associated issues such as frailty, cognitive impairment, and multimorbidity. The White Paper on Geriatric Traumatology provides guidance for establishing interdisciplinary clinical processes that significantly improve the quality of care and contribute to a sustainable increase in survival time for these patients (Aigner et al. 2021) (see Fig. 23.5).

Preoperative risk evaluation prior to necessary surgical interventions, through comprehensive medical history and physical examination, are the strongest predictors for the occurrence of perioperative complications. In this context, assessment of cognitive impairment in these patients is mandatory. Prophylaxis and treatment of delirium, as well as accompanying multidisciplinary measures, help to minimize postoperative risks, especially in cognitively impaired patients.

Prevention of postoperative delirium is carried out in intensive care units for patients requiring postoperative intensive care, and otherwise on peripheral wards. This is achieved by establishing a delirium care nurse, who provides postoperative nursing and therapeutic support as well as cognitive stimulation for older and cognitively impaired patients, in order to reduce the risk of postoperative delirium.

23.5 Outlook

The particular vulnerability of geriatric patients, especially after severe trauma, has become increasingly recognized in recent years in the context of demographic change. The goal of the German Society for Trauma Surgery and the German Society for Geriatrics is to establish interdisciplinary and interprofessional units (Geriatric Trauma Centers) throughout Germany by 2025, which recognize and foster the strengths of all team members (Aigner et al. 2021).

For virtually all older patients, treatment will not be completed upon discharge from acute care or inpatient rehabilitation. Unfortunately, outpatient follow-up care still exhibits significant deficits and gaps at present. Our healthcare system is therefore called upon to optimize these interfaces and to close the identified gaps promptly. However, Germany is still at the beginning of this process of improving these interfaces (Aigner et al. 2021).

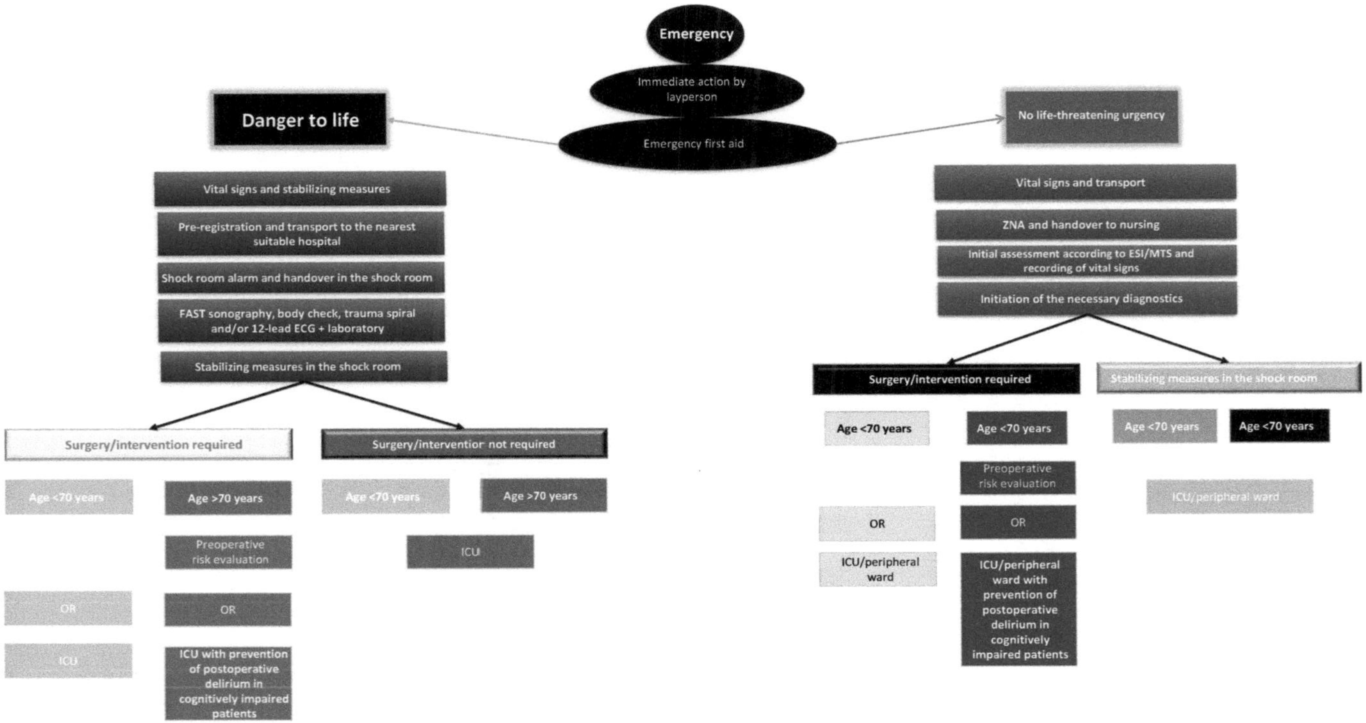

Fig. 23.5 Standardized protocol for emergency medical care in geriatric patients. (Own illustration)

References

Aigner R, Anderson P, Arnim C, v, Bales G, Bartl C, Bliemel C, Böcker W, Bollheimer C, Bork H, Bücking B, Bühl K, Burkhardt H, Coburn M, Denkinger M, Dreinhöfer K, Ernst F, Eschbach D, Eschweiler G, Friess T (2021) In: Liener UC, Becker C, Rapp K, Raschke MJ, Kladny B, Wirtz DC (Hrsg) Weißbuch Alterstraumatologie und Orthogeriatrie. Kohlhammer, Stuttgart

Deutsche Gesellschaft für Unfallchirurgie (2019) Weißbuch Schwerverletztenversorgung: Empfehlungen zur Struktur, Organisation, Ausstattung sowie Förderung von Qualität und Sicherheit in der Schwerverletztenversorgung in der Bundesrepublik Deutschland. Berlin. https://www.traumanetzwerk-dgu.de/fileadmin/user_upload/dgu-weissbuch_schwerverletztenversorgung_2020_3._Auflage.pdf. Zugegriffen am 18.01.2023

Deutsche Krankenhausgesellschaft e.V. (2019) DKG-Empfehlung für die Weiterbildung Notfallpflege. https://www.dkgev.de/fileadmin/default/Mediapool/2_Themen/2.5._Personal_und_Weiterbildung/2.5.11._Aus-_und_Weiterbildung_von_Pflegeberufen/Notfallpflege/DKG-Empfehlung_Weiterbildung_Notfallpflege.pdf. Zugegriffen am 18.01.2023

Erste Hilfe (2004) Lebensrettende Sofortmassnahmen am Unfallort, 2. Aufl. Österreichisches Rotes Kreuz (ÖRK)

Gilboy N, Tanabe P, Travers DA (2005) The Emergency Severity Index Version 4: changes to ESI level 1 and pediatric fever criteria. J Emerg Nurs 31(4):357–362. https://doi.org/10.1016/j.jen.2005.05.011

Grossmann FF, Delport K, Keller DI (2009) Emergency Severity Index: Deutsche Übersetzung eines validen Triageinstruments. Notfall + Rettungsmedizin 12(4):290–292. https://doi.org/10.1007/s10049-009-1156-7

Hodgetts TJ, Mahoney PF, Russell MQ, Byers M (2006) ABC to <C>ABC: redefining the military trauma paradigm. Emerg Med J 23(10):745–746. https://doi.org/10.1136/emj.2006.039610

Mackway-Jones K (Hrsg) (2011) Verlag Hans Huber Programmbereich Pflege. Ersteinschätzung in der Notaufnahme: Das Manchester-Triage-System, 3. Aufl. Huber

Mackway-Jones K, Marsden J, Windle J (2011) Ersteinschätzung in der Notaufnahme: Das Manchester-Triage-System. Deutsche Ausgabe übersetzt und bearbeitet von Krey J, Moecke HP (Hrsg.) 3., überarbeitete und ergänzte Aufl. Hans Huber, Bern

Wölfl CG, Bouillon B, Lackner CK, Wentzensen A, Gliwitzky B, Gross B, Brokmann J, Hauer T (2008) Prehospital Trauma Life Support (PHTLS): Ein interdisziplinäres Ausbildungskonzept für die präklinische Traumaversorgung [Prehospital Trauma Life Support (PHTLS): an interdisciplinary training in preclinical trauma care]. Unfallchirurg 111(9):688–694. https://doi.org/10.1007/s00113-008-1466-0

Pharmacotherapy, Polypharmacy, and Adherence

24

Daniel Diehl

Contents

24.1 Polypharmacy—Development of the Concept

Chronic diseases today represent the greatest challenge for global healthcare. In particular, non-communicable diseases such as cardiovascular diseases, diabetes, or cancer account for an increasing proportion of worldwide deaths (Lim et al. 2012; Murray et al. 2012). In European healthcare systems, this trend is manifested as a decline in mortality rates combined with an aging population and an increasing prevalence of multimorbidity (see Contribution 6).

Polypharmacy refers to the simultaneous use of various medications by an individual to treat one or more health problems. The term is primarily associated with older or multimorbid individuals who often require many medications to manage chronic diseases

D. Diehl (✉)
Fakultät für Gesundheit, Lehrstuhl für Parodontologie,
Universität Witten/Herdecke, Witten, Germany
e-mail: Daniel.Diehl@uni-wh.de

D. Schmitz et al. (eds.), *Chronic Care—Science and Practice*,
https://doi.org/10.1007/978-3-662-72298-5_24

and age-related conditions. The term does not refer exclusively to prescription drugs, but explicitly includes over-the-counter medications and dietary supplements. Unfortunately, to this day, there is no universally accepted definition of polypharmacy, which significantly impairs the assessment of safety aspects in clinical pharmacotherapy by all healthcare professionals (Masnoon et al. 2017).

Common definitions of polypharmacy range from purely numerical counts—the use of more than five medications is the most common here—to therapy duration, and even to descriptive definitions that include attributes such as "minor," "moderate," "major," and "excessive" polypharmacy. However, the contextless, specific number of medications taken is not necessarily an indicator of the appropriateness of therapy, since in principle all medications may be clinically necessary and suitable for the patient. Neither the presence of specific comorbidities nor the possible presence of patient-specific adverse drug reactions is taken into account in this way.

By adding therapy duration to the classic definition, it is possible to more precisely delineate polypharmacy patients; however, this has no clinically relevant impact on harm minimization, as the time specifications themselves are often based only on the dispensing dates of the medications and not on an evidence-based approach to identifying inappropriate therapies.

To account for the relationship between an increased number of prescribed medications and the likelihood of adverse drug reactions and harm, polypharmacy should more accurately be characterized by the use of more medications than would be clinically appropriate given the existing comorbidities. To accurately describe the group that, in the context of polypharmaceutical therapy, exhibits a negative risk-benefit ratio, the term polypharmacy is therefore expanded by the attributes "appropriate" and "inappropriate."

24.2 Epidemiology

The prevalence of polypharmacy in the literature is highly heterogeneous, which is understandable given the variable definitions of the problem. Depending on the definition of polypharmacy, age, gender, and region, the figures range from 4% to 90% (Guillot et al. 2020; Khezrian et al. 2020).

Within the cohort study "Services and Health for Elderly in Long Term care" (SHELTER), it was shown that of 4,000 people with an average age of 83.6 years, at least 49.9% take more than 5, and another 24.3% take at least 10 medications simultaneously (Zazzara et al. 2023). According to an analysis of data from the Survey of Health, Ageing, and Retirement (SHARE), which was based on 34,232 patients with an average age of 75 years, the Europe-wide prevalence of polypharmacy is 52%.

Between 2010 and 2013, the epidemiology of polypharmacy in Sweden was investigated in a large, prospective, register-based cohort study with 1,742,336 patients. Here, a prevalence (use of five or more medications) of 44%, and 11.7% (use of 10 or more medications) was found. The incidence rate of "excessive" polypharmacy was 8.0 per

100 person-years, and that of newly developed polypharmacy was 19.9 per 100 person-years (Morin et al. 2018).

In the Berlin Aging Study, Steinhagen-Thiessen and Borchelt (1999) examined the relationship between morbidity, medication use, and functional limitations in old age. The aim of the study was to understand how medical problems and prescription medications affect functional limitations in people aged between 70 and 100 years. The prevalence of patients taking more than 5 medications was reported as 53.7%. Due to the questionnaire design, this study was also the first to show that many of the regularly taken medications were not prescribed by a doctor but were purchased independently (Steinhagen-Thiessen and Borchelt 1999). These so-called "over-the-counter drugs" (OTC) lead to a worsening of the cumulative risk of adverse drug interactions in the context of inappropriate polypharmacy and have since been taken into account in strategies to avoid polypharmacy.

24.3 Causes of Inappropriate Polypharmacy

Polypharmacy frequently affects older adults and is therefore often defined as an independent geriatric syndrome. However, this is not an adequate classification, as polypharmacy is not a problem exclusive to older people (Wehling et al. 2010). Younger individuals can also be multimorbid and thus have an equally high risk for inappropriate polypharmacy. This is also reflected in the results of a randomized, multicenter study in Europe. Among 3,904 study participants, not only was no association found between age and polypharmacy, but rather a decreasing prevalence was observed in people over 85 years of age. The group of authors instead found a very strong association with frailty, multimorbidity, obesity, as well as poor physical and mental health status. It therefore appears that only the increased occurrence of these risk factors in advanced age creates the impression that age per se is a risk factor for inappropriate polypharmacy (Rieckert et al. 2018).

To ensure the quality of evidence-based medicine in practice, disease-specific clinical guidelines are developed and regularly updated. In their efforts to comply with these recommendations for their patients, physicians may prescribe a large number of medications. For people with multiple chronic conditions, however, strict adherence to disease-specific recommendations and treatment goals carries a high risk of inappropriate polypharmacy. In the study by Dumbreck et al. (2015), the recommendations of several National Institute for Health and Care Excellence (NICE) guidelines regarding adverse drug reactions and drug-drug interactions were thoroughly examined. The investigation showed that while drug interactions are addressed, discrepancies were found both in the proposed changes to prescribing regimens and in the specific interactions mentioned (Dumbreck et al. 2015).

The often fragmented care of chronically ill and multimorbid patients, resulting from a lack of coordination and communication between prescribing physicians across different areas of the healthcare system, leads to a multitude of prescribing errors. The care of chronically ill patients often involves various independent institutions. Under these circumstances, it is not surprising that there are frequently barriers to interdisciplinary communication regarding the pharmacotherapeutic plan (McCarthy et al. 2017). However, due to this lack of coordination, the likelihood of duplicate prescriptions, drug interactions, and inappropriate medication use increases. A retrospective study in Hubei Province, China, found a 2.4-fold increased risk of inappropriate polypharmacy in patients who visited different healthcare facilities for various conditions (Wang et al. 2021).

Many medications have adverse effects (AEs) or interact with other drugs. If these AEs are mistakenly interpreted as independent disease entities, this can lead to inappropriate pharmacotherapy even when pharmacological treatment is guideline-compliant. This phenomenon was described by Rochon and Gurwitz as the prescribing cascade (Rochon and Gurwitz 1997). Prescribing cascades have far-reaching consequences and are influenced by a number of factors (see Fig. 24.1). These include the misclassification of negative drug side effects as diseases, poor communication between healthcare providers, as well as appropriate but poorly monitored polypharmacy. Unnecessary medications, in turn, increase the risk of inappropriate polypharmacy and thus the risk of serious adverse drug interactions. A large cohort study showed that up to 9.5% of patients treated with calcium channel blockers for arterial hypertension were subsequently prescribed a diuretic to treat edema (Savage et al. 2020).

24.4 Consequences of Inappropriate Polypharmacy

Adverse Drug Reactions (ADR)

Polypharmacy raises serious issues regarding drug interactions and ADRs. The likelihood of experiencing ADRs, i.e., unfavorable and severe drug reactions, increases with the intake of additional medications. These can range from mild side effects such as nausea or dizziness to more severe ones, such as allergic reactions or intoxications. A positive correlation between the number of medications taken and the probability of ADRs has been repeatedly demonstrated in research. An analysis of the population database by Guthrie et al. (2015) found that polypharmacy was strongly associated with a higher

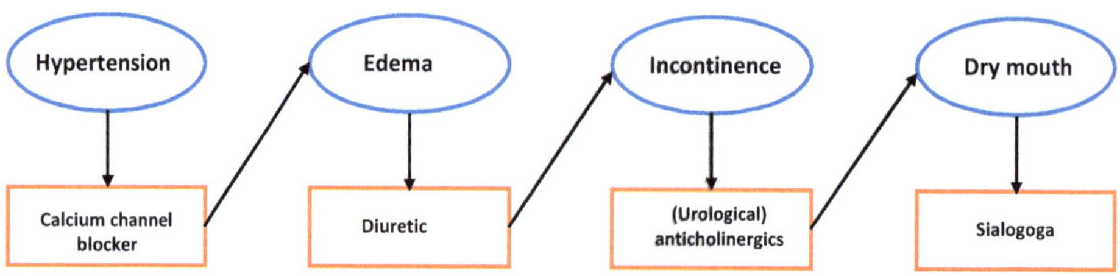

Fig. 24.1 Example of a possible prescribing cascade in a patient with arterial hypertension

incidence of adverse drug reactions. In the cohort of older patients, the prevalence of ADRs is 10%, with the risk increasing dramatically due to advanced age, chronic diseases, and polypharmacy (Alhawassi et al. 2014). However, the high prevalence of ADRs in the elderly population is not a consequence of age itself, but rather of phenomena associated with advanced age, such as multimorbidity and polypharmacy (Field et al. 2004).

Drug Interactions
Adverse drug interactions (Drug-Drug Interactions, DDI) represent a special type of ADR, as they do not occur in connection with a defined active substance. With more than 2,500 identified drug combinations, there is a long list of possible DDIs; however, not all potential interactions are clinically significant (Baxter and Preston 2010). Drug interactions can be modeled and occur in 5.6% of cases when two medications are taken, but in 100% of cases when seven medications are taken simultaneously (Karas 1981). The actual prevalence of potential DDIs is therefore difficult to determine and, depending on context and study methodology, ranges between 0.8% and 90.6%. In contrast, clinically detectable interactions that lead to hospitalization are much rarer, at 1.2–2% (Fokter et al. 2010; Zheng et al. 2018).

Pharmacokinetic Drug Interactions
The absorption of orally administered drugs is largely determined by gastrointestinal function. Medications with anticholinergic effects or opioids can reduce motility, which may delay or completely block the absorption of other drugs. Dopamine receptor antagonists and various parasympathomimetics, on the other hand, increase motility, thereby enhancing the absorption of other medications. These changes in transit time must be carefully monitored and taken into account, as they can have a significant impact on the onset of action and serum concentration of medications.

The metabolism of drugs in the liver is the cause of a wide variety of interactions. Primarily, six CYP450 enzymes are responsible for the breakdown of various drugs. Knowledge of the specific CYP450 enzymes involved in the metabolism of a drug can help predict and avoid drug interactions. In particular, CYP3A4 and CYP2D6 together metabolize more than 70% of drugs metabolized in the liver, and interactions with these enzymes often lead to clinically relevant ADRs. Factors such as age, liver function, or diseases also exert strong influences on CYP450 metabolism.

Interactions involving CYP450 enzymes occur through inhibition or enhancement of the respective enzyme function, with the majority of clinically relevant, life-threatening interactions being due to inhibition of CYP450 enzymes. Enzyme inhibition usually occurs when several drugs must be metabolized by the same enzyme, leading to slowed metabolism and thus increased concentrations of both drugs in the blood or tissue. The most relevant interaction in the context of chronic care concerns CYP3A4, as this isoenzyme is responsible for the metabolism of many drugs used in the treatment of chronic diseases. These include, among others, benzodiazepines, immunosuppressants, calcium channel blockers, macrolide antibiotics, as well as anticoagulants such as phenprocoumon and apixaban. Approximately 830 million defined daily doses of anticoagulant medications were taken in 2020, usually for the treatment of chronic diseases and conditions. Interactions at CYP3A4 can lead to increased levels of anticoagulants in the blood, which in rare cases can result in severe bleeding. According to a population-based study on fatal ADRs, bleeding accounts for nearly 80% of fatal ADRs (Wester et al. 2007).

Pharmacodynamic Interactions
When the effect of one drug directly alters the effect of another, this is referred to as a pharmacodynamic interaction. These interactions occur frequently and can have both synergistic and antagonistic effects. Such synergisms can be either intentional or unintentional. For example, additive pharmacodynamic effects are often utilized in drug-based cancer therapy or in the treatment of diabetes mellitus (e.g., sulfonylureas and metformin). The deliberate combination of antihypertensive medications (e.g., ACE inhibitors and beta-blockers) also aims to enhance their overall effect. Conversely, unintended interactions can also occur. Serotonin syndrome, triggered by the combination of tramadol and selective serotonin reuptake inhibitors, for example, is a potentially life-threatening drug reaction characterized by high body temperature and muscle spasms.

The American Medical Directors Association (AMDA) and the American Society of Consultant Pharmacists (ASCP) have developed a guideline to help members of the interdisciplinary healthcare team recognize the clinical symptoms of drug interactions more quickly. The researchers examined the therapeutic significance, potential for harm, frequency of interactions, and prescribing frequency of various medications in nursing homes. This enabled the creation of a list of the ten most common drug interactions and their symptoms, which staff in chronic healthcare should focus on (see Fig. 24.2).

24.5 Polypharmacy and Adherence

During the treatment of chronic diseases, the long-term use of medications is widespread. Although pharmacotherapy has been proven to improve life expectancy and quality of life, studies consistently show that people with chronic illnesses take only 50–60% of their prescribed medications (Laufs 2011). This non-adherence represents a significant burden on the global healthcare system and is observed in industrialized countries around the world.

The WHO estimates that improving pharmacotherapeutic adherence would have a greater impact on global health than the development of novel drugs. Especially in the field of cardiovascular diseases, poor adherence is often associated with significantly increased mortality (Gehi et al. 2007). However, non-compliance with medication pre-

Drug 1	Drug 2	Interaction potential	Avoidance
ACE inhibitors	Potassium dietary supplements	ACE inhibition leads to reduced aldosterone aldosterone production and reduced potassium excretion. potassium excretion. Risk of hyperkalemia	Before treatment with an ACE inhibitor Determine potassium level (> 5.0 mmol/l). Monitor dietary supplements
	Spirinolactone	Hyperkalemia may occur as both drugs can increase the serum potassium concentration	
digoxin	Amiodarone	Amiodarone can reduce the clearance of digoxin, which can lead to digoxin intoxication. The digoxin dosage must be halved and digoxin blood levels must be monitored	Digoxin dosage must be halved and digoxin blood levels must be monitored
	Verapamil	Bradycardia and potential heart block are caused by the slowing of myocardial contraction and conduction due to pharmacodynamic synergistic effects	Digoxin levels should not exceed 2.6nmol/L
Theophylline	Fluoroquinolones	Possible epileptogenic effect; possible theophylline toxicity; inhibition of hepatic metabolism of theophylline by quinolones.	Gatifloxacin, levofloxacin and moxifloxacin are fluoroquinolones that do not show strong interactions with theophylline
Vitamin K antagonists	Macrolides	Macrolides inhibit CYP3A4 metabolism and the subsequent excretion of warfarin from the body. Risk of bleeding!	Alternative antibiotics Check INR values regularly Dose adjustment of phenprocoumon
	NSAID	NSAIDs irritate the stomach and promote erosion of the protective gastric mucosa, which favors the development of gastrointestinal bleeding. NSAIDs also reduce the cohesive properties of blood platelets, which are necessary for clotting	Avoid if possible. Alternatives to classic NSAIDs are: Acetaminophen or Coxibe
	Phenytoin	Possible increased effect of warfarin and/or phenytoin	INR monitoring. Watch out for bleeding
	Fluoroquinolones	Risk of bleeding due to increased effect of vitamin K antagonists.	Microbiological tests for targeted antibiotic therapy. Alternative antibiotic if necessary
	Sulfonamides	increases the effect of warfarin. This may be more noticeable in people who are malnourished. Sulfamethoxazole can prevent the metabolism of warfarin and lead to a displacement of the warfarin protein.	Reduction of the phenprocoumon dose by 50 % during therapy

Fig. 24.2 List of the ten most dangerous drug interactions in long-term care. (*Source:* https://paltc.org/top-10-particularly-dangerous-drug-interactions-paltc)

scriptions also causes unnecessary healthcare costs, estimated at €10 billion annually (Laufs 2011).

Adherence is defined as the extent to which a patient's behavior matches the instructions and therapeutic recommendations of their physician/therapist. This is a multifactorial phenomenon. It is important to understand that while taking a tablet on time and correctly may seem simple, it is in reality a complex process. Scheduling appointments, obtaining prescriptions, filling medications at the pharmacy, taking medications as prescribed, ensuring timely supply of follow-up prescriptions, and adequate monitoring by healthcare professionals are essential adherence factors in which patients, healthcare providers, and the healthcare system are equally involved.

Patient-related factors

The most important patient-related factors for non-adherence are adverse effects, memory problems, and financial constraints. Other factors contributing to non-adherence include low literacy and lack of confidence in the effectiveness of the treatment.

Polypharmacy presents an additional obstacle. The self-management of multiple medications, each with its own dosing regimen, quickly leads to overwhelm. As a result, patients become frustrated and less motivated to adhere to complex dosing schedules. Systematic reviews of chronic diseases have shown that higher dosing frequency and more complex therapeutic regimens equally lead to poorer adherence, whereas patients who take their medications only once daily demonstrate significantly higher adherence rates (Coleman et al. 2012; Saini et al. 2007). Accordingly, medications with a low number of adverse effects and daily dosing should, under appropriate circumstances, have their dosing frequency reduced to improve adherence (WHO 2003).

Individual health literacy, i.e., the ability to understand and use health information to secure support from the healthcare system, is one of the most important predictors of non-compliance with medication regimens. At 54.4%, a considerable proportion of the adult population in Germany lacks sufficient knowledge to navigate the healthcare system. Low health literacy is even more prevalent in certain population groups—including those with chronic illnesses (73%), the elderly (66%), people with a migration background (71%), and those with low socioeconomic status (78%)—than in the general population (Schaeffer et al. 2017).

Healthcare system-related factors

Understanding the package insert of a medication and correctly interpreting the information requires a high level of health literacy. Ideally, patients should receive the necessary information for the safe and appropriate use of medications when communicating with physicians or pharmacists. However, studies show that these conversations are often incomplete or even completely forgotten (Tarn et al. 2006). Many patients appear not to know, after a hospital stay, what the prescribed amount of new medications is and what adverse effects to expect (Makaryus and Friedman 2005).

The previously mentioned fragmentation of the healthcare system also promotes non-adherence, especially during the transition from inpatient to outpatient care. Discrepancies between treatment plans at the interface of different healthcare facilities often lead to unnecessary hospitalizations.

24.6 Strategies to Improve Adherence

Essentially, three strategies can contribute to improving adherence, which, when combined, show far better effects than when used alone (Spoelstra et al. 2015)

1. Individual counseling

   Effective communication between healthcare providers and patients is of critical importance. Educating patients about their medications, their purpose, possible side effects, and the importance of adherence improves overall health literacy, which could increase adherence in the long term by 11–36% (Laufs et al. 2011). It can be helpful to ask patients about their knowledge and beliefs regarding medications before providing education. Open-ended questions are used to understand the patient's adherence practices, build trust, and address any barriers.

Behavioral strategies such as self-monitoring, linking new and established behaviors, and positive reinforcement are also well-studied options for establishing adherence strategies. Where possible, family members, pharmacy staff, and nursing staff should be included in the motivational strategies used, as adherence can decline again without regular re-motivation (Lee et al. 2006).

2. Adjustment of pharmacotherapy

   Improving medication regimens includes the use of individual pill boxes and weekly blister packs to organize daily doses and simplifying the dosing schedule to once-daily administration. The number of tablets to be taken daily correlates significantly with adherence (Claxton et al. 2001). Therefore, all prescribers should prefer medications that can be taken once daily whenever possible.

   Medication regimens should be regularly reviewed for potential drug interactions and duplicate prescriptions to reduce inappropriate polypharmacy. This is especially important at the interface between different healthcare facilities.

3. Aids and technology

   Behavioral recommendations for adherence to pharmacotherapeutic measures should also integrate the use of reminder cues into the daily routine. Reminder cues can be linked to fixed and regular daily activities such as going to the bathroom, certain meals, or bedtime. An example of a reminder cue is the prominent placement of the medication package next to the coffee machine or toothbrush. Modern technologies and inventions can provide professional support in managing non-adherence. For example, mobile phone reminders or electronic pill boxes can significantly improve adherence. Furthermore, modern apps, coupled with smart pill boxes, can provide real-time feedback to patients and healthcare providers, thereby ensuring adequate monitoring of medication intake (Granger and Bosworth 2011).

Adherence to pharmacological therapies is crucial for high-quality healthcare. However, it requires a combination of educational and behavioral strategies as well as regular, patient-specific reviews of therapy by all parties involved. Adherence should be addressed on multiple levels, including patient education, physician compliance with guidelines, and support from the healthcare system.

References

Alhawassi TM, Krass I, Bajorek BV, Pont LG (2014) A systematic review of the prevalence and risk factors for adverse drug reactions in the elderly in the acute care setting. Clin Interv Aging 9:2079–2086. https://doi.org/10.2147/CIA.S71178

Baxter K, Preston CL (2010) Stockley's drug interactions, Bd 495. Pharmaceutical Press, London

Claxton AJ, Cramer J, Pierce C (2001) A systematic review of the associations between dose regimens and medication compliance. Clin Ther 23(8):1296–1310

Coleman CI, Limone B, Sobieraj DM, Lee S, Roberts MS, Kaur R, Alam T (2012) Dosing frequency and medication adherence in chronic disease. J Manag Care Pharm 18(7):527–539

Dumbreck S, Flynn A, Nairn M, Wilson M, Treweek S, Mercer SW et al (2015) Drug-disease and drug-drug interactions: systematic examination of recommendations in 12 UK national clinical guidelines. BMJ 350:h949

Field TS, Gurwitz JH, Harrold LR, Rothschild J, DeBellis KR, Seger AC et al (2004) Risk factors for adverse drug events among older adults in the ambulatory setting. J Am Geriatr Soc 52(8):1349–1354

Fokter N, Mozina M, Brvar M (2010) Potential drug-drug interactions and admissions due to drug-drug interactions in patients treated in medical departments. Wien Klin Wochenschr 122(3–4):81–88

Gehi AK, Ali S, Na B, Whooley MA (2007) Self-reported medication adherence and cardiovascular events in patients with stable coronary heart disease: the heart and soul study. Arch Intern Med 167(16):1798–1803

Granger B, Bosworth H (2011) Medication adherence: emerging use of technology. Curr Opin Cardiol 26(4):279–287

Guillot J, Maumus-Robert S, Bezin J (2020) Polypharmacy: a general review of definitions, descriptions and determinants. Therapies 75(5):407–416. https://doi.org/10.1016/j.therap.2019.10.001

Guthrie B, Makubate B, Hernandez-Santiago V, Dreischulte T (2015) The rising tide of polypharmacy and drug-drug interactions: population database analysis 1995–2010. BMC Med 13(1):1–10

Karas S (1981) The potential for drug interactions. Ann Emerg Med 10(12):627–630. https://doi.org/10.1016/S0196-0644(81)80085-6

Khezrian M, McNeil CJ, Murray AD, Myint PK (2020) An overview of prevalence, determinants and health outcomes of polypharmacy. Ther Adv Drug Saf 11:2042098620933741

Laufs U (2011) Medikamentenadhärenz bei chronischen Erkrankungen. Der Nervenarzt 82(2):153–158

Laufs U, Böhm M, Kroemer H, Schüssel K, Griese N, Schulz M (2011) Strategien zur Verbesserung der Einnahmetreue von Medikamenten. DMW-Dtsch Med Wochenschr 136(31/32):1616–1621

Lee JK, Grace KA, Taylor AJ (2006) Effect of a pharmacy care program on medication adherence and persistence, blood pressure, and low-density lipoprotein cholesterol: a randomized controlled trial. Jama 296(21):2563–2571

Lim SS, Vos T, Flaxman AD, Danaei G, Shibuya K, Adair-Rohani H et al (2012) A comparative risk assessment of burden of disease and injury attributable to 67 risk factors and risk factor clusters in 21 regions, 1990–2010: a systematic analysis for the Global Burden of Disease Study 2010. Lancet 380(9859):2224–2260

Makaryus AN, Friedman EA (2005) Patients' understanding of their treatment plans and diagnosis at discharge. Paper presented at the Mayo clinic proceedings

Masnoon N, Shakib S, Kalisch-Ellett L, Caughey GE (2017) What is polypharmacy? A systematic review of definitions. BMC Geriatr 17:1–10

McCarthy C, Clyne B, Corrigan D, Boland F, Wallace E, Moriarty F et al (2017) Supporting prescribing in older people with multimorbidity and significant polypharmacy in primary care (SPPiRE): a cluster randomised controlled trial protocol and pilot. Implement Sci 12(1):99. https://doi.org/10.1186/s13012-017-0629-1

Morin L, Johnell K, Laroche M-L, Fastbom J, Wastesson JW (2018) The epidemiology of polypharmacy in older adults: register-based prospective cohort study. Clin Epidemiol 10:289–298

Murray CJL, Vos T, Lozano R, Naghavi M, Flaxman AD, Michaud C et al (2012) Disability-adjusted life years (DALYs) for 291 diseases and injuries in 21 regions, 1990–2010: a systematic analysis for the Global Burden of Disease Study 2010. Lancet 380(9859):2197–2223. https://doi.org/10.1016/S0140-6736(12)61689-4

Rieckert A, Trampisch US, Klaaßen-Mielke R, Drewelow E, Esmail A, Johansson T et al (2018) Polypharmacy in older patients with chronic diseases: a cross-sectional analysis of factors associated with excessive polypharmacy. BMC Fam Pract 19(1):113. https://doi.org/10.1186/s12875-018-0795-5

Rochon PA, Gurwitz JH (1997) Optimising drug treatment for elderly people: the prescribing cascade. BMJ 315(7115):1096–1099

Saini SD, Schoenfeld P, Kaulback K, Dubinsky MC (2007) Effect of medication dosing frequency on adherence in chronic diseases. The American journal of managed care 15(6):22–33

Savage RD, Visentin JD, Bronskill SE, Wang X, Gruneir A, Giannakeas V et al (2020) Evaluation of a common prescribing cascade of calcium channel blockers and diuretics in Older Adults With Hypertension. JAMA Int Med 180(5):643–651. https://doi.org/10.1001/jamainternmed.2019.7087

Schaeffer D, Vogt D, Berens E-M, Hurrelmann, K (2017) Gesundheitskompetenz der Bevölkerung in Deutschland: Ergebnisbericht

Spoelstra SL, Schueller M, Hilton M, Ridenour K (2015) Interventions combining motivational interviewing and cognitive behaviour to promote medication adherence: a literature review. J Clin Nur 24(9–10):1163–1173

Steinhagen-Thiessen E, Borchelt M (1999) Morbidity, medication, and functional limitations in very old age. In: The Berlin aging study: aging from 70 to 100. Cambridge University Press, New York, S 131–166

Tarn DM, Heritage J, Paterniti DA, Hays RD, Kravitz RL, Wenger NS (2006) Physician communication when prescribing new medications. Arch Int Med 166(17):1855–1862

Wang J, Feng Z, Dong Z, Li W, Chen C, Gu Z et al (2021) Does having a usual primary care provider reduce polypharmacy behaviors of patients with chronic disease? A retrospective study in Hubei Province, China. Frontiers Pharmacol 12

Wehling M, Burkhardt H, Frölich L (2010) Arzncitherapie für Ältere, Bd 2. Springer, Berlin

Wester K, Jönsson A, Spigset O, Hägg S (2007) Spontaneously reported fatal suspected adverse drug reactions: a 10-year survey from Sweden. Pharmacoepidemiol Drug Saf 16(2):173–180

WHO (2003) Adherence to long-term therapies: evidence for action. World Health Organization, Genf

Zazzara MB, Villani ER, Palmer K, Fialova D, Corsonello A, Soraci L et al (2023) Frailty modifies the effect of polypharmacy and multimorbidity on the risk of death among nursing home residents: results from the SHELTER study. Front Med 10. https://doi.org/10.3389/fmed.2023.1091246

Zheng WY, Richardson L, Li L, Day R, Westbrook J, Baysari M (2018) Drug-drug interactions and their harmful effects in hospitalised patients: a systematic review and meta-analysis. Eur J Clin Pharmacol 74:15–27

Technical Support Systems in Individual Care

25

Beate Radzey

Contents

25.1 What are Technical Support Systems in Individual Care?

There is no clear definition of what constitutes technical support systems in the context of chronic care. The term is often used synonymously with concepts that are no less loosely defined, such as Smart Home or Ambient Assisted Living (AAL). While the target group for Smart Home is less clearly defined, AAL describes the aim of enabling primarily older people to live independently in their own homes with the help of supportive

B. Radzey (✉)
Leitung LANDaufwärts, Göppingen, Germany
e-mail: beate.radzey@vinzenz-sd.de

D. Schmitz et al. (eds.), *Chronic Care—Science and Practice*,
https://doi.org/10.1007/978-3-662-72298-5_25

assistance systems. The term *digitalization in care* is more closely linked to the context of nursing. This refers to the use of technologies to meet care requirements and ultimately improve quality of life. Support can be provided either to people with chronic limitations themselves or to caregivers. In the case of the person in need of care, the goal is to compensate for limitations, facilitate daily life, increase comfort and safety, and promote participation and activity. If the focus is on caregivers, technology can directly support care activities or help make care processes, management, and knowledge transfer more effective (Kunze and König 2017).

25.2 Smart Home and Technical Assistance Systems—A Connected Home

Living labs clearly demonstrate how security, comfort, and energy efficiency solutions from the field of home automation go hand in hand with assistive technical solutions and are networked into an intelligent home: A camera transmits an image of the person at the front door to a display inside the apartment, blinds and lights can be controlled via tablet, temperature sensors regulate the heating, wall cabinets can be lowered at the push of a button, or a flashing light signals the doorbell. The vision is that the home unobtrusively and intelligently compensates for the residents' limitations. More and more providers in elderly care are using these solutions in senior-friendly serviced apartments. Installation in individual households, however, remains the exception.

25.3 Monitoring and Rehabilitation: Focus on Safety and Care

When the monitoring of a person is the main focus, these are also referred to as monitoring systems: Sensors record health, behavioral, and environmental data, and in an emergency, a caregiver is automatically notified. For example, inactivity detectors combined with a door contact check whether the person is present in the apartment and trigger an alarm if there is no movement for an unusually long period. Monitoring of medical parameters up to and including video surveillance also falls within this area. Here, ethical and data protection concerns become more apparent and must be adequately addressed and taken seriously (Niemeijer et al. 2010).

In the context of chronic care, technical support systems are also relevant that enable networking between care sectors as well as rehabilitative measures in the home environment. The focus here is on providing good and effective care with fewer personnel resources, especially in structurally weak regions. At the same time, the person in need of care can save time and travel. For example, long-term telemedical support for people with chronic illnesses can be provided in the form of digitally offered exercises and therapies, check-ups, and consultations.

25.4 Slow Adoption of Technical Support Systems

The adoption of new technologies in the context of care has progressed less rapidly than in other areas of life. While, in general, a more open attitude toward technology in care can be observed compared to a few years ago (Scorna 2021), there is still a gap between supply and demand. The development of and research into technical support systems continues unabated, but their actual implementation in institutions and private households remains hesitant.

In practice, it is primarily documentation and security systems that have become established, especially in inpatient care, and to a much lesser extent in outpatient settings. Digital media for communication and entertainment are also used in inpatient contexts (Haug 2021). Since the use of assistive technologies is still seen as an important future strategy in view of demographic change and the care crisis, there is great interest in achieving a real breakthrough.

25.5 Barriers to the Use of Technology

There are a variety of hurdles to establishing technical support systems in individual care. The main ones include:

25.5.1 Technical and Organizational Shortcomings

First, technical prerequisites such as the widespread availability of reliable Wi-Fi systems must be ensured. Another technical shortcoming is the often lacking standardization of systems, resulting in insufficient compatibility between different manufacturers and application areas (Haug 2021). On the organizational level, institutions lack digitalization strategies regarding the equipment and use of technical support systems.

25.5.2 Lack of Evidence of Effectiveness

Technical support systems inevitably need to be examined from an economic perspective as well. “In order to assess the potential and risks as well as the benefits and costs of such assistive technologies, methodologically sound evaluation studies are needed to provide evidence of their effectiveness” (Mähs 2021, p. 330) and to meet the complexity of the systems. For example, can different fall detection technologies (radar, IR sensor, fall detector) be compared with each other? Does it make a difference whether users have cognitive impairments or not?

In a climate of cost containment and economization, technology will only find its place if there is valid evidence of its effectiveness and, as a result, financing models can be presented so that payers are encouraged to support these systems (Meyer 2016).

25.6 Users in Focus: Acceptance and Effectiveness

To promote the use of technology, it is above all necessary to involve the target groups even more consistently in development. Particular attention should also be paid to the people receiving care. The needs of their environment are still at the forefront. For example, the largest number of technologies used in the field of dementia are still primarily aimed at increasing safety in the home (Lorenz et al. 2019).

Demonstrated effectiveness and product testing with the target group already during the development phase would increase acceptance among users themselves (Palmdorf et al. 2021). This could help avoid situations where the shortcomings of the technology only become apparent too late, such as a non-intuitive user interface that results in a long learning curve (Scorna 2021).

In summary, Weber succinctly describes the central issue as follows: "Anyone who wants to use more technology in care must, not least, organize the design and implementation of age-appropriate assistance systems as a bottom-up process; there must be a shift from 'technology push' to 'demand pull.'" (2021, p. 25)

25.7 User-oriented Development and Focus on the Setting

A prerequisite for user-oriented development is the understanding that the entire context in which the technology is used must be considered. Technical support systems are only understood as sociotechnical systems if they are embedded in different contexts that influence them. Consequently, there is not just one large target group for a technical support system: Needs are heterogeneous and, for example, depend on the specific impairment or care situation.

25.8 Further Focus: Consulting, Training, and Implementation

Given the confusing array of available options, support is also needed in selecting suitable technical systems. Training programs are necessary for professionals, relatives, and those affected, as well as for digitalization experts within institutions. Technical consulting services and product guides must be further expanded and networked. For example, the Fraunhofer Institute is developing a comparison portal for platform solutions for nursing homes, while the technical consulting center for digital assistance in the city of Hanover addresses users in their own homes.

Assistive technologies are merely tools. The realization of their potential for users is closely linked to the quality of the implementation process. The introduction of each technical innovation must be accompanied by a social innovation (Gaugler et al. 2021). This includes, for example, analyzing the context of use, discussions with those involved, recording and adapting processes, training in the use of the technology, and designating those responsible for the system or its components. The deployment of technical systems should be participatory from the outset.

25.9 Always Keep in Mind: Ethical and Data Protection Assessment

Anyone who focuses on the user during the development and implementation of technology will also continuously incorporate ethical considerations. Ienca et al. (2018) call for a proactive approach in which the ethical perspective is integrated into the development process from the very beginning. In Germany, the MEESTAR procedure (see contribution 54) was developed to implement such an approach in the field of age-appropriate assistance systems (Manzeschke et al. 2013).

In a technological world, technology can and must also support us in caring for people with chronic illnesses. However, technical systems are not a stand-alone solution, but rather a component of a holistic support strategy. The focus must be on strategic proposals for the targeted establishment of technical solutions in the everyday lives of those affected, as well as on expanding systematic evaluations of their actual benefits in care practice.

References

Gaugler JE, Zmora R, Mitchell LL, Finlay J, Rosebush CE, Nkimbeng M, Peterson CM (2021) Remote activity monitoring for family caregivers of persons living with dementia: a mixed methods, randomized controlled evaluation. BMC Geriatr 21(1):715. https://doi.org/10.1186/s12877-021-02634-8

Haug S (2021) Nutzung, Planung und Bewertung digitaler Assistenzsysteme in der Pflege: Ergebnisse einer Befragung von Führungskräften in ambulanten und stationären Einrichtungen. In: Frommeld D, Scorna U, Haug S, Weber K (Hrsg) Gute Technik für ein gutes Leben im Alter? Akzeptanz, Chancen und Herausforderungen altersgerechter Assistenzsysteme. Transcript Verlag, Bielefeld, S 185–213

Ienca M, Wangmo T, Jotterand FA, Kressig RW, Elger B (2018) Ethical design of intelligent assistive technologies for dementia: a descriptive review. Sci Eng Ethics 24(4):1035–1055. https://doi.org/10.1007/s11948-017-9976-1

Kunze C, König P (2017) Systematisierung technischer Unterstützungssysteme in den Bereichen Pflege, Teilhabeunterstützung und aktives Leben im Alter. In: Hämmerle I, Kempter G (Hrsg) Umgebungsunterstütztes Leben: Beiträge zum Usability Day XV. Papst Science Publishers, S 15–21

Lorenz K, Freddolino PP, Comas-Herrera A, Knapp M, Damant J (2019) Technology-based tools and services for people with dementia and carers: mapping technology onto the dementia care pathway. Dementia 18(2):725–741. https://doi.org/10.1177/1471301217691617

Mähs M (2021) Anforderungen an die Evaluation von altersgerechten Assistenztechnologien aus gesundheitsökonomischer Sicht. In: Frommeld D, Scorna U, Haug S, Weber K (Hrsg) Gute Technik für ein gutes Leben im Alter? Akzeptanz, Chancen und Herausforderungen altersgerechter Assistenzsysteme. Transcript Verlag, S 317–339

Manzeschke A, Weber K, Rother E, Fangerau H (2013) Ethische Fragen im Bereich Altersgerechter Assistenzsysteme. Berlin. https://www.interaktive-technologien.de/service/publikationen/ethische-fragen-im-bereich-altersgerechter-assistenzsysteme. Zugegriffen am 21.07.2023

Meyer S (2016) Technische Unterstützung im Alter – was ist möglich, was ist sinnvoll? Expertise zum Siebten Altenbericht der Bundesregierung. Retrieved from Deutsches Zentrum für Altersfragen. https://nbn-resolving.org/urn:nbn:de:0168-ssoar-49980-9. Zugegriffen am 27.07.2023

Niemeijer AR, Frederiks BJ, Riphagen II, Legemaate J, Eefsting JA, Hertogh CM (2010) Ethical and practical concerns of surveillance technologies in residential care for people with dementia or intellectual disabilities: an overview of the literature. Int Psychogeriatr 22(7):1129–1142

Palmdorf S, Stark AL, Nadolny S, Eliass G, Karlheim C, Kreisel SH, Dockweiler C (2021) Technology-assisted home care for people with dementia and their relatives: scoping review. JMIR Aging 4(1):e25307. https://doi.org/10.2196/25307

Scorna U (2021) Digitale Technik in der ambulanten und stationären Pflege: Eine Interviewstudie zum Einfluss des Pflegepersonals auf die Einführung digitaler Assistenzsysteme. In: Frommeld D, Scorna U, Haug S, Weber K (Hrsg) Gute Technik für ein gutes Leben im Alter? Akzeptanz, Chancen und Herausforderungen altersgerechter Assistenzsysteme. Transcript, S 215–232

Weber K (2021) Gute Technik für ein gutes Leben?! In: Frommeld D, Scorna U, Haug S, Weber K (Hrsg) Gute Technik für ein gutes Leben im Alter? Akzeptanz, Chancen und Herausforderungen altersgerechter Assistenzsysteme. Transcript Verlag, S 11–26

What If? Social Design as a Competence Enhancement in Interdisciplinary Teams in the Context of Chronic Care

26

Diana Cürlis and Carolin Schreiber

Contents

26.1 Design and Chronic Care—is there a fit?

Interprofessional cooperation, especially in the form of multiprofessional teams pursuing a synergistic or integrative treatment mode, is considered a significant quality feature in all areas of care, including medical rehabilitation (Körner and Bengel 2004). This article aims to encourage consideration of designers and (participatory) design methods as a way to expand competencies for interdisciplinary teams in the context of chronic care.

The term *design* is not protected and is used for a wide variety of things: from *nail design* to *designer yachts*, the range is broad, suggesting that design is primarily about *beautification* or *styling*. Another perspective on design comes from the historical devel-

D. Cürlis (✉) · C. Schreiber
Münster School of Design (MSD), FH Münster University of Applied Sciences, Münster, Germany
e-mail: diana.cuerlis@fh-muenster.de

C. Schreiber
e-mail: carolin.schreiber@fh-muenster.de

D. Schmitz et al. (eds.), *Chronic Care—Science and Practice*,
https://doi.org/10.1007/978-3-662-72298-5_26

opment of division of labor through industrialization: designers create products that are mass-produced. Alternatively, design is associated with advertising.

However, design has always been capable of more—and the call for a responsible attitude in design is not a recent development. As early as the 1970s, there was clear criticism of the discipline from within its own ranks. Viktor Papanek, an Austrian-American designer, postulated in his 1971 polemic "Design for the Real World" an approach to design that places the real needs of people at its center. He also called for an interdisciplinary orientation of design as well as an alignment of the design disciplines with research and other sciences.

The responsible design attitude postulated by Papanek is what the authors of this article strive to fulfill by practicing a form of design in which things are not designed *for* a user or person, but *with* people. This ensures that real needs are addressed, rather than imposing design solutions from above.

26.2 Social Design: Design in the Context of Societal Challenges

This conviction forms the basis for viewing design as *social design*. Social design is not a sharply defined term. The authors subsume under it primarily the aspects of participatory design, which in turn is oriented toward a participatory research style as described by Hella von Unger (2014). Participatory design and participatory research share the dual objective of simultaneously understanding and changing social reality, as well as empowering co-researchers.

What is specific to participatory design are the explicitly creative tools and methods that are used. Elisabeth Sanders speaks of make-tools and distinguishes three categories: *telling*, *enacting*, and *making* (Sanders 2013). Depending on the objective (or the resources of the co-designers), for example, 2D or 3D collages may be used, cards are sorted according to preferences, or in design theater, products are acted out and scenarios are tested.

One advantage of design methods is that through joint drawing, building, and testing, communication can be fostered even where, for example, cognitive limitations make verbal exchange difficult.

Furthermore, visualizations or prototypes[1] help to make even abstract phenomena or visions tangible in the truest sense of the word. Translating concepts into something tangible is especially important when design laymen are to participate in developing design solutions.

[1] A prototype is understood as an initial approximation of a solution to be designed, which is not yet final in form but already allows for testing of its properties.

This type of participatory design is also often referred to as co-design. For the authors, the consistent participatory and qualitative orientation is a decisive criterion for a social design practice.[2]

The following two examples will outline the potential of a *social design practice*.

26.3 Dementia Things—Participatory Design with People with Dementia

The model project Dementia Things was funded by the Stiftung Wohlfahrtspflege NRW over a period of four years (2018–2022). The interdisciplinary research team consisted of designers (communication design, industrial design, social design), dementia experts (elderly care, social work, gerontology), and a sociologist who provided social science support for the project. Among other things, the project addressed the following question: *How can the lives of people with dementia and their caregiving relatives (in the home context) be improved through participatory design interventions and design empowerment?*

The project comprised two phases. The first phase focused on immersion in the field. In this phase, each designer teamed up with a dementia expert to form a competence team, which then worked together with a person with dementia and a caregiving person. In total, 14 households with a person with dementia were recruited, who were willing to welcome the competence teams into their homes and participate in the project through regular meetings.

The collaboration usually lasted several months, with the longest lasting almost a year. Initially, the competence teams aimed to get to know the people with dementia and their caregiving relatives in their everyday situations. Gradually, individual concerns, needs, and wishes were jointly identified and formulated, and some challenges and difficulties were uncovered.

To address these needs—or to improve a problematic situation—the so-called DementiaThings were developed in a participatory manner. A DementiaThing is a type of everyday aid that is designed *with* a person with dementia (see Fig. 26.1).

[2] Human-centered design can also be participatory, as by definition it is intended to place people at the center. However, this involvement often occurs only sporadically or is primarily based on quantitative market research mechanisms.

Universal design calls for a universal design for all, for example, products that work for both blind and sighted people. The idea of creating more inclusive products or environments is, in itself, absolutely commendable. However, not all specific needs can be addressed with a one-fits-all solution without risking that the universal solutions become so complex that the resulting complexity can, in turn, be exclusionary.

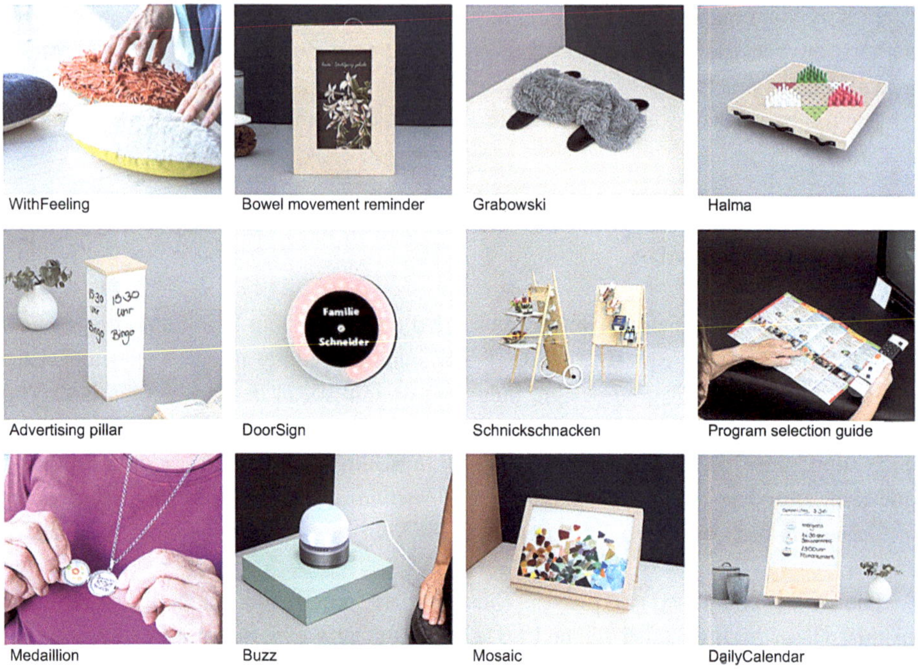

Fig. 26.1 Overview of some DementiaThings

The most important foundation for the participatory design processes was a resource-oriented perspective on the co-designers with dementia.

Fundamentally, many DementiaThings allow for a broader context of use. The *Day-Calendar* and the *Medallion* address the need for security by improving orientation within the daily structure. The *BowelMovementReminder* addresses safety in relation to one's own bodily functions.

The *Mosaic* also originated from a "hyper-personalised (designing for one) co-design approach" (Wilkinson and Hendriks 2022, p. 77) and was developed for a man with dementia who could no longer pursue his beloved hobby—stained glass work.

Nevertheless, various application contexts and other target groups are conceivable, even beyond cognitive impairments. Creating a mosaic is fun, has a calming and meditative effect, and particularly successful compositions can be displayed for one's own enjoyment and that of others.

In addition to focusing on the participatory design of everyday aids, the project also included a second level: the development of a training concept for caregivers. This targeted both caregiving relatives and nursing students, who, through the teaching of participatory design methods and raising awareness of the added value of design interventions in everyday care, are to be empowered to proactively address the challenges of caregiving.

To this end, the design processes leading to a DementiaThing within families were documented and evaluated. These findings formed the basis for a multimedia training concept,[3] consisting of a handbook, a video series, and a virtual dementia companion in the form of a chatbot, which addresses the psychological well-being of caregiving relatives by providing guidance on self-care techniques.

In the DementiaThings project, design had an impact on several levels:

On the one hand, tailored design outcomes—the DementiaThings—contribute to greater well-being in everyday life or can minimize friction.

On the other hand, design had an effect at the process level: a resource-oriented perspective on the co-designers with dementia is both a prerequisite and a result of a successful design process, and thus has positive effects on the relational level.

Thirdly, it was shown that design methods are excellently suited to enabling a form of communication even beyond cognitive impairments.

Finally, the project has an impact through the training media developed, in terms of design empowerment—that is, enabling caregivers by imparting design methods.

26.4 Interdisciplinary Student Semester Project *Palliative Care and Design*

In the summer semester of 2023, the authors, together with colleagues from the university, initiated and taught an interdisciplinary project between the Departments of Health and Design at FH Münster. In this tandem project, master's students from the field of Palliative Care worked together with master's students from the Design program on shared questions related to complex interventions. To this end, the students formed interdisciplinary working teams. The design students were able to participate in some seminars with their fellow students from Palliative Care in order to familiarize themselves with the domain. Due to curricular structures and the tight schedule of the part-time program, unfortunately, there was no opportunity for the Palliative Care students to attend the design seminars in return. However, within the Palliative Care seminars, space was created for interdisciplinary collaboration, and beyond that, the tandem teams met during their self-study time.

The Palliative Care students came from very different health and nursing professions and had, in some cases, only limited prior contact with the field of Palliative Care. The prospective designers therefore engaged with a wide range of focal points, depending on the prior experience brought by their team partners from the Health Department.

As a result, projects included, among others, a game to destigmatize the topic of dying, or a concept for a well-being-oriented occupational therapy treatment for palliative care patients. Here, with the help of various objects and a documentation tool, the

[3] Further information available at www.demenz-dinge.com.

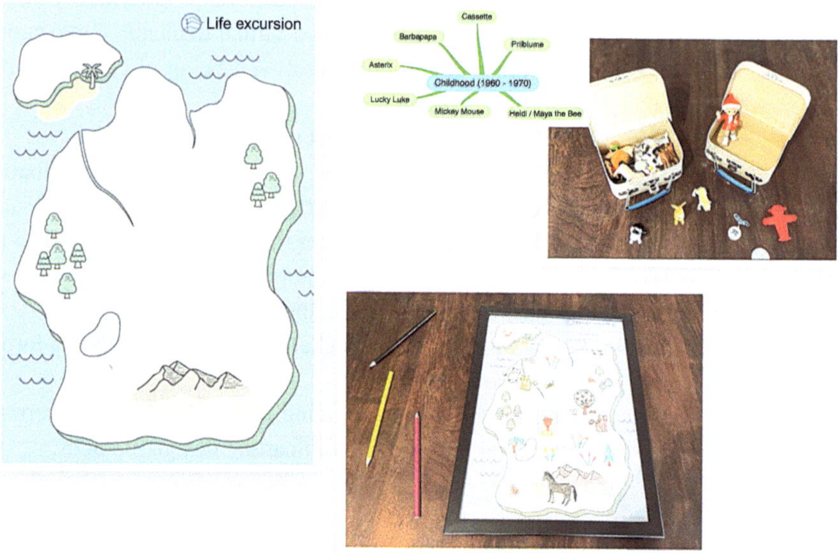

Fig. 26.2 Project Life Excursion: Suitcase and poster, adaptation of genogram work (courtesy of Tobias Brägelmann)

appropriate stimuli are gradually identified in order to tailor the treatment entirely to the person's preferences.

In the "Lebensausflug" (Life Excursion) project, the principle of genogram work was adapted (see Fig. 26.2). A genogram visually represents a person's family relationships. Unresolved, formative events or conflicts with relatives can also be noted. In the Life Excursion project, there are small suitcases with various objects that could relate to the person's age or origin, for example, a suitcase with objects reminiscent of the GDR. These are intended to encourage storytelling through the objects. Various *theme suitcases* can be tried out one after another. There is also a poster with a map on which hospice guests (with relatives or caregivers) can note biographically important dates or events, as well as wishes.

From the joint evaluation, three aspects seem to be of particular importance in the context of this contribution.

1. Outstanding were those projects in which the tandem teams had a close connection to the respective stakeholders, either through field access or through intensive interdisciplinary exchange.
2. The designers managed to immerse themselves very empathetically in the unfamiliar domain.

3. The Palliative Care students found it more difficult to engage in an interdisciplinary project team with designers than vice versa.[4]

26.5 Potential of Social Design in the Context of Chronic Care

The two examples illustrate the impact that social design, in the sense of participatory design, was able to achieve in the context of dementia and palliative care. In both projects, designers worked successfully in inter- and transdisciplinary teams with experts from the respective domains. In both projects, the design outcomes as well as the participatory design processes generated clear added value for those affected.

Design theorist Horst Rittel coined the term “wicked problems” in the 1960s (see contribution 56), referring to highly complex issues that cannot be understood from a single perspective. It is therefore justified that there is a call for inter- and transdisciplinary teams to address these multifaceted challenges. The classification of chronic disease as a “wicked problem” is widely accepted. Depending on how one operationalizes the term “single perspective,” it is worth discussing to what extent the disciplines currently involved in chronic care are already sufficiently broad to meet the challenges as effectively as possible.

Designers and design methods show great potential to generate diverse added value in the complex environment of chronic care:

- whether at the process level or as a design outcome
- whether as an object or artifact, or as a changed social practice
- whether as a solution to a problem or as an enhancement of subjective well-being

Design can focus on the affected individual, but can also initiate or accompany change processes at the structural, institutional, or even normative level.

In doing so, design can not only generate insights as a research method that explain a situation and describe the state that *is*. Design always has a projective character and asks: What *could* be, and in the design process describes “the emergence of what does not yet exist.” (Aicher 1991, p. 196). The design does not remain in a description of what is possible, but to a certain extent also involves the creation of what is possible (Bieling 2019).

With regard to person-centered care, design, in the sense of the social design approach presented and as an extension of an inter- and transdisciplinary care team, can help to

[4]The professor from the Health Department suggested that this might be due to a kind of customer-oriented attitude on the part of the designers. The authors argue that design (in contrast to art) does not create things solely from within itself, but always exists in close exchange with other disciplines. From this, one could conclude that designers are well equipped for collaboration in inter- or transdisciplinary teams.

sensitively identify "what is needed or wanted" and at the same time open up perspectives on "what is possible."

References

Aicher O (1991) die welt als entwurf – Schriften zum Design. Ernst & Sohn, Berlin

Bieling T (2019) Inklusion als Entwurf: Teilhabeorientierte Forschung Über, Für Und Durch Design. Birkhauser, Basel

Körner M, Bengel J (2004) Teamarbeit und Teamerfolg bei multi- und interdisziplinären Teams in der medizinischen Rehabilitation. Die Rehabilitation 43(6):348–357

Sanders E (2013) Perspectives on Participation in Design. In: Mareis C, Held M, Joost G (Hrsg) Wer gestaltet die Gestaltung? Praxis, Theorie und Geschichte des partizipatorischen Designs. transcript Verlag, Bielefeld S 65–78

Von Unger H (2014) Partizipative Forschung: Einführung in die Forschungspraxis. Springer VS, Wiesbaden

Wilkinson A, Hendriks N (2022) The emerge of empathy: through designing for one. In: Rodgers P (Hrsg) Design research for change: caring for people living with dementia. Routledge, New York pp 77–90

Digital Assistance Systems for the Care of Chronically Ill Persons

27

Peter Rasche, Theresa Sophie Busse, Ina Carola Otte and Horst Christian Vollmar

Contents

P. Rasche (✉)
Hochschule Niederrhein, Krefeld, Deutschland
e-mail: Peter.Rasche@hs-niederrhein.de

T. S. Busse · I. C. Otte · H. C. Vollmar
Ruhr-Universität Bochum, Abteilung für Allgemeinmedizin – Fach 15, Anke Prange MA 1/61, Bochum, Deutschland
e-mail: Theresa.Busse@ruhr-uni-bochum.de

I. C. Otte
e-mail: Ina.Otte@ruhr-uni-bochum.de

H. C. Vollmar
e-mail: horst.vollmar@ruhr-uni-bochum.de

D. Schmitz et al. (eds.), *Chronic Care—Science and Practice*,
https://doi.org/10.1007/978-3-662-72298-5_27

27.1 Assistance Systems

An assistance system (also referred to as assistive technology or assistive technology device) is a collection of technical aids, devices, software, or systems developed to support people with various types of limitations or needs. These systems aim to improve users' independence, mobility, communication, safety, and quality of life. Assistance systems can be used in many different areas, including healthcare, education, the workplace, daily life, and leisure (Luthe et al. 2022).

The range of assistance systems is very broad and is oriented toward the field of application and the individual needs of the target group. Assistance systems initially include well-known aids such as wheelchairs or hearing aids. However, due to digitalization, digital assistance systems are now also available, such as smartwatches for fall detection or home automation systems for targeted support in one's own home. These range from automated lighting to refrigerators that reorder supplies independently. Due to this wide range of applications and the associated level of support, assistance systems are found in various fields. Notably, the areas of Ambient Assisted Living or Active Assisted Living and Digital Health should be mentioned here (Luthe 2022). Ambient Assisted Living describes the use of assistive technologies to design the home environment in a way that promotes health and aims at health prevention. The term Digital Health refers to various digital assistance systems used therapeutically or actively in healthcare provision.

27.2 Ambient Assisted Living

The term Ambient Assisted Living or Active Assisted Living (AAL) refers to technologies and services designed to support and improve people's daily lives (Luthe 2022). This particularly applies to the lives of older people and individuals with physical and cognitive impairments (Wallhoff and Bruns 2023). The technologies used range from environmental sensors to communication and information platforms. AAL aims to improve quality of life and promote the autonomy of patients. In addition, AAL is also used to support caregivers. The goal here, alongside the physical and psychological relief of caregivers, is to increase the efficiency of care by integrating supportive technologies into everyday (nursing) routines. Here, too, prevention and health promotion are the main focus.

27.2.1 Historical Context of the Term in German-Speaking Countries

The term AAL was first coined in the early 2000s and has since developed into an important concept in healthcare and nursing. In Germany and the German-speaking region, AAL has established itself as a response to the growing challenge of demographic change, where the population is increasingly aging and the demand for supportive services and technologies is rising. In recent years, the German federal government has increasingly promoted the topic of AAL to drive innovation in the field of assistive technologies (Beyer-Wunsch 2021).

27.2.2 Current Trends Related to the Term *Ambient Assisted Living*

1. **Connected Health Monitoring:** Modern AAL technologies enable continuous monitoring of health parameters such as heart rate, blood pressure, and movement. This data can be transmitted in real time to caregivers or relatives to enable early response to changes in health status.
2. **Smart Home Integration:** AAL systems integrate seamlessly into the home environment and utilize smart home technologies, such as intelligent lighting, thermostats, or security systems. This enables a comfortable and safe environment for older people and individuals with impairments.
3. **(Assistance) Robots:** Advances in robotics have led to the development of assistive robots capable of performing simple tasks such as handing over objects or providing support with mobility. These robots can promote independence and social interaction.

These trends demonstrate the close connection between the AAL field and the topic of health and health care. It can also be noted that assistance systems, such as smart home solutions, make it easier for people with chronic illnesses to live long-term with a condition in their own homes as well as in care facilities (Hüning et al. 2022). The focus here is on maintaining patient autonomy. However, since these systems are not aimed at treating or explicitly compensating for limitations resulting from a chronic illness, further research areas on digital assistance systems need to be explored in the context of this contribution.

27.3 Digital Health

The research area of Digital Health focuses on the use of digital technologies, information and communication technologies (ICT), and electronic media to support and improve healthcare, prevention, diagnosis, treatment, and aftercare (Lorenz et al. 2022). It is a broad field of research that also includes the study of the development and use of digital assistance systems. These systems are designed for the diagnosis, treatment, and long-term support of people with chronic illnesses, with a particular focus on the care, support, and nursing of this target group.

Digital Health solutions are used in two settings: the home setting and the clinical setting. In the home setting, applications are used independently by patients. In the clinical setting, on the other hand, the applications primarily serve to support the work of healthcare providers. The aim of this support is to increase the efficiency of their work or to reduce the physical and psychological strain resulting from their professional activities.

27.3.1 Digital Health in the Home Setting

Assistance systems used in the home environment within the field of Digital Health enable, among other things, the continuous collection of health data, such as blood pressure, heart rate, and blood glucose levels (Lorenz et al. 2022). This allows changes in the course of illness to be detected early and therapeutic measures to be taken. This contributes to improved treatment and the prevention of complications.

Concrete examples include:

1. **Telemedicine solutions:** Telemedicine enables cooperation and communication between patients and providers across geographic distances. People with chronic illnesses can independently record their health data such as blood pressure, blood glucose levels, or heart rate at home and transmit them to their physicians. Contact with nursing staff for wound care is also a possible use case in the context of telecare. This form of cooperation enables continuous monitoring and regular, individualized adjustment of treatment plans.
2. **Smart health apps:** There is a wide range of mobile apps designed to support people with chronic illnesses in self-managing their health. These apps can provide medication reminders, enable symptom tracking, and record nutrition or physical activity.
3. **Implantable medical devices:** Some chronic conditions require continuous monitoring of internal bodily functions. Implantable medical devices such as pacemakers or insulin pumps can help stabilize and improve the health of people with chronic illnesses and enable them to lead a more self-determined life.
4. **Intelligent wearables:** Wearable devices such as smartwatches or fitness trackers can be used to track physical activity, sleep patterns, and heart rate. This information can help patients and providers assess the course of illness and make adjustments.
5. **Environmental health monitoring:** Sensor-based technologies can be installed in the home environment to record movement patterns and activities. These data can be used to detect changes in behavior that may indicate potential health problems. For example, a sudden lack of activity could indicate a deterioration in health status, or sensors could detect abrupt movements that may occur during falls.

These examples illustrate how Digital Health can help improve the care and support of people with chronic illnesses. Digital Health enables closer monitoring, early intervention, and facilitates self-management of health in everyday life.

27.3.2 Digital Health in the Clinical Setting and Inpatient Long-Term Care

Assistance systems in the clinical setting within the field of Digital Health usually support not only the patients themselves but also medical providers (Luthe et al. 2022). Due to the increasing shortage of skilled nursing staff and the physical challenges associated with nursing, solutions are continuously being developed to support both professional and informal caregivers in carrying out their tasks (Braeseke et al. 2022). Examples of Digital Health systems used in clinical settings and inpatient care include:

1. **Electronic patient records (EPR):** These systems enable healthcare professionals to electronically record, retrieve, and collaboratively use all relevant patient data. This simplifies documentation and facilitates access to important information. They are also used in outpatient settings.
2. **Medication management systems:** These systems help ensure the safe administration of medications. They can monitor dosages, check for interactions, and send medication reminders to providers and/or patients.
3. **Remote monitoring systems:** By using sensors and wearables, patients can be monitored over distances. Nursing professionals receive alerts or notifications when there are changes in health status, enabling early intervention. Nursing staff can also use telemedicine platforms to request medical consultations via video call, which can improve inpatient care.
4. **Care robots:** Robots can be used in care to take over simple tasks such as mobilizing and positioning patients or delivering medications. They can also serve as social companions for patients.
5. **Speech recognition and processing:** This technology enables nursing professionals to capture spoken information and convert it into text. This can facilitate documentation and communication.
6. **Hospital information and management systems:** These systems support the planning, coordination, and monitoring of care processes in hospitals and other facilities.
7. **Data analytics and artificial intelligence:** By analyzing large volumes of data, patterns can be identified that may be helpful in the diagnosis, treatment, and prevention of diseases.

Assistance systems in the clinical and inpatient care sector are primarily intended to support the work of on-site providers. They are designed to help improve the quality of patient care and make everyday work more efficient and less burdensome.

27.4 Ethical, Legal, and Social Aspects Surrounding Assistance Systems

The use of digital assistance systems in the care of people with chronic illnesses raises complex ethical and legal questions that must be carefully considered. Below, various key areas that should be taken into account when implementing these systems are presented and explained as examples. Important topics in the context of deploying such systems include data protection, data security, and privacy (Luthe et al. 2022). On the one hand, this is due to the collection of health-related data and the resulting increased need for protection in accordance with the General Data Protection Regulation. On the other hand, it is due to the technology used. A voice assistant is continuously active in order to respond when prompted. An example of this is the command *"Hey Siri!"* or saying the word "*Computer!*". Another key area is accessibility and equity. The implementation of assistance systems should be inclusive and not create a digital divide. In this context, such systems should also strengthen the autonomy and self-determination of their users. This can be achieved by ensuring that users retain control over their decisions and thus over the assistance system. With regard to the professional use of assistance systems, questions of liability and responsibility must also be addressed. In the event of malfunctions or incorrect diagnoses by assistance systems, it must be clear who bears responsibility. The issue of liability risk should also be clarified before a system is deployed. Fundamentally, the key area of trust and acceptance must also be considered (Luthe et al. 2022). In order to realize the benefits of assistance systems, patients and caregivers must trust in their accuracy and reliability and perceive the system as a means of reducing their own workload. Overall, the use of assistance systems requires a balanced consideration of these aspects to ensure the best possible support for people with chronic illnesses.

27.5 Financing of Assistance Systems

It is important to emphasize that the financing of digital assistance systems varies depending on individual needs, medical condition, level of care, and other factors. It is advisable to consult the relevant authorities, such as long-term care insurance funds, health insurance providers, physicians, or the Federal Office for Social Security, to obtain detailed information about the specific conditions and possibilities for cost coverage.

The simplest way to cover costs is for users to finance the assistance system themselves. Examples include smartphones, voice assistant systems, or smart home solutions. In addition, cost bearers such as long-term care insurance, health and nursing care funds, or social welfare agencies may also be considered for financing. However, financing by one of these institutions is generally linked to a specific legal mandate and requires compliance with specific formal requirements by the manufacturers of the systems. Cost coverage usually requires proof that the system is medically necessary and cost-efficient.

27.6 Acceptance of Assistance Systems

In addition, the question arises as to the acceptance of digital technologies among those affected. The acceptance of digital assistance systems is a decisive factor for their successful use (Braeseke et al. 2022). It depends on how well users embrace the technology and integrate it into their daily lives.

Factors influencing acceptance:

1. **Usefulness and Benefit:** Assistance systems should provide a clear benefit and meet the needs of users. If the technology is perceived as helpful, the likelihood of acceptance increases.
2. **Ease of Use:** The user interface and interaction with the system should be intuitive and easy to understand. Complex or difficult-to-use systems can lead to frustration and rejection.
3. **Availability of Support and Training:** Users need support when introducing and using new technologies, as digital and health literacy can vary. Providing training and technical support can enhance digital and health literacy and thus increase acceptance.
4. **Trust and Security:** Data protection and data security are crucial. Users must trust in the security of their data and feel protected against misuse.
5. **Adaptability:** The ability to adapt the assistance system to individual needs can increase acceptance. The better the technology matches personal preferences, the more likely it is to be accepted.

Overall, the acceptance of digital assistance systems strongly depends on prior experience, perceived benefit, user-friendliness, and trust in the technology. Careful design, consideration of users' needs, and clear communication are crucial to achieving high acceptance.

27.7 Participatory Development of Assistance Systems

The development of digital assistance systems is demanding and should be designed in a participatory manner. Future users (patients, providers, and relatives) should be involved early in the development process to understand their needs, requirements, and preferences and to incorporate them into the design of the assistance system from the outset. It is also important to involve users at multiple points during development to keep them engaged throughout the process and to be able to consider comprehensive requirements. This leads to the development of assistance systems that are better tailored to the needs and living circumstances of users, thereby increasing acceptance and adherence. In this context, adherence refers to the use of the systems—in the sense of using them with the correct "dose" ("use as it is designed" (Kernebeck et al. 2021, p. 1279)). This includes the respective frequency, intensity, duration, and type of system use. Approaches such as gamification (learning with playful elements), for example, can increase adherence. Close collaboration between technology developers, researchers, and future users is key to success.

27.8 Summary

Digital assistance systems are widely present in our everyday lives and are becoming increasingly important. This is also evident in the context of care and daily life for people with chronic illnesses. Nevertheless, it cannot yet be said that digital assistance systems are in widespread use across Germany. Despite problems in care resulting from illness, staff shortages, and rising costs, the challenges in the healthcare sector are diverse, and digital assistance systems are not yet being used on a broad scale to address them. Rather, the trend shows that assistance systems developed for the general public (such as speech recognition systems like Siri or Alexa) are being adapted for use in care.

The use of digital assistance systems requires not only acceptance of the technology but above all the competence and knowledge to use them (safely). This calls for initiatives to enhance the skills of patients, relatives, and providers in order to promote the ability to use these systems and to reduce barriers to their use.

Overall, it is clear that digital assistance systems have great potential to improve the care and support of people with chronic illnesses. They can contribute to early detection and treatment and enhance quality of life. At the same time, their use requires careful consideration of benefits and potential risks, as well as individual adaptation to the needs of those affected. Ongoing development and research in this field are crucial to finding the best solutions for the successful implementation of digital assistance systems in the chronic care context.

References

Beyer-Wunsch P (2021) Reichweite und Nomenklatur der AAL-Technologien. In: Sailer M, Mahr A (Eds) Active Assisted Living. Springer VS. https://doi.org/10.1007/978-3-658-34335-4_3

Braeseke G, Pflug C, Lingott N, Pörschmann-Schreiber U (2022) Technische Assistenzsysteme in der pflegerischen Versorgung. In: Luthe EW, Müller SV, Schiering I (Eds) Assistive Technologien im Sozial- und Gesundheitssektor. Gesundheit. Politik – Gesellschaft – Wirtschaft. Springer VS. https://doi.org/10.1007/978-3-658-34027-8_26

Hüning N, Schack E, Steinhart I (2022) Smart Home zur Unterstützung des Alltags von Menschen mit Beeinträchtigung. In: Luthe EW, Müller SV, Schiering I (Eds) Assistive Technologien im

Sozial- und Gesundheitssektor. Gesundheit. Politik – Gesellschaft – Wirtschaft. Springer VS. https://doi.org/10.1007/978-3-658-34027-8_32

Kernebeck S, Busse TS, Ehlers JP, Vollmar HC (2021) Adhärenz digitaler Interventionen im Gesundheitswesen: Definitionen, Methoden und offene Fragen. Bundesgesundheitsbl 64:1278–1284. https://doi.org/10.1007/s00103-021-03415-9

Lorenz T, Pleger M, Schiering I (2022) Smart Devices als Assistive Technologien. In: Luthe EW, Müller SV, Schiering I (Eds) Assistive Technologien im Sozial- und Gesundheitssektor. Gesundheit. Politik – Gesellschaft – Wirtschaft. Springer Fachmedien Wiesbaden

Luthe EW (2022) Rechtliche Rahmenbedingungen assistiver Technologien im Gesundheits- und Sozialsektor. In: Luthe EW, Müller SV, Schiering I (Eds) Assistive Technologien im Sozial- und Gesundheitssektor. Gesundheit. Politik – Gesellschaft – Wirtschaft. Springer VS. https://doi.org/10.1007/978-3-658-34027-8_18

Luthe EW, Müller SV, Schiering I (Eds) (2022) Assistive Technologien im Sozial- und Gesundheitssektor. Springer Fachmedien Wiesbaden

Wallhoff F, Bruns FT (2023) Assistive Technologien. In: Groß M, Hennig B, Kappel S, Wallhoff F (Eds) Assistive Technologien, technische Rehabilitation und Unterstützte Kommunikation. Springer. https://doi.org/10.1007/978-3-662-64118-7_1

Part III

Organizational Level of Chronic Care: Fundamental Aspects, Institutional Forms of Care, and Self-Determined Living

Migration and Chronic Care 28

Patrick Brzoska and Yüce Yilmaz-Aslan

Contents

28.1 Background

The population of Germany and other European countries includes a significant proportion of people with a migration background. This group differs from people without a migration background in several health-related aspects. On average, they experience certain chronic diseases more frequently than people of the same age without a migration background. These differences can be attributed to social and health-related influences to

P. Brzoska (✉) · Y. Yilmaz-Aslan
Witten/Herdecke University, Faculty of Health, School of Medicine, Health Services Research, Witten, Germany
e-mail: Patrick.Brzoska@uni-wh.de

Y. Yilmaz-Aslan
e-mail: Yuece.Yilmaz-Aslan@uni-wh.de

D. Schmitz et al. (eds.), *Chronic Care—Science and Practice*,
https://doi.org/10.1007/978-3-662-72298-5_28

which people with a migration background are exposed. While some of these influences are positive, stressful working conditions, an unfavorable social situation, and discrimination act as negative factors contributing to health disadvantages. Healthcare facilities are often unable to address these challenges comprehensively, resulting in people with a migration background facing barriers at all stages of the care process that hinder their access to services and may negatively affect care outcomes. This article illustrates these issues using the nursing care and rehabilitation sectors as examples. It also demonstrates why, in addition to migration background, other diversity characteristics must be considered in order to sustainably enable user-oriented care for the entire population.

28.2 The Health of People with a Migration Background in Germany

The population of Germany is constantly changing. More than 22.3 million people, and thus more than a quarter of the population, now have a migration background (Federal Statistical Office 2022). This means that they themselves or their parents immigrated to Germany from another country.[1] People with a migration background are highly heterogeneous due to their diverse cultural, religious, and linguistic backgrounds. People of Turkish descent and German resettlers ([Spät-]Aussiedler/innen) are among the largest groups with a migration background in Germany.

Data on the health of people with a migration background are limited. Available survey studies and routine data from social insurance providers suggest that, in particular, older people with a migration background have a higher prevalence of certain chronic diseases such as type 2 diabetes mellitus. With regard to other diseases, such as some oncological conditions, there are also health advantages, which are reflected, among other things, in lower incidence rates. In terms of work-related morbidity, non-German nationals—a subgroup of people with a migration background who are often the only group identifiable in health reporting data—have a higher risk of occupational accidents, occupational diseases, and reduced earning capacity. This can be explained by the employment profiles of people with a migration background, which expose them more frequently to stressful working conditions. Individuals who come to Germany as refugees are also exposed to additional specific physical and psychological burdens. They have often experienced violence in their countries of origin and have frequently undergone a traumatic journey of fleeing their home country. These experiences also contribute to a significantly higher prevalence of mental disorders such as depression and post-traumatic stress disorder among them (Brzoska and Razum 2015).

---

[1] For a critical discussion of the term migration background, see, among others, Federal Government Expert Commission on the Framework Conditions for Integration Potential *(2021). Shaping Immigration Society Together. Berlin: Federal Chancellery.*

28.3 Utilization and Outcomes of Healthcare Services

Available studies indicate that people with a migration background differ from those without a migration background in their use of healthcare services. In particular, primary and secondary prevention services such as dental or cancer screening examinations are used less frequently by them. There are also differences in the area of nursing care, where people with a migration background primarily make use of financial assistance and provide care themselves, and only rarely use professional outpatient nursing care services (Yilmaz-Aslan et al. 2021). Although the data situation in the field of rehabilitation is more inconsistent, studies also suggest that some population groups with a migration background make less use of rehabilitative care services. These differences cannot be explained solely by the influence of socioeconomic or health-related factors (Brzoska and Razum 2015).

Similar to the utilization of care, there are also differences in care outcomes. People with a migration background who use healthcare services are not only less satisfied with their care, but on average also achieve less favorable care outcomes (Brzoska and Razum 2015). In the field of rehabilitation, this is reflected, for example, in a higher risk of reduced earning capacity after rehabilitation, poorer self-rated treatment outcomes, or an unfavorable social-medical assessment at the end of rehabilitation. For instance, a study based on routine data from the German Pension Insurance for the years 2006–2016 among individuals who completed rehabilitation for musculoskeletal and connective tissue diseases showed that patients with citizenship from Turkey or the successor states of former Yugoslavia had, during the period mentioned, an approximately 50% higher statistical chance of completing rehabilitation with an unfavorable outcome (adjusted odds ratio [aOR] = 1.56; 95% CI = 1.45–1.67 and aOR = 1.52; 95% CI = 1.41–1.65, respectively) (Brzoska et al. 2023).

28.4 Barriers in Healthcare

A wide range of quantitative and especially qualitative studies have identified challenges and barriers faced by people with a migration background in the healthcare system. These affect needs-based and user-oriented care, which can negatively affect access to care and its outcomes. Challenges become apparent, for example, in problems with communication and interaction between healthcare users and healthcare staff, which are due to insufficient information about available services, limited health literacy, and lack of language skills. In addition to language and information deficits, problems in communication and interaction can also arise from a lack of sensitivity on the part of healthcare facilities to the needs and care expectations of people with a migration background, for example regarding concepts of illness and treatment. Both overt and covert discrimination experienced by people with a migration background in the healthcare system also have a detrimental effect on care (Brzoska and Razum 2015).

28.5 Sustainable Implementation of User-Oriented Care Considering Intersectional Differences

To ensure user-oriented healthcare for people with a migration background, providing specialized services for selected population groups with a migration background is not enough. This approach does not do justice to the heterogeneity of the population group, nor to the fact that other diversity characteristics, independent of migration background, can also be associated with inequalities in care. As shown in the aforementioned study by Brzoska et al. (2023), for example, women had a higher statistical chance than men of completing rehabilitation with a negative outcome (aOR = 1.11; 95% CI = 1.08–1.13). Furthermore, rehabilitation patients with low socioeconomic status had a higher chance of an unfavorable rehabilitation outcome than those with high socioeconomic status (aOR = 1.13; 95% CI = 1.10–1.17). The study also demonstrated that diversity characteristics can interact with each other (intersectionality). For example, the differences between men and women as well as between rehabilitation patients with low and high socioeconomic status partially decreased with age, while the differences between German and non-German nationals increased with age. An exploratory analysis of the interaction between gender, nationality, and age also showed that among men, differences between German nationals on the one hand and nationals from Turkey and a successor state of former Yugoslavia on the other existed across all age groups and tended to increase with age. Among women in both groups, the differences also increased with age, but only became pronounced from the age of 45 onwards.

This example shows that inequalities in healthcare are not caused by a single factor, but that many determinants are involved, some of which interact with each other. Consequently, it is not enough to consider only selected diversity characteristics such as migration status in the design of care in order to provide appropriate healthcare to all population groups. Instead, healthcare facilities must implement strategies and frameworks that take into account the diversity of needs and expectations and their interactions as a whole. Through such an intersectional approach, they can better implement user-oriented care, which can lead to higher satisfaction with care and better care outcomes. Healthcare facilities are aware of this necessity, as surveys in various healthcare sectors show (e.g., Aksakal et al. 2023b). However, suitable strategies to promote diversity-sensitive care are rarely used (Aksakal et al. 2023b). This is also due to the lack of practical overviews of suitable tools that can be used for this purpose. In a recent project, this limitation for rehabilitative care in Germany was addressed by developing the DiversityKAT manual with tools and recommendations that can support rehabilitation facilities in implementing diversity-sensitive care approaches (Aksakal et al. 2023a). These tools include, for example, diversity-sensitive mission statements, diversity training, mentoring programs, the employment of diversity officers, the use of needs assessment forms, or the deployment of interpreters. The selection of specific diversity-sensitive care strategies depends on the particular characteristics and goals of the respective healthcare facilities. These must be determined as part of a needs assessment.

A diversity-sensitive approach should also take into account that healthcare personnel themselves are characterized by diversity. Diversity-sensitive human resource management strategies can help address challenges arising from limited German language skills, lack of knowledge of the German healthcare system, or differences in training content in countries of origin. At the same time, the potential associated with a different cultural background and foreign language skills can be leveraged to optimize care processes and facilitate more user-oriented care.

28.6 Conclusions

Compared to people without a migration background, people with a migration background are often disadvantaged in terms of their health and socioeconomic factors. In the healthcare system, they encounter barriers that can negatively affect access to care and care outcomes. In order to make care more user-oriented for the entire population and improve opportunities for participation, it is crucial to remove these barriers and sensitize healthcare facilities to the needs and expectations of their diverse users. The implementation and evaluation of appropriate strategies play a central role in this process. In the long term, only diversity-sensitive services will enable sustainable care for the entire population, including people with a migration background.

References

Aksakal T, Mader M, Annac K, Erdsiek F, Korn M, Padberg D, Idris M, Yilmaz-Aslan Y, Razum O, Brzoska P (2023a) Handreichung zu Umsetzungsmöglichkeiten diversitätssensibler Versorgung in der Rehabilitation. https://www.deutsche-rentenversicherung.de/SharedDocs/Downloads/DE/Experten/reha_forschung/forschungsprojekte/handreichung_diversitykat.html. Deutsche Rentenversicherung Bund, Berlin

Aksakal T, Erdsiek F, Yilmaz-Aslan Y, Mader M, Padberg D, Razum O, Brzoska P (2023b) Umsetzungsstrategien einer diversitätssensiblen Gesundheitsversorgung und Unternehmensführung: Eine bundesweite postalische Befragung von Rehabilitationseinrichtungen. Die Rehabilitation 62:40–47

Brzoska P, Razum O (2015) Erreichbarkeit und Ergebnisqualität rehabilitativer Versorgung bei Menschen mit Migrationshintergrund. Bundesgesundheitsbl Gesundheitsforsch Gesundheitsschutz 58:553–559

Brzoska P, Annac K, Yilmaz-Aslan Y (2023) Intersectional differences in health care outcomes among patients with musculoskeletal disorders in Germany. Reports 6:20

Statistisches Bundesamt (2022) Bevölkerung und Erwerbstätigkeit: Bevölkerung mit Migrationshintergrund: Ergebnisse des Mikrozensus 2021. (Fachserie 1 Reihe 2.2)

Yilmaz-Aslan Y, Aksakal T, Annac K, Razum O, Özer-Erdogdu I, Tezcan-Güntekin H, Brzoska P (2021) Diversität in der Pflege am Beispiel von Menschen mit Migrationshintergrund. In: Bonacker M, Geiger G (Eds) Migration in der Pflege: Wie Diversität und Individualisierung die Pflege verändern. Springer, Heidelberg, pp 155–171

Transculturality, Cultural Appropriateness, Cultural Sensitivity, and Cultural Competence in Health Care

29

Heike Becker and Manfred Fiedler

Contents

29.1 Concept of Culture

Before we approach the keywords in the heading within the text, it is necessary to first clarify what is meant by culture in this contribution.

This text is based on the expanded concept of culture by Hilmar Hoffmann, encapsulated in the formula *Culture for all*. He places everyday culture on an equal footing with high culture, as it is, for example, experienced in museums and operas (Hoffmann 1981). "For culture is how people live and how they relate to their fellow human beings" (Hoffmann 1990, p. 58). This understanding includes all forms of everyday social interaction,

H. Becker (✉)
Faculty of Health, Witten/Herdecke University, Witten, Germany
e-mail: heike.becker@uni-wh.de

M. Fiedler
Department of human medicine, Witten/Herdecke University, Witten, Germany
e-mail: manfred.fiedler@uni-wh.de

D. Schmitz et al. (eds.), *Chronic Care—Science and Practice*,
https://doi.org/10.1007/978-3-662-72298-5_29

such as living culture, food culture, work culture, and consequently also the culture of health, illness, and their care settings (see Contribution 37).

Accordingly, the subjective, culturally appropriate (cultural) design of care settings (see Contributions 16 and 17) is closely intertwined with the respective biography and identity of those affected. Nevertheless, as explained in the following text, biography and identity must be distinguished from one another.

Biographical research considers a person's biography as a self-description or description by others, which is expressed orally or in writing in formal or informal contexts and documented according to the given framework conditions.

Thus, a person's biography is an active (re)interpretation and construction of the past, which may be subject to societal or institutionalized patterns, some of which have also been internalized during the socialization process, in order to narrate one's own life story. Ideally, this enables the person to attain interpretive authority and, beyond that, orientation in their actions and life plans (Rosenthal 2014).

Identity, on the other hand, is only formed through communication—including nonverbal communication such as gestures and facial expressions—and interaction with other people in different normative systems, action contexts, and their respective contradictions. Thus, it is subject to a constant dynamic process of change, adjustment, and adaptation, in order to achieve a balance between the demands and expectations of others and individual needs (Krappmann 2010).

The building blocks of identity are coherence, authenticity, recognition, resources, agency, and narration, whose balance is fundamental in everyday identity work. A successful identity emerges when a person has found their own measure within this dynamic context (Keupp et al. 2013) (see Contribution 37).

29.2 On the Understanding of Culture and Cultural Sensitivity in the Health Sciences Discourse

Over the past 20 years, at least in terms of terminology, cultural sensitivity has become established in the German healthcare landscape. In light of increasing migration, for example due to displacement, it has gained importance, as demonstrated by the project in North Rhine-Westphalia funded by the Robert Bosch Foundation to promote cultural competence among physicians, nurses, and medical assistants (Bartig 2023; Kassenärztliche Vereinigung Nordrhein 2018).

Although the concept of culture is understood in a rather colorful and diverse way in international scientific discourse, in Germany we primarily encounter it with regard to ethnic, national, and geographic origin (German Ethics Council 2010). While this definition of the term acknowledges that people's cultural (self-)definition is of particular importance in dealing with illness and health, on the other hand, this narrowing of the concept of culture focuses on human difference through otherness. In turn, it assumes that for locals, the non-foreign, care requirements are identical within certain boundaries and thus are each *culturally* appropriate.

Evidence for this can be found in epidemiological analyses of health data for migrants compared to the native (in the broadest sense, of German descent) population, which show significantly poorer values, for example regarding life expectancy or specific morbidity (Razum and Neuhauser 2008).

Longitudinal studies, taking into account socio-economic data such as income or educational level, indicate that care outcomes also vary greatly within the culturally differentiated social groups (migrants—non-migrants) (Razum and Wenner 2016; Wadenpohl 2017). In other words, even regardless of migration background, health opportunities are unequally distributed.

A twofold hierarchy of social health opportunities becomes apparent: in the social cross-section as a differentiation between migrants and non-migrants, and in the socio-cultural longitudinal section for socio-economically defined social strata (Bailey et al. 2017; Brownson et al. 2021; Kapadia et al. 2022).

One might now simply assume that, in the case of longitudinal differentiation, we are dealing exclusively with socio-economically determined working and living conditions, which are considered restrictions on the realization of a health-promoting lifestyle. This is an overly simplistic conclusion. Nevertheless, socio-economic factors undoubtedly play an extraordinarily significant role (Henseke 2018).

Spatially distributed living situations (Weisser 1978) or milieus, differing from the class-differentiating concept of milieu (Wippernann 2009), are particularly relevant when medical and nursing care takes place in the home environment and intervenes in or enters into action-oriented communication with the everyday contexts of life, such as family, neighborhood, and circle of friends.

Against this background, focusing solely on ethnic and/or religious otherness does not suffice to meet the requirements of an effectiveness-oriented healthcare system. A society therefore consists of a politically guiding, intended culture with a normative character depending on its strictness (dominant culture (Beichelt 2003)), and a multitude of lived cultures, which possess both familiar and unfamiliar (foreign) characteristics among themselves. This real plurality or diversity of lifestyles and life worlds is better captured by a non-normative definition of culture, as well as by a comprehensive concept of emergence.

In the context considered here, the focus is on recognizing a group-related rather than a society-related concept of culture, which emphasizes difference (diversity). This includes, in addition to religion and ethnicity, sexual orientation, socio-economic aspects (e.g., income, education, career orientation), as well as spatial influences on cultural experience (e.g., degree of urbanization, neighborhood/milieu).

This group-based differentiation is important for approaching an understanding of culturally sensitive care in healthcare, as it acknowledges the diversity within modern societies as a working basis.

29.3 Cultural Sensitivity, Cultural Competency, or Cultural Equity—Differentiating Concepts in Healthcare Provision

In the immigration countries of the USA and Canada, it is not surprising that one encounters not only a wide range of culturally differentiated care concepts. There is also a greater number of group-specific prevalence studies, for example on heart failure, obesity, or specific types of cancer. Furthermore, a variety of different concepts can be found that aim to address the requirements for appropriate healthcare arising from the plurality of culturally influenced life worlds.

In contrast, German concepts are more practice-oriented and focus primarily on barriers to accessing services, particularly those related to language and unfamiliarity (for migrants).

It is therefore important to make a terminological distinction and to relate each term to a fundamental conceptual understanding.

In the Anglo-American literature, three fundamental terms can essentially be distinguished: 1. Cultural Sensitivity 2. Cultural Competency 3. Cultural Equity. These can be translated as cultural sensitivity, cultural competency, and cultural equity, respectively.

The terms cultural sensitivity and cultural competency are often used synonymously; in particular, what is understood in German as cultural sensitivity is also described in Anglo-American contexts with the term cultural competency. While in German-language literature, cultural competency is usually understood as an element of personnel development, that is, as personal capability or qualification (Droste et al. 2015), in Anglo-American literature, institutional or organizational capability is also described with cultural competency (Betancourt 2002), instead of the term cultural sensitivity, which is used less frequently. Cultural equity, as a system-level concept, is almost absent from German-language literature. Cultural equity thus refers to the cultural appropriateness of systemic structures and services.

These three definitions make it possible to capture the fundamental levels of healthcare provision: on the one hand, the service provision level, which concerns culturally appropriate, needs-based care structures that enable non-discriminatory access; on the other hand, the organizational or institutional level, which is organizationally sensitive in dealing with diversity; and finally, the level of health professions, which, in the sense of a person-centered understanding, have developed competencies to deal with cultural diversity in their professional practice.

References

Arbeitskreis Migration und öffentliche Gesundheit, Unterarbeitsgruppe Krankenhaus (2015) Das kultursensible Krankenhaus: Ansätze zur interkulturellen Öffnung. Praxisratgeber, Berlin

Bailey ZD, Krieger N, Agénor M, Graves J, Linos N, Bassett MT (2017) Structural racism and health inequities in the USA: evidence and interventions. Lancet 389(10077):1453–1463. https://doi.org/10.1016/S0140-6736(17)30569-X

Bartig S (2023) Gesundheit von Menschen mit ausgewählten Staatsangehörigkeiten in Deutschland – Ergebnisse der Studie GEDA Fokus. Vorab-Onlinepublikation. https://doi.org/10.25646/11089

Betancourt JR (2002) Cultural competence in health care: emerging frameworks and pracitical approaches. Field report

Brownson RC, Kumanyika SK, Kreuter MW, Haire-Joshu D (2021) Implementation science should give higher priority to health equity. Implement Sci 16(1):28. https://doi.org/10.1186/s13012-021-01097-0

Deutscher Ethikrat (Hrsg) (2010) Migration und Gesundheit: Kulturelle Vielfalt als Herausforderung für die medizinische Versorgung

Droste M, Gün AK, Kiefer H, Koch E, Naimi I, Reinecke H, Wächter M, Wesselman E (2015) Das kultursensible Krankenhaus: Ansätze zur interkulturellen Öffnung, 2. Aufl. Praxisratgeber erstellt vom bundesweiten Arbeitskreis Migration und öffentliche Gesundheit, Unterarbeitsgruppe Krankenhaus, Berlin

Henseke G (2018) Good jobs, good pay, better health? The effects of job quality on health among older European workers. Eur J Health Econ 19(1):59–73. https://doi.org/10.1007/s10198-017-0867-9

Hoffmann H (1981) Kultur für alle: Perspektiven und Modelle. Fischer, Frankfurt am Main

Hoffmann H (1990) Kultur als Lebensform. Fischer, Frankfurt am Main

Kapadia D, Zhang J, Salway S, Nazroo J, Booth A, Villarroel-Williams N, Bécares L, Esmail A (2022) Ethnic inequalities in healthcare; a rapid evidence review. Final report V7. https://www.nhsrho.org/wp-content/uploads/2022/02/RHO-Rapid-Review-Final-Report_v.7.pdf

Kassenärztliche Vereinigung Nordrhein (2018) Kultursensible Versorgung: Ärzte, Zahnärzte, MFA und Pflegende erproben interprofessionelles Fortbildungskonzept [Pressemitteilung] (14. März). Bielefeld. https://www.kvno.de/60neues/2018/pm_kultursensible-versorgung/index.html

Keupp H, Ahbe T, Gmür W, Höfer R, Mitzscherlich B, Kraus W, Strauss F (2013) Identitätskonstruktionen: Das Patchwork der Identitäten in der Spätmoderne, 5. Aufl. Rowolt, Hamburg

Krappmann L (2010) Soziologische Dimensionen der Identität: Strukturelle Bedingungen für die Teilnahme an Interaktionsprozessen, 11. Aufl. Klett-Cotta, Stuttgart

Razum O, Neuhauser H (2008) Migration und Gesundheit: Schwerpunktbericht der Gesundheitsberichterstattung des Bundes. Gesundheitsberichterstattung des Bundes. Robert-Koch-Inst. http://nbn-resolving.de/urn:nbn:de:0257-1002227

Razum O, Wenner J (2016) Social and health epidemiology of immigrants in Germany: past, present and future. Public Health Rev 37:4. https://doi.org/10.1186/s40985-016-0019-2

Reichelt T (2003) Herrschaftskultur: ein Konzept zur kulturwissenschaftlichen Öffnung der Vergleichenden Politikwissenschaft. Berliner Debatte Initial 14(1):60–74

Rosenthal G (2014) Biographieforschung. In: Bauer N, Blasius J (Hrsg) Handbuch Methoden der empirischen Sozialforschung. Springer, Wiesbaden, pp 509–520

Wadenpohl S (2017) Gesundheit und Bildung von Kindern im Sozialraum: Integrierter Gesundheits- und Bildungsbericht 2017. Recklinghausen

Weisser G (1978) Beiträge zur Gesellschaftspolitik: Philosophische Vorfragen – beratende Sozialwissenschaft – soziale Sicherung – Mitbestimmung – Verteilungs- und Vermögenspolitik – Ordnungspolitik – besonders Einzelwirtschaftspolitik (Katterle S, Mudra W, Neumann L, Neumann LF Hrsg). Verlag Otto Schwartz & Co, Göttingen

Wippernann C (2009) Lebensstile und Milieus: Einflüsse auf die Gesundheit. In: Schumpelick V (Hrsg) Herder Taschenbücher. Volkskrankheiten: Gesundheitliche Herausforderungen in der Wohlstandsgesellschaft; Beiträge des Symposiums vom 4. bis 7. September 2008 in Cadenabbia; [„Cadenabbia-Gespräche Medizin – Ethik – Recht“ in der Villa La Collina. Herder, pp 143–156

Structured Care: Prevention—Cure—Rehabilitation—Long-Term Care

30

Manfred Fiedler

Contents

30.1 Definition of Terms

Healthcare systems are structured both functionally and in terms of inherent care relationships. This segmented care is characterized by the fact that, within the various functional sectors of care, professional actors operate in different institutions with specific care responsibilities. The respective service contents and objectives differ accordingly.

For recipients of services, this segmentation can lead to interfaces that impair the continuity of care (see Contribution 31). Nevertheless, the segmented structure of a healthcare system does provide orientation for those involved, as responsibilities and thus points of contact—such as on the side of insurers and for patients—are organized.

What is special about segmented care is not only its functional and professional significance on the side of service provision and providers, but also that, based on this structure, financial regulations (remuneration structures) and, furthermore, substantive

M. Fiedler (✉)
Department of human medicine, Witten/Herdecke University, Witten, Germany
e-mail: manfred.fiedler@uni-wh.de

D. Schmitz et al. (eds.), *Chronic Care – Science and Practice*,
https://doi.org/10.1007/978-3-662-72298-5_30

responsibilities in the sense of institutional leadership on the part of payers or service providers are linked. This means that different social insurance providers are responsible for different areas of care within the segmented structure of the healthcare system. For example, statutory long-term care insurance is responsible for long-term nursing care, and statutory accident insurance is responsible for the care of individuals harmed by occupational activities. This segmentation among social insurance providers is associated with an entitlement to benefits in a care sector according to the type and scope of services (see Contribution 41).

30.2 Segmented Care: Between Horizontal and Vertical Segmentation

Generally, a distinction is made between horizontal and vertical segmentation. In horizontal segmentation, we differentiate according to the functional and professional tasks and contents of care, that is, between (nursing) long-term care, curative (acute) care, or rehabilitation. These are often also regulated by special laws. In contrast, these fields of care are vertically segmented into institutional sites of care, essentially the major care settings.

On the horizontal, professional-functional level, we differentiate between curative/acute care, rehabilitation, and long-term care (see Fig. 30.1). On the vertical level, we usually distinguish between the levels of home-based, outpatient, semi-inpatient, and inpatient care. In the systemic segmentation, there are indeed intermediate forms, such as short-term care within long-term care.

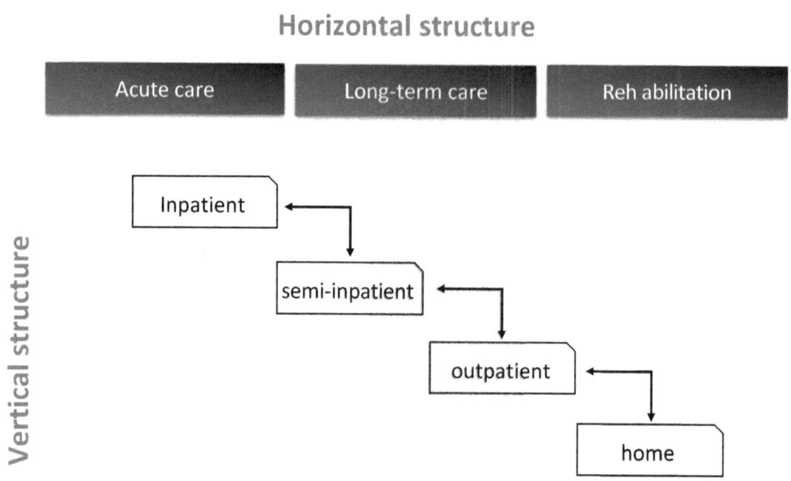

Fig. 30.1 Horizontal—Vertical Segmentation

This means that, vertically, we ask about the degree of institutionalization and the spatial context of care, i.e., how closely it is organized to the everyday life of those affected.

While in horizontal segmentation, services can be provided simultaneously, for example in the context of long-term care and curative care, in vertical segmentation, services are provided as part of a treatment chain. They are not delivered simultaneously, but sequentially, related to the disease or life phase, in a (structured) sequence of interventions, such as a treatment chain.

For example, the transition from home-based to inpatient long-term care is a life-phase-related change, as home care can no longer be organized on a permanent basis. Treatment chains in the sense of transitions from outpatient to inpatient care and back to outpatient care are found in curative care.

30.3 Care Sectors in Structured Healthcare Provision

The following provides a brief introduction to the individual care sectors.

1. **Prevention as a Principle of Preventing or Delaying Disease**
Prevention aims to avert disease itself or its manifestation. The focus is on both individual and group-related risk for disease, as well as the means of disease prevention.

Prevention is less a clearly defined service area, which is why it is not easily assigned to a specific sector within structured healthcare provision. On the one hand, prevention is a goal, for example in the form of health objectives with varying spatial and social group relevance. On the other hand, it is a fundamental societal field of action, particularly in the area of public health (e.g., food safety, environmental protection) and occupational health and safety. The main aim here is to reduce prevalence and incidence.

Primary prevention includes measures and services that prevent the onset of diseases (Rosenbrock 2008). The early detection of disease is called secondary prevention, which aims to influence the severity of the disease course or to avoid chronicity. This also includes the goal of preventing recurrence (tertiary prevention). Traditionally, these are targeted rehabilitative and therapeutic services aimed at the physical and psychological strengthening of those affected following acute treatment.

Furthermore, we distinguish between structural prevention and behavioral prevention. Structural prevention concerns requirements for health protection in areas not directly assigned to the healthcare system. For example, in occupational health and safety, there is an obligation to prevent work-related illnesses and accidents. In occupational health and safety, we distinguish a hierarchy of measures. First comes the design of the work environment, the avoidance of health-damaging and the creation of health-promoting conditions in work processes. If structural prevention measures are insufficient, person-related measures, such as the use of protective equipment (as in infection wards in hospitals), and finally behavioral preventive measures through work instructions or staff training become necessary.

Beyond this, structural prevention is particularly relevant to social and living environments, especially as public health (see contribution 48). Behavioral prevention, in turn, is particularly significant for measures related to individuals' lifestyle and everyday experiences. For this context of preventive measures and programs, identifying risk groups and risk behaviors is crucial.

2. **Curative Care**

Curative care (acute care) encompasses all services and interventions aimed at curing an existing disease where possible or improving the health status affected by the disease. Curative services account for the largest share of total healthcare expenditures. Approximately two-thirds of all healthcare spending is directly allocated to acute care.

In acute care, a distinction is made between primary care, secondary care, and acute inpatient care (see Fig. 30.2).

In Germany, primary care refers to general practitioner and family medicine, which usually also includes pediatric and gynecological care. This definition is due to the structure of the German healthcare system and only partially corresponds to the international understanding of primary care. In other countries, an initial consultation with a physician is not necessarily required at the start of treatment. Hospitals or individuals with medical qualifications may also be the first point of contact in the event of an acute illness.

Secondary care includes specialist medical care or specialized physician services (Klein-Hitpaß and Leber 2012). Looking more closely at what this means, we see that

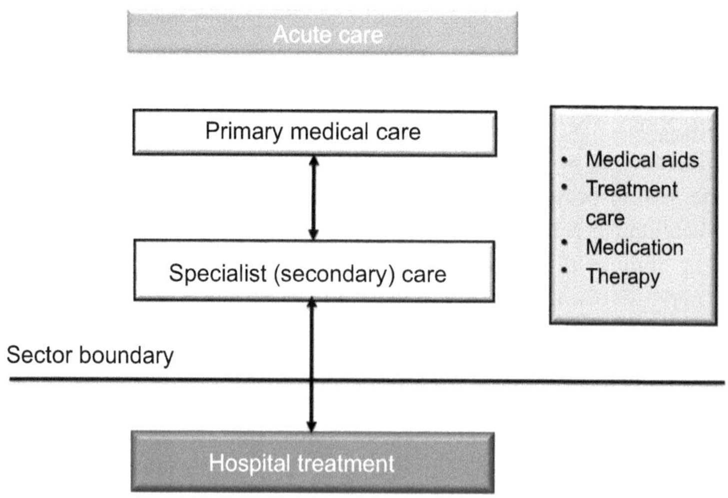

Fig. 30.2 Acute Care Structure. (Own illustration)

specialist care is usually provided by referral from primary care physicians or a primary care facility. Internationally, secondary care is often closely linked to inpatient care. Outpatient specialists routinely work at or in connection with hospitals. In Germany, hospital physicians can only participate in outpatient care if they are authorized to do so or act in a private medical capacity. Outpatient activities by hospital physicians can reduce interface issues between secondary care in inpatient settings, such as for post-discharge care. Another possibility is for primarily outpatient physicians to work as attending physicians at hospitals.

Inpatient acute care includes the treatment of all somatic, psychiatric, and psychosomatic patients in inpatient facilities (hospitals) who, for professional or patient safety reasons, cannot be treated on an outpatient basis.

This division between primary, secondary, and inpatient care is a vertical one, meaning it usually does not occur simultaneously but rather through transitions between the levels.

3. **Rehabilitation**

Rehabilitation aims, primarily through therapeutic measures, to compensate for disease-related physical, social, mental, and psychological consequences and to restore individuals to a state as close as possible to their pre-illness condition.

We generally distinguish between medical, occupational, and social rehabilitation. Medical rehabilitation focuses on restoring the physical, mental, and everyday abilities lost due to illness so that those affected can lead as independent a life as possible, with little or no external support. Occupational rehabilitation (Stöbe-Blossey et al. 2021) additionally aims at reintegration into the workplace, while social rehabilitation (Simeon 2014) seeks to increase opportunities for social participation that have been limited by illness or accident.

Rehabilitation can be provided on an outpatient, day clinic, or fully inpatient basis within the vertical structure. The different goals and forms result in differentiated relationships with other care sectors, such as follow-up treatment after acute care or rehabilitation to stabilize or improve the situation of people in need of care.

4. **Long-Term Care**

The term long-term care is rather uncommon in Germany. Internationally, however, it is referred to as *Long Term Care* and means the care of people who require continuous, long-term support. In Germany, this refers to nursing services provided at home or in institutional long-term care settings. Medical or therapeutic services are not included under this term. As previously mentioned, the basic vertical structure is usually seen as a life-phase-related transition. Nevertheless, there are types of care, such as short-term care, where people are cared for in an inpatient facility due to the temporary, short-term absence of professional home care or informal caregivers. Temporary inpatient or outpatient care may also become necessary if, following an acute medical intervention, transitional care is required before further treatment in another setting.

30.4 Chronically Ill People in the Segmented Care System

The needs of chronically ill people cut across the segmentation of the healthcare system. From a social policy perspective, Herder Dorneich refers to socio-economic regulatory cycles within the healthcare sector (Herder-Dorneich 1986). In addition to the relevance under social law, it should be noted that those affected constantly move between functional and professional regulatory cycles, each of which is governed by specific guidelines, quality standards, and, in detail, different approaches to illness and the illness situation. A chronically ill person has care needs in the area of rehabilitation, in the sense of improving or at least stabilizing their health status. He or she has needs in the area of clinical and outpatient acute care, as well as ongoing diverse care needs in different settings within the segments of the healthcare system, especially in cases of multimorbidity (see Contribution 09).

For many, specialist care takes on the character of primary care, as they are permanently dependent on specialized care due to their illness.

However, in today's healthcare system, these different regulatory cycles are not automatically interconnected. As a rule, there is also no coordinated, planned overall intervention for chronically ill people. Future challenges therefore concern the better institutional integration of those involved in segmented care, in the sense of overcoming not only sectoral boundaries but also functional and professional boundaries. In addition, for chronically ill people, there is the particularity that their illness always has an impact on their daily lives. Chronically ill people must not only cope with the illness itself, but also integrate it into their everyday lives, which requires care contexts oriented toward their living environment. Therefore, it is also necessary to consider areas of care that are neither financially nor structurally connected to the segmented healthcare system.

References

Herder-Dorneich P (1986) Theorie der sozialen Steuerung, die Theorie der Scheine, 1. Aufl. Nomos-Verl.-Ges., Baden-Baden

Klein-Hitpaß U, Leber W-D (2012) Spezialärztliche Versorgung – Plädoyer für eine Neuordnung. In: Klauber J, Geraedts M, Friedrich J, Wasem J (Hrsg) Ökonomie. Krankenhaus-Report 2012: Schwerpunkt: Regionalität, 1. Aufl. Schattauer GmbH Verlag für Medizin und Naturwissenschaften, S 206–236. https://bem.wido.de/fileadmin/Dateien/Dokumente/Publikationen_Produkte/Buchreihen/Krankenhausreport/2012/Kapitel%20mit%20Deckblatt/wido_khr2012_kap13.pdf. Zugegriffen am 03.10.2023

Rosenbrock R (2008) Primärprävention – was ist das und was soll das? (WZB Discussion Papers SP I 2008-303). Wissenschaftszentrum Berlin für Sozialforschung, Berlin

Simeon M (2014) Soziale Rehabilitation. In: Strubreither W, Neikes M, Stirnimann D (Hrsg) Klinische Psychologie bei Querschnittlähmung: Psychologische und psychotherapeutische Interventionen bei psychischen, somatischen und psychosozialen Folgen, 1. edn. Wien, Springer, pp 42–46

Stöbe-Blossey S, Brussig M, Drescher S, Ruth M (2021) Schnittstellen in der Sozialpolitik: Analysen am Beispiel der Felder Berufsorientierung und Rehabilitation, 1. edn. Springer eBook Collection. Springer Fachmedien, Wiesbaden

Care Interfaces and Transitions in the Care of people with chronic conditions

31

Daniela Schmitz, Simone Hatebur and Manfred Fiedler

Contents

31.1 Definition, Emergence, and Impact of Interfaces

Individuals with chronic diseases pass through various facilities and their respective professional groups during the course of their illness. In multi- and interprofessional as well as cross-sectoral care, interfaces and transitions are of particular importance, as infor-

D. Schmitz (✉) · M. Fiedler
Department of human medicine, Witten/Herdecke University, Witten, Germany
e-mail: Daniela.Schmitz@uni-wh.de

M. Fiedler
e-mail: manfred.fiedler@uni-wh.de

S. Hatebur
Faculty of Health, Witten/Herdecke University, Witten, Germany
e-mail: simone.hatebur@uni-wh.de

D. Schmitz et al. (eds.), *Chronic Care—Science and Practice*,
https://doi.org/10.1007/978-3-662-72298-5_31

mation loss and lack of information transfer can lead to disruptions in care (see Contribution 11). Interfaces can take on three forms: transition, interference, and diffusion (Stöbe-Blossey et al. 2021). Transitions describe interfaces characterized by a change in the responsible institution, which can result in gaps and disruptions in service delivery. These interfaces require successive processing strategies, whereby cases are transferred to the next institution with the necessary information, such as the condition of the patients and to ensure continuity of therapeutic procedures, as is the case with discharge management. In interfering interfaces, areas of responsibility of different institutions overlap, which can lead to conflicts and contradictions in care. For work at these interfaces, simultaneous processing strategies based on coordination are helpful. Interfaces with the character of diffusion are characterized by distributed or unclear responsibilities and a lack of linkage, which can result in problems being shifted and goals being neglected. Interfaces also arise when involved individuals are expected to consider the goals of other organizations in their actions, as is the case with cross-sectional tasks such as diversity and gender equality (Stöbe-Blossey et al. 2021). Sensitive processing strategies are considered a solution for dealing with differences, by taking into account the goals of other organizations within one's own institutional context.

Interfaces can arise due to changes in the life circumstances of those receiving care, such as threatened employability or transition into retirement, and from problem-solving between involved institutions (Stöbe-Blossey et al. 2019). Interface problems then occur when changing sectors of care, for example between outpatient and inpatient care or vice versa. Interfaces also exist systemically between different service systems (see Contribution 30). Even though the German Social Code Book V (SGB V) fundamentally stipulates the avoidance of interfaces in § 11 (4): "Insured persons are entitled to care management, particularly to solve problems during transitions between different areas of care. (translation from German)" Nevertheless, interfaces still arise in terms of subject matter and personnel. At these transitions, information must be passed from one system to the next, and errors often occur due to insufficient, incorrect, contradictory, redundant, or delayed information. Fig. 31.1 illustrates exemplary interfaces:

The emergence of care interfaces is due, on the one hand, to the segmented care and sectoral separation of the healthcare system (see Contribution 30) and, on the other hand, to temporal and personnel framework conditions. Care processes are defined within each organization: if a process crosses different organizations or organizational units, an interface exists (Wendt 2020). From the perspective of those involved in the care process, points of contact between individuals also result in interfaces. These points of contact can be characterized as functional, organizational, or personal interfaces, depending on whether the point of contact lies between different functional units, organizational units or areas of responsibility, or in the involvement of different individuals within a process. Interfaces can also arise within a single organization between different functional areas and individuals, such as in a hospital between medicine, nursing, and administration. The background for the multitude of interfaces in care is the increasing prevalence of chronic diseases and multimorbidity among older people, which necessitates numerous

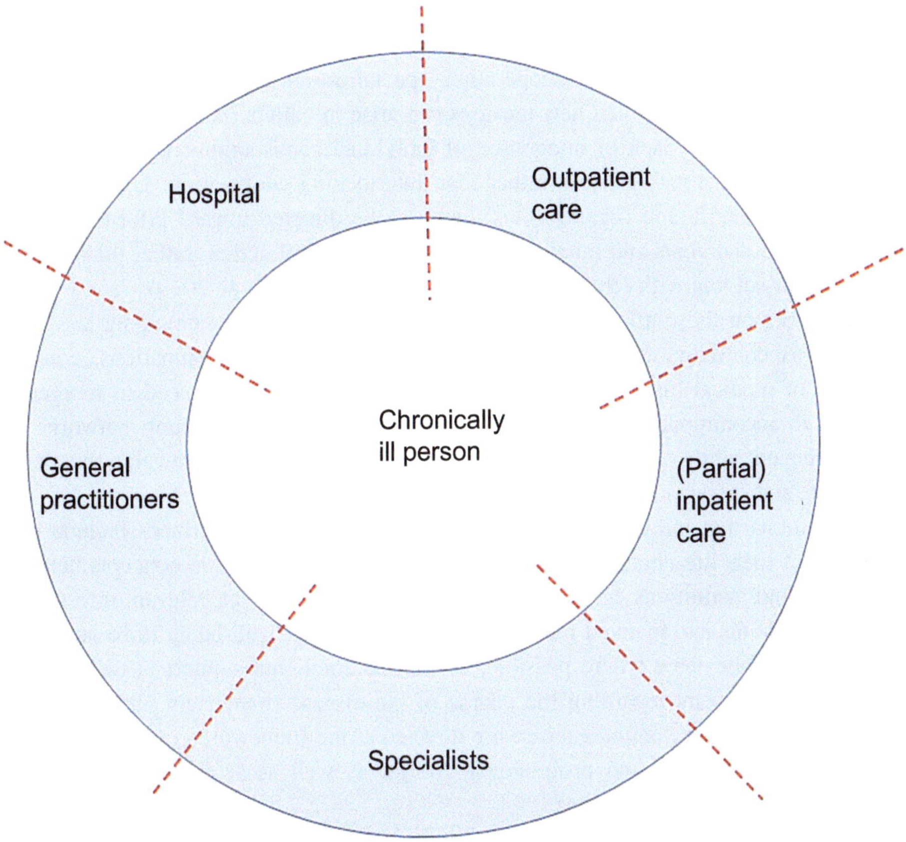

Fig. 31.1 Exemplary interfaces in the care of people with chronic conditions (Own illustration)

actors in the treatment process. The care system is rather acutely medical and episodic in orientation and, as a result of rationality logics, increasing technical potential, further differentiation of institutional structures, and increasing specialization of actors, leads to disruptions in care for those affected (Höhmann 2009).

The impact of interfaces is evident for both those affected and service providers. Individuals involved in care lose sight of the overall situation of the patients, as they view the present problem from the logic of their actions within their institution and see themselves less as a link in a chain of care (Feuerstein 1993). One consequence is communication barriers between professionals and patients. If it is not possible to align one's own professional action strategies with the coping requirements of those affected, gaps, errors, and problems can arise, for example in compliance. Ultimately, this leads to wasted resources in the system. Especially with a focus on chronic diseases and multimorbidity, professional action must take into account the unpredictability and long-term nature of disease courses and the different phases for interventions. Due to the increasing specialization of professions, these are effective in their specific areas, but with regard to the overall course of action, they are only limitedly effective because of the numerous interfaces. For interprofessional cooperation, specialization also leads to a fragmentation of responsibility, in which new tensions can arise in collaboration. From an organizational perspective, a lack of integration of individual contributions leads merely to a sequence of professional services rather than interlocking cooperation. Ultimately, the self-interest of actors and organizations may also be directed toward prioritizing their own organizational goals and maximizing their own scope of action, rather than seeking joint problem-solving with other organizations (Stöbe-Blossey et al. 2019).

The impact on those affected is seen in long treatment courses, changing and often perceived as contradictory treatment arrangements, redundant examinations, constant repetition of medical history during treatment, uncertainty, and the need to reorganize daily life to accommodate the illness. In the long term, personal support networks are also challenged, while economic follow-up problems arise, and withdrawal, a threatened self-image, and social isolation loom (Feuerstein 1993).

Expectations that individuals with chronic diseases have of interfaces include consideration of their life concepts and dignity, coordinated intervention concepts between individuals and institutions, as well as regular exchange of current, relevant information about health status and planned measures. They expect their well-being to be supported and symptoms alleviated where possible, as well as emotional support in dealing with uncertainties and fears regarding the course of the disease (Feuerstein 1993). In summary, expectations for continuous care are directed at the framework conditions of care, at individual institutions and professional groups, as well as at the respective actors involved in the course of treatment.

31.2 Concept of Interface Analysis

Interfaces exist in the healthcare system on multiple levels. At the macro level, there are procedural guidelines for working at interfaces, and structurally, there are framework conditions for goals and tasks within the system. At the meso level, interfaces between organizations in the healthcare system are considered, as well as existing agreements for cooperation and networking between them. At the micro level, it is the individual actors in the care process, their scope of action, their interactions with each other, and contacts with the recipients (Stöbe-Blossey et al. 2019). These three levels are mutually interconnected and create prerequisites and consequences for action.

Feuerstein systematically addressed interfaces in healthcare and developed the concept of interface analysis. The starting point of his observations on interfaces is an excess of highly specialized individual services and too few services oriented toward the entire course of treatment. The success of treating chronic diseases lies in ensuring that what is necessary for treatment is done at the right time, in the designated place, and to the appropriate extent (Feuerstein 1993). Often, patients encounter a multitude of technical examination procedures, different institutions and their respective departments, as well as a large number of actors who sometimes act relatively independently of each other during the course of treatment. The increasing use of technologies and apparatus-based diagnostics also leads to a shift in attention away from the person of the patient and toward data: "*The person of the patient, the sociobiographical background of the illness, and the psychological resources for coping with the disease move out of the center of medical perception. The less time the physician can devote to direct conversation with the patient, the greater the dominance of so-called hard data within the framework of the diagnosed clinical picture (translation from German)*" (Feuerstein 1993, p. 45). Technology thus becomes a new interface and requires exchange and communication about data as well as their integration into processes and organizations. This leads to a dominance of technology-centered forms of therapy, viewing disease as a measurable deviation of organic functions (Feuerstein 1993), and thus also to a technology spiral in which the extent of technical application often bears little relation to therapeutic relevance (e.g., individual health services (IGeL)), yet the use of technology is associated with increased significance. From the system's perspective, interface problems do not lead to a decline in demand for system services, so these issues still persist.

Feuerstein's concept of interface analysis serves to decode complex systems and their interfaces in order to identify dysfunctional effects at different levels and to understand their consequences for patients and the system (Feuerstein 1993).

- The analysis of interface problems: on the factual level, this involves the sequencing of medical-technical interventions. If these are poorly coordinated, those affected experience a lack of orientation and support, leading to confusion during the course of treatment and in coping with illness. The result can be a lack of compliance and low effectiveness of the resources used.
- The analysis at the personal level considers the increasing specialization and division of labor, especially among healthcare professionals. For those affected, this means a multitude and frequent change of contact persons. For the system, there is a need to transfer information between individuals to achieve smooth coordination in treatment.
- The analysis at the institutional level focuses on the consequences of professional specialization in the healthcare system, which, for example, leads to new departments, specialized clinics, or specialized facilities. For those affected, this increasingly results in transitions between treatment settings. The coexistence of different (quality) standards can lead to duplicate examinations as well as contradictory interventions.
- The analysis of interfaces at the temporal level focuses on the chronological sequence of services. In the course of treatment, problems can arise if diagnostics are not performed in a timely manner, due to temporal discrepancies between curative interven-

tion and rehabilitation, or fundamentally due to discontinuities and idle periods in the treatment process between consecutive treatment steps. For those affected, this can, for example, reduce rehabilitation potential, lead to disease manifestation, and unnecessarily prolong the illness phase.
- Interface problems at the conceptual level are evident, for example, in incompatible professional role models that can hinder integrated care processes. Those affected are confronted with different interpretations of their illness and encounter different treatment concepts. In the system, this leads to friction in actions and in the implementation of integrated care concepts.

There are three approaches to analyzing interfaces: a process-oriented analysis from the system perspective, a process-oriented analysis from the patient perspective, and a point-specific analysis of selected interfaces. Methodologically, Feuerstein describes three approaches for each analysis: surveys, observations, and document analyses.

Process-Oriented Analysis from the System Perspective
This form of interface analysis is the most complex variant, aiming to comprehensively map interfaces in the system in the form of processes. Interfaces at different levels can be the subject of analysis: interfaces at the micro, meso, and macro levels of the system; interfaces in the factual as well as social and temporal context of the treatment process; and in the context of collaboration between professions, between institutions, and interfaces with technology. The aim is to capture the sequences and interlocking of services across the entire care chain and their disruptions. The results should provide insights into the linkage of services, personnel deployment, task structures, workflows, use of technology, and formal cooperation structures.

Process-Oriented Analysis from the Patient Perspective
The analysis from the patient perspective offers a way to describe all services linearly from the viewpoint of the patients. The subject of analysis is thus all actions in the care chain that are visible from the patients' perspective or that take place within their perceptual range. The results should provide indications of weaknesses in the interaction of individual actions and in the use of resources. Ultimately, the aim is to identify problems in the transfer of information, in treatment structures, in the interpretation and communication of diagnostic and therapeutic data, in conversations with patients, and overall in the continuity and integration of care.

Point-Specific Analysis of Interfaces
In this variant, typical process structures and stages in treatment courses, or particularly problematic or frequent interface problems, are selected as the subject of analysis. One or more levels can be examined methodologically through surveys, observation, or analysis of documents in the course of treatment.

31.3 Dealing with Interfaces and Solution Approaches

Central to dealing with interfaces in everyday professional life is knowledge about the responsibilities, tasks, and accountabilities of other professions involved in the treatment process, as well as a shared language based on a common understanding. Feuerstein (1993) identifies three strategies for dealing with interfaces: interface design, interface management, and interface avoidance.

31.3.1 Strategies for Dealing with Interfaces

Interface design focuses on a technology-oriented approach and involves the design of technology at the human-technology interface. This means that technology is better adapted to functional conditions. Furthermore, there is a progressive technologization of individual elements of the system, with the aim of better interlinking the treatment process and structures. However, technology continues to act as a perceptual filter. As a result, patients are perceived in measurable dimensions of illness, while social aspects are rather neglected (Feuerstein 1993). Thus, technology-centered strategies for dealing with interfaces may offer advantages in terms of efficiency and cost, but they increase the distance to patients and do not address all levels of interface management.

Interface management, on the other hand, is a strategy for the social handling of interfaces and their respective characteristics. It aims to provide results, materials, data, or information needed for further process handling (Wendt 2020). Problematic situations are solved creatively to manage interfaces. The professions involved strive to mediate between services and institutions, but even so, they cannot address all levels of interface management.

Avoiding interfaces requires a change in existing structures of care by better interlinking institutions and reorganizing care in terms of content, social aspects, and timing. Although there are legal, administrative, economic, and professional-cultural obstacles, integrated, coordinated care concepts can provide a common basis for understanding and treatment concepts.

31.3.2 Cooperative Forms of Care

Solution approaches are concepts of cooperative forms of care, generally also discussed as integrated care. The term is used inconsistently and essentially describes care concepts that, beyond formal legal requirements, aim for holistic, interdisciplinary, and cross-sectoral care (Hellmann 2021). Cross-sectoral care refers to the organizational integration of outpatient and inpatient services. Interdisciplinary forms of cooperative care include care centers, such as outpatient health centers or primary care centers, where different professional care services (e.g., rehabilitative, medical, nursing, or social) and professions cooperate institutionally. Professional networks, as spatially collaborating but organizationally independent service providers (e.g., diabetes networks or dementia networks), are increasingly being established for chronic diseases with ongoing complex care requirements. Disease Management Programs (DMPs) have been established in Germany, enabling people with chronic diseases to receive quality-assured, continuous care within the DMP network of participating professions, based on individual therapy plans and goals, and to be closely supported in parallel.

A content-oriented solution approach is clinical pathways, which describe disease-/diagnosis-specific treatment processes. Clinical pathways construct the sequence of treatment steps and the structural collaboration to make information available to the professional groups involved (Wendt 2020). Where guidelines exist, clinical pathways should be guideline-based. In the past, clinical pathways were designed for the clinical setting. More recently, outpatient and cross-sectoral clinical pathways are also being developed (Hellmann 2021).

The goal of cooperative forms of care is to combine medical, nursing, therapeutic, and social responsibilities in a functionally and economically sensible way in order to achieve better quality and greater needs-based care, as well as to optimize the use of scarce resources (Wendt 2020). For the implementation of such concepts, legal and financial framework conditions at the structural level, influencing factors at the level of individual organizations, as well as routines, responsibilities, and tasks at the level of the actors must be taken into account.

31.4 Example: Interfaces in Rehabilitation

Rehabilitation serves to eliminate the consequences of illness, restore physical, mental, cognitive, and social abilities, and, as tertiary prevention, to prevent recurrence. It can be understood as a complex intervention, as it is highly person-centered and carried out with the involvement of various professions. Rehabilitation goals in terms of medical, occupational, and social rehabilitation depend on the specific disease and its background, which also includes the social-biographical characteristics and life-world context of those affected. This diversity of content is also reflected in the social law responsibilities of the social insurance providers, which are determined by the indication, rehabilitation goals, and the rehabilitative procedure. At the same time, a general effectiveness can be established for certain rehabilitation procedures. However, the highly case-specific indication does not allow for an assessment of effectiveness related to the individual therapeutic measure (Lübke 2015), which is why repeated assessments over time by the actors involved in the rehabilitation process are necessary to determine effectiveness.

In Germany, the most common rehabilitation measures are those following a stroke and those following joint replacement procedures as part of degenerative musculoskeletal processes, which represent the underlying conditions that justify rehabilitation measures after acute clinical intervention. These are accompanied by health conditions that impair the rehabilitation process, such as cardiovascular diseases, severe overweight or obesity, chronic pain, cognitive or mobility impairments.

Following the acute intervention, appropriate early rehabilitative measures are already required in the clinical setting to prepare those affected for subsequent inpatient rehabilitation. This is particularly important for stroke patients, as rehabilitation goals can be jeopardized by delays. Priorities regarding the type and timing of therapeutic intervention to prevent permanent consequences of illness must therefore be set early, both in the clinical setting and with regard to the transition to subsequent inpatient rehabilitation. In terms of interface design, the following challenges arise: the timing coordination of services, especially in connection with acute medical intervention; internal organization regarding multiprofessional collaboration; and the transition to the inpatient rehabilitation clinic. In the transition, questions such as the timing of the transfer relative to the clinical stay, whether those affected can temporarily live at home, and what support services are necessary in this phase (e.g., organizing fall prevention for patients with joint replacement) play a role. Finally, it is important that the need for measures determined by the rehabilitative indication is qualitatively clarified between the professionals of the involved institutions. Although the social service or discharge management of hospitals is usually responsible for this, they often act more as mediators, working on the timing dimension of transitional interfaces.

Especially for older, multimorbid patients, subsequent ongoing outpatient rehabilitation is required to secure the therapy outcome. In Germany, this is initiated by office-based specialists and assessed and, if necessary, secured with regard to the rehabilitation goal. In terms of content, those affected experience not only institutional transition, but also a crossing of sector boundaries, which represents a different regulatory cycle both qualitatively and in terms of professional responsibility.

Complex interventions, as are the norm in the healthcare of chronically ill and often multimorbid people, are characterized by a multitude of interfaces. Interface analysis and management are established, for example, in the form of discharge management and increasingly as case management in the acute clinical setting. Cross-sectoral forms, such as comprehensive quality networks for rehabilitation, are largely the exception. For people with chronic diseases, forms of sustained cooperation are necessary, which, however, like today's dementia networks, should not be structured as exceptional and voluntary alongside established structures and care processes, but should become an integral part of the regional health system.

References

Feuerstein G (1993) Systemintegration und Versorgungsqualität: Über Schnittstellen im Behandlungsgeschehen und ihre Bedeutung für die Analyse und Gestaltung komplexer Versorgungsstrukturen. In: Badura B, Feuerstein G, Schott T (Hrsg) System Krankenhaus: Arbeit, Technik und Patientenorientierung. Juventa, Weinheim/München, pp 41–67

Hellmann W (2021) Kooperative Versorgungsformen: Chance für den ländlichen Raum. KU Gesundheitsmanagement. Mediengruppe Oberfranken, Bamberg

Höhmann U (2009) Voraussetzungen und Möglichkeiten einrichtungs- und berufsgruppenübergreifender Kooperation zur Verbesserung der Versorgungsqualität pflegebedürftiger Menschen. In: Stemmer R (Hrsg) Qualität in der Pflege trotz knapper Ressourcen? Schlütersche, Hannover, pp 11–28

Lübke N (2015) Explorative Analyse vorliegender Evidenz zu Wirksamkeit und Nutzen von rehabilitativen Maßnahmen bei Pflegebedürftigen im Hinblick auf eine mögliche Anwendbarkeit im Rahmen der Feststellung des Rehabilitationsbedarfs bei der Pflegebegutachtung. G3 Gutachten im Auftrag des Medizinischen Dienstes des Spitzenverbandes Bund der Krankenkassen e.V. (MDS) online verfügbar: https://md-bund.de/fileadmin/dokumente/Publikationen/GKV/Rehabilitation/Gutachten_Reha_bei_Pflegebeduerftigkeit_KCG.pdf

Stöbe-Blossey S, Brussig M, Ruth M, Schulz SE (2019) Der komplexe Sozialstaat: Eine Heuristik zur Rekonstruktion von Schnittstellen. Soz Fortschr 68:749–768

Stöbe-Blossey S, Brussig M, Drescher S, Ruth M (2021) Schnittstellen in der Sozialpolitik: Analysen am Beispiel der Felder Berufsorientierung und Rehabilitation. Springer VS, Wiesbaden

Wendt J (2020) Prozessoptimierungen und Schnittstellenmanagement in der Gesundheitsversorgung. In: Leal W (Eds) Qualitätsmanagement in der Gesundheitsversorgung. Springer, Berlin/Heidelberg, pp 55–72

Human Resource Development and Staffing Needs Considering the Care of Chronically Ill People

32

Manfred Fiedler

Contents

32.1 Healthcare Provision and Personnel Development

Healthcare services, as person-related services, are highly labor-intensive. Additionally, working with people in a field of existential importance, which can be critical in individual cases, places high demands on the qualifications and competencies of the involved health professions. This applies not only to the specific professional actions but also to the relationship between the professional and those affected and their social networks, as well as the particular conditions of the respective care settings.

Fundamentally, the personnel employed, in terms of both qualification and number, is a component of structural quality. Inadequate or insufficiently qualified personnel poses a risk to patients and is often to be assessed as organizational negligence on the part of those responsible for staffing. This is especially true where binding external staffing requirements exist.

M. Fiedler (✉)
Department of human medicine, Witten/Herdecke University, Witten, Germany
e-mail: manfred.fiedler@uni-wh.de

D. Schmitz et al. (eds.), *Chronic Care—Science and Practice*,
https://doi.org/10.1007/978-3-662-72298-5_32

The debate about the academization of nursing professions, for example, is justified not only by a generally more professional and normative connotation, but also by the better process competence of academically qualified individuals (Görres et al. 2019), and, on the other hand, by better patient outcomes (Kutney-Lee et al. 2013).

Minimum requirements set by professional associations for centers or facilities, especially in inpatient acute care—such as for emergency departments or perinatal centers—as well as legal regulations in Germany like the Nursing Staff Minimum Staffing Regulation (PUGV) for patient-related minimum staffing in so-called *nursing-sensitive* areas, or the Psychiatry Personnel Regulation (PsychPV), are all aimed at ensuring the safety of those affected.

Demographic developments are intensifying the skilled labor shortage that has been observed for years. Traditional personnel recruiting, especially in structurally weak, rural regions, is reaching its limits. The development of in-house personnel has three objectives: adapting to care requirements, retaining existing staff, and ultimately supporting recruitment by offering opportunities for individual development.

32.2 Understanding Personnel Development

The understanding of personnel development (PD) is diverse (Meifert 2010). Especially in healthcare institutions, it was primarily equated with more or less structured in-house training and continuing education. This resulted in a systematic in the sense of the need for personnel development, when companies were exploring their desired training offerings. Continuing education, for example in the area of advanced nursing training, was traditionally offered and only limitedly adapted to operational requirements. Expenditures for personnel development in this sense were often considered organizational hygiene, particularly through self-care offerings, and not infrequently were seen mainly as a cost factor with limited approval. Even in the medical field, where continuous education was mandatory for maintaining qualifications, it was not consistently pursued at the organizational level and was often supported by supplying health companies, especially pharmaceutical companies.

Thus, PD was often not understood as strategic, i.e., aligned with goal-oriented organizational development. Since many healthcare institutions also lacked quantitative and qualitative personnel planning and personnel controlling aligned with this, PD remained insignificant for a long time.

Due to primarily external requirements resulting from the shortage of skilled workers, the establishment of external specifications regarding staffing levels and qualifications, as well as the continuously developing and changing guidelines and professional standards related to care processes—especially the nursing expert standards—PD has increasingly become a core entrepreneurial task.

The understanding applied here is an integrative one. While personnel planning is generally seen as a prerequisite for PD, no distinction is made between quantitative and qualitative personnel needs and their development. PD asks which personnel are needed, when, and in what number, as well as the means to ensure the achievement of future-oriented personnel goals.

1. Organizational Development and Personnel Development
   If we identify organizational development (OD) as a continuous process of innovative change in organizational structures and processes to address operational challenges (see contributions 43 and 46), then PD is a fundamental component of this. At the same time, OD is an important prerequisite for systematic personnel development.
   The interaction between OD and PD is based on the entrepreneurial understanding of OD and the underlying hierarchical structures.
   In organizations with strong hierarchical structures, OD is a top-down initiated process. In this case, PD is based on OD. Changes are planned, and then the necessary personnel are developed accordingly.
   If OD is understood and initiated as a participatory process, PD is a prerequisite component of OD. We first ask what is needed to initiate and implement change.
   PD and OD are thus interrelated, in the sense that PD is both a prerequisite for and a result of organizational change processes.
   This is also related to the fact that, in healthcare organizations, formal professional qualifications and competencies are of particularly high importance. (Inversion). At the same time, we are dealing with a multiprofessional field of action, in which the collaboration of different professions is crucial for the outcome. Change processes, therefore, cannot be sustainably implemented without involving the respective professional competencies and, on the other hand, without the cooperation of the involved professions.
   This can indeed be observed as an effect of OD processes shaped by external consulting firms. The competencies introduced by these firms initiate change processes for a limited period, usually with pre-agreed goals. After the consulting assignment ends, organizations often revert to previous negotiation processes, with the result that the renewed organization is not lived out permanently by those involved, and the achieved economic and non-economic improvements dissipate.
   PD thus represents not only a person-centered development effort but also a targeted action to qualify an organization for change. In this understanding, it concerns both *staff mix* and *skill mix* (Dubois and Singh 2009) as tasks of PD.
   Especially in healthcare organizations, and with regard to the particularly acute shortage of skilled workers there, PD not only serves the organizational function of supporting OD but also promotes the personal development of employees. It is precisely here that the often still existing legitimacy gap of PD becomes apparent, which also manifests as a contradiction between supporting organizational goals and promoting individual goals of employees (Jung 2009). This contradiction is due, not least, to the fact that in-house training measures always also involve the competencies of employees in their respective work contexts and, in this sense, indirectly focus on specific organizational development goals.

2. Personnel Development and Competence Development
   In this context, personnel development (PE) refers to the field of competence development. The term competence itself is quite diffuse, as it has become deeply embedded in everyday language and thus has lost some of its technical specificity. Additionally, the concept of competence is ambiguous (Huber 2004).
   Etymologically, competence can be traced back to the Latin *competere*, which means *to strive for (together), to achieve*. *Competens*, in turn, means *appropriate, lawful*.
   These linguistic backgrounds give rise to the two essential meanings of the term competence. Historically, competence first emerged as an authorized sphere of action, as the lawful authority of a person to do, decide, or initiate something. Later, it evolved into the idea of joint striving or competition, which is reflected in the English word "competition."
   The understanding relevant to PE here, however, is quite recent and was initially seen as competitive, that is, as the comparative positioning of one's own abilities against those of others in carrying out activities and tasks. Only later did the understanding of competence as the ability to pursue and achieve goals (together and with others) develop, and subsequently, in relation to acquired qualifications and knowledge, to be able to appropriately apply these in practice.
   Two terms are also associated with competence: 1. Abilities, as capabilities that develop through and within the person themselves; 2. Skills, on the one hand as technical proficiencies and, with the sometimes specific understanding of personality-related (soft) skills, as special abilities acquired by the person themselves.
   In German-speaking countries, the competence model of Lehmann and Nieke is often referenced in training (see Fig. 32.1):
   Referring to these five types of competence includes, as a core competence, the ability to act in a goal-oriented manner, but can be seen as a classic subdivision. In theory and practice, however, there are a multitude of other competence concepts, such as leadership competence or cultural competence; outside the corporate context, for example, terms like health competence, digital competence, or media competence are used.
   Since some of these competence concepts are increasingly used in the corporate/professional context, it makes sense in the corporate context to initially keep the concept of competence more open and to define competence development with regard to operational requirements, and for those requirements that are not yet specific to the company, to focus on personal development.
3. Quantitative Personnel Development—Personnel Planning
   Personnel planning is directly linked to the quantitative development of employees by occupational group necessary for operational performance. In healthcare, this is referred to as personnel requirements calculation or personnel requirements determination. This is also due to the fact that personnel deployment and personnel deployment planning are usually carried out decentrally, which often makes it necessary to set the area-specific full-time equivalent number in advance by agreement as a

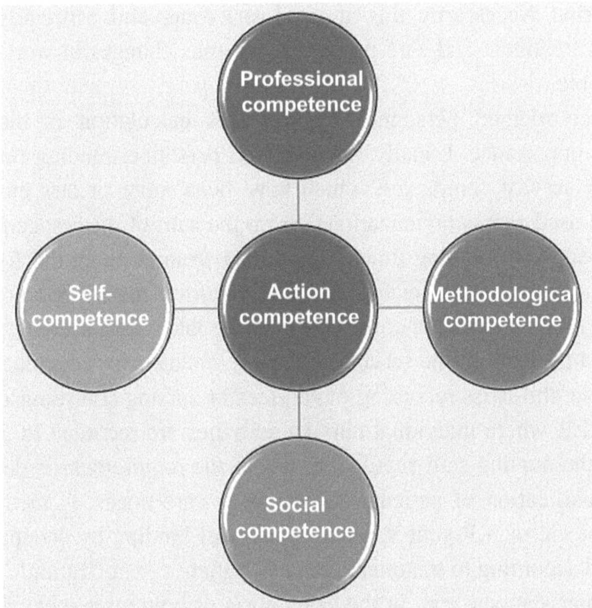

Fig. 32.1 Competence model. (Own illustration based on Lehmann and Nieke n.d., p. 2)

framework. In many areas of healthcare, budgets or remuneration are also negotiated between payers and service providers. Evidence of personnel and personnel requirements serve as benchmarks and legitimation for the amount of the budget or remuneration.

Finally, quantitative and qualitative planning, deployment, and documentation of deployed personnel in healthcare play an increasingly important role as part of external quality assurance, which, for example, in the case of the PUGV, can lead to the closure of service areas and/or loss of revenue, or, as in the case of perinatal centers, is a structural prerequisite for recognition. Especially with this type of structural requirement, not only is the occupational group specified, but also a profession-specific specialized further training or additional qualification.

Personnel planning thus answers the question of which personnel are needed, in what number, and when. This task requires close cooperation between personnel controlling, recruiting, and development.

Personnel requirements calculation is based on different approaches, which can only be outlined very briefly here. In healthcare, four principal methods can be distinguished, which are often used simultaneously in practice:

- The oldest method is calculation based on reference figures. The basis for personnel deployment is, for example, the expected number of occupied care beds, the number of patients treated, or, as in food services, the number of catering days in a given period. Necessarily, this figure is very rough and, especially with regard to changes in treatment and care processes and thus changes in work intensity, rigid and inflexible.

- Performance-oriented personnel requirements calculation is therefore gaining increasing importance. Usually, standardized personnel binding times for specific services or service complexes, which have been more or less empirically determined, are used across organizations. From the sum of the respective services and the total personnel binding times determined from them in the form of hours or minutes, the performance-related personnel requirement can be calculated.
  The effort required for data collection must be taken into account, which depends on the level of detail of the services to be documented for personnel measurement. For example, the swiss recording of services in nursing (Leistungserfassung in der Pflege – LEP, where individual nursing activities are recorded in great detail, differs from the nursing staff regulation, where the requirement is determined based on the classification of patients according to care needs. A method of medium detail is the German PsychPV, where personnel binding by occupational group is determined according to treatment area and patient categorization.
  For new interventions, e.g., in the calculation of home treatment (inpatient-equivalent services) for psychiatric patients, such data are not available, so personnel binding must be specifically determined based on activity-related, work-analytical time recording.
  The problem with these methods is, on the one hand, the accuracy of the documented services, and on the other, their differentiation. For example, technical innovations influence personnel binding. In the early days of cross-sectional imaging diagnostics, scan times were relevant triggers for personnel binding. Technological advances have significantly reduced scan times, so that, for example, positioning times for immobile and/or overweight patients have become highly significant for personnel binding.
- Revenue-based personnel requirements measurement is a recent concept that has gained importance through the introduction of externally determined remuneration rates. Based on the shares calculated for individual occupational groups in external remuneration, the revenue share can be broken down to the respective institution and compared with the institution's own personnel costs. For services remunerated on a lump-sum basis, such as in emergency care or outpatient care, general lump-sum calculations are applied with regard to the involved professional staff.
  The disadvantage here is that this does not actually reflect real personnel requirements, but only the financed personnel, and the result also depends on the institution-specific average personnel costs and the particular structural and service (volume) characteristics of the institution.
- In the structural or workplace-based personnel measurement method, as the last approach, the number of positions to be filled over time is used as the benchmark. Here, the focus is on the time-related binding of employees, on the one hand due to

working time models, but also structural and qualitative requirements that are specific to the institution (e.g., travel times) or, for example, to ensure the necessary staffing for irregular service demand in 24/7 care.

This issue is particularly important when there is a specialized professional need that must be met continuously, but to ensure coverage, a higher number of qualified professionals is essential. An example is ensuring the care of high-risk births through continuous specialist medical presence for timely intervention in obstetrics.

In particular, the structural method highlights a dilemma in healthcare. The more specific a care requirement is, and the more unique and specialized the characteristics of the professionals needed for it, the less they can be represented by standardized personnel requirements methods.

4. Theoretical References: Human Capital—Human Resource Development

   Personnel development (PE) is justified both in terms of business management references and in terms of personal aspects with the concept of human capital. When Bourdieu speaks of cultural capital (see contribution 37), which represents an aspect of a person's social position, the primarily economic understanding (Thoma 2006) of human capital is at least a related concept. As *personal assets*, acquired qualifications, abilities, and skills represent a personal asset that distinguishes the individual in terms of their potential for economic gain (income and wealth). At the company level, the retention of highly qualified employees also represents a non-activatable capital that strengthens the company's development potential. In this respect, PE represents an investment, because qualified personnel serve to maintain and increase monetary value. A renowned physician attracts referrals, highly qualified employees make better use of technical equipment. The development and retention of personal assets relevant to business success is defined as Human Resource Development (Nafukho et al. 2004).

   This functionalization of personal characteristics at the company level has ethical implications, as it reduces the value of people in general to their economic function and ultimate value creation. At the same time, it undermines the societal value of personal characteristics by reducing them to business utility. In the words of Nafukho et al., it concerns the effect on the "well-being of organizations, communities, and societies" (Nafukho et al., p. 549). At the same time, it must be considered that the antagonism between competitive competence and shared business goals, especially in healthcare organizations, can have contradictory effects. Where interprofessional collaboration is required for successful care, competitive behavior can be counterproductive (Nafukho et al. 2004).

   Aside from this criticism, human capital theory has a strong connection to reality, both as a societal consensus on the value of education and qualification, and as a consequence for distribution policy, in the sense that these *intangible* assets are an important aspect of the unequal distribution of social opportunities.

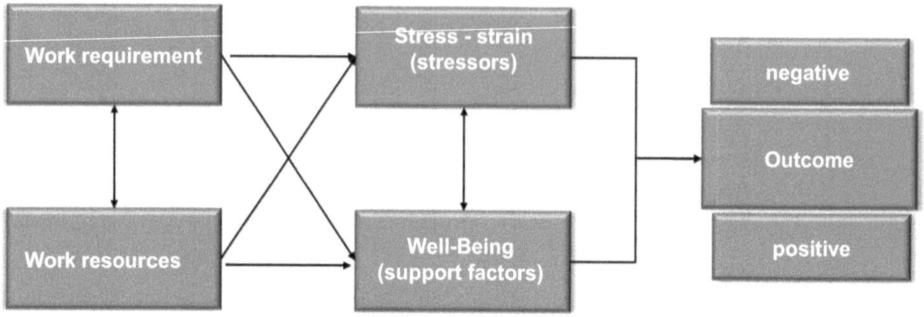

Fig. 32.2 Job Demand Resources Model according to Schaufeli and Taris (2014)

5. Work Science Approaches
   The discussion about working conditions in almost all care settings and healthcare institutions highlights another aspect of PE beyond the traditional business management function. PE is an instrument for working on employee well-being. The theoretical basis can be the Job Demand-Resources Model (Schaufeli and Taris 2014), which, unlike classic strain-stress models that are situational-analytical in nature, establishes a coherent relationship between work-related demands, work-related resources, as well as stressors and promoting factors (see Fig. 32.2).
   The understanding of work resources in the form of qualifications, skills, and personnel resources is closely related to the competence model. At the same time, in terms of analyzing stressors as working conditions and work organization, connections can be made to organizational development (OE), which there is represented as organizational coping competence (resilience), and in terms of PE, measures can be developed that promote personal competence/resilience to cope with work demands and critical work situations.

32.3 Requirements and Competencies

The aforementioned connection of PE to the Job Demand-Resources Model can also be found in the methodology of competence or potential analysis (Gunkel 2014; Prien et al. 2003). Potential analysis involves assessing personal resources and competencies, usually in relation to specific requirements of a job or field of activity. While the term competence analysis generally refers more to assessing suitability for a task or job and thus falls more into the field of recruiting, potential analysis also focuses on employees who are already working in company contexts and are to be further developed through PE measures, or for whom it is to be assessed what development needs they have in order to better or more appropriately meet the requirements of their field of activity.

Classic personnel assessments tend to refer to general competencies without direct reference to the field of work, whereas PE-related potential analyses require a task- or job-related requirements profile. Such a requirements profile differs from classic job or position descriptions, which, in addition to formal qualifications, usually describe tasks or job content. Such job descriptions thus serve not only for recruiting but also for classification within a compensation or pay scale system.

Requirements profiles go further in this respect, as they, in consideration of job-related work requirements, ask not only about the formal qualifications but also about the necessary competencies and personal characteristics and abilities, and compare these in the form of the requirements profile with the existing competencies of an employee or even a team.

The goal of matching can be suitability, but above all the team- or person-specific PE needs. In this respect, competence analysis represents a complex strengths-weaknesses analysis of employee teams.

Like any procedure used under business management conditions, potential analysis also has contradictions. When used as a personnel selection tool in hierarchical organizations, it risks undermining the trust base that is necessary for honest participation and thus the accuracy of the results, especially since it also asks about invisible personal characteristics.

No less important, as with any assessment procedure, is the fundamental question of whether the selected items for assessing potential are reliable in relation to the requirements profile. This methodological reliability is not always guaranteed, for example, if subjective assessments are made along a Likert scale and these are later presented as a point value or, much better, as a competence field analysis. Finally, a feedback loop is fundamentally required for the final evaluation in order to classify the result in an employee-related and participatory manner, which is almost imperative in light of the above. Potential analyses are not exact miracle instruments, but, after all, a useful tool for employee-oriented PE.

32.4 Personnel Requirements for the Care of Chronically Ill People

The care of chronically ill people is a complex field of action. The requirements in this field of work are very diverse. In addition to individual workplaces, there are mono-professional as well as multi-professional team-based work contexts. Even where inter-professional collaboration does not take place directly, there are interprofessional work relationships. In addition, health work always involves emotional labor, which requires balancing one's own emotions in relation to the emotions and reactions of those affected and their social networks. Personal milieus and cultural self-definitions of those affected and their relatives, and the associated approaches to illness, suffering, and dying in the care context, also play a significant role. Professionally, we speak of interprofessionality, cultural competence, and interpersonal skills, and finally of coping competence. The aforementioned instruments and perspectives of PE can be a supportive tool for employees in the care of chronically ill people to fulfill their role in wellbeing.

References

Dubois C-A, Singh D (2009) From staff-mix to skill-mix and beyond: towards a systemic approach to health workforce management. Human Res Health 7:87. https://doi.org/10.1186/1478-4491-7-87

Görres S, Silke Böttcher S, Schumski L (2019) Rationaler Personaleinsatz in der Alten- und Langzeitpflege. In: Jacobs K, Kuhlmey A, Greß S, Klauber J, Schwinger A (Hrsg) Springer eBook Collection: Bd. 2019. Pflegereporrt: Mehr Personal in der Langzeitpflege – aber woher. Springer, Berlin-Heidelberg, pp 137–157

Gunkel L (2014) Akzeptanz und Wirkung von Feedback in Potenzialanalysen: Eine Untersuchung zur Auswahl von Führungsnachwuchs. Springer VS, Wiesbaden. https://search.ebscohost.com/login.aspx?direct=true&scope=site&db=nlebk&db=nlabk&AN=1073663. https://doi.org/10.1007/978-3-658-04505-0

Huber HD (2004) Im Dschungel der Kompetenzen. In: Staatliche Akademie der Bildenden Künste Stuttgart (Hrsg) Visuelle Netze: Wissensräume in der Kunst. Hatje Cantz, Ostfildern-Ruit, pp 15–29

Jung K (2009) Krankenhäuser brauchen eine integrierte Personalentwicklung: Stand und Perspektiven einer integrierten Personalentwicklung an den Universitätsklinika Deutschlands, Österreichs und der Schweiz [Dissertation]. Leuphana UniversitätLüneburg, Lüneburg

Kutney-Lee A, Sloane DM, Aiken LH (2013) An increase in the number of nurses with baccalaureate degrees is linked to lower rates of postsurgery mortality. Health Aff (Project Hope) 32(3):579–586. https://doi.org/10.1377/hlthaff.2012.0504

Lehmann G, Nieke W (o.J.) Zum Kompetenzmodell. Universtität Bayreuth. sinus.uni-bayreuth.de/fileadmin/sinusen/PDF/modul10/text-lehmann-nieke.pdf. Accessed 03.07.2018

Meifert MT (2010) Was ist strategisch an der strategischen Personalentwicklung? In: Meifert M.T (Hrsg) Strategische Personalentwicklung: Ein Programm in acht Etappen; Bonusmaterial im Web, 2., überarb. u. akt. Aufl., pp 3–28. Springer, Berlin/Heidelberg

Nafukho FM, Hairston N, Brooks K (2004) Human capital theory: implications for human resource development. Human Res Devel Int 7(4):545–551. https://doi.org/10.1080/1367886042000299843

Prien EP, Schippmann JS, Prien KO (2003) Individual assessment: as practiced in industry and consulting. Applied psychology series. L. Erlbaum Associates. https://search.ebscohost.com/login.aspx?direct=true&scope=site&db=nlebk&db=nlabk&AN=83858. Accessed 29.03.2023

Schaufeli WB, Taris TW (2014) A critical review of the job demands-resources model: implications for improving work and health. In: Bauer GF, Hämmig O (Eds) Bridging occupational, organizational and public health: a transdisciplinary approach, 1. Aufl. Springer, Dordrecht, pp 43–68

Thoma D (2006) Die Theorie des Humankapitals zwischen Kultur und Ökonomie. Z Wirtsch Unternehmensethik (ZfWU) 7(3):301–323

Interpreprofessional Action and Competencies for Interprofessional Collaboration

33

Daniela Schmitz and Jan-Hendrik Ortloff

Contents

33.1 Forms of Interprofessionality

Interprofessional describes a permanent, institutionalized, and rule-based form of exchange between members of two or more professions whose competencies may overlap (for a distinction from the terms multiprofessional and transprofessional, see Contribution 04 and Contribution 56, respectively). Generally, interprofessional refers to collaboration in the clinical context between medicine, nursing, and therapy professions. The literature uses various terms, such as interprofessional action, interprofessional collaboration, interprofessional cooperation or collaboration, as well as interprofessional learning or interprofessional education (Walkenhorst et al. 2015). Underlying these are three perspectives:

D. Schmitz (✉) · J.-H. Ortloff
Department of human medicine, Witten/Herdecke University, Witten, Germany
e-mail: Daniela.Schmitz@uni-wh.de

J.-H Ortloff
e-mail: Jan-Hendrik.Ortloff@uni-wh.de

D. Schmitz et al. (eds.), *Chronic Care—Science and Practice*,
https://doi.org/10.1007/978-3-662-72298-5_33

1. the learning or education for interprofessional collaboration (interprofessional education = IPE), which is implemented among learners from two or more professions and in which the participants learn with, about, and from each other, as well as
2. the competencies acquired from this for successful collaboration (interprofessional collaboration = IPC), and also
3. the consideration of everyday practice (interprofessional practice = IPP), which requires collaboration among professions. The starting point for this was the theses on cooperation by the German Medical Association from 1997 as well as the report on cooperation and responsibility by the Council of Experts from 2007. There is currently no universally valid, consistent use of the different terms.

Interprofessional education (IPE) is intended to prepare for interprofessional practice (IPP) in the profession and to enable goal-oriented cooperation (IPC) in order to ensure safe patient care (WHO 2010). In German-speaking countries, there are various concepts for IPE, "but there is still a lack of viable and sustainable concepts that support educational institutions in developing their own interprofessional concepts and the necessary structures for them (translation from German)" (Kaap-Fröhlich et al. 2022, p. 15). In addition, IPE must also take place as a regular, training-accompanying process rather than as a one-off event. For this purpose, the idea of "Learning together to work together for better health" has been proclaimed since 2010 in the Framework for Action on Interprofessional Education & Collaborative Practice of the World Health Organization. Meta-analyses can demonstrate positive effects of IPE on attitudes, knowledge, and understanding of roles. Generally, informal opportunities for contact, small groups, and prior professional experience have a supportive effect. It remains unclear which factors positively influence learning outcomes among the different professional groups. There is also a lack of demonstrable causality that IPE leads to a fundamental measurable improvement in patient care in practice. Often, key figures such as length of stay or deaths within a certain period are used. Further studies are needed to capture the concrete effects of IPE on professional practice. However, studies can only ever examine partial aspects and often limit themselves to measuring attitudes toward IPE and other professional groups. Proven outcomes of interprofessional education are found primarily in the area of changed perceptions of joint learning, changed attitudes toward IPE or other professions, and the generation of knowledge about other professions (Reeves et al. 2017).

The positive impact and effectiveness of IPE for different health professions is also demonstrated by Guraya and Barr. In their systematic review and meta-analysis on the integration of IPE learning units, they identify improved acquisition of knowledge about collaboration skills as well as more positive attitudes of learners toward IPC. Furthermore, job satisfaction increases and stereotypes are reduced (Guraya and Barr 2018).

Interprofessional collaboration is generally defined by five fundamental terms: reciprocal exchange among professions, joint action by all participants, shared power, mutual dependence, and dynamic processes (D'Amour et al. 2005). For this interprofessional field of practice, corresponding competencies should be acquired by all participants.

33.2 Frameworks and Competencies for Interprofessional Collaboration

Competency frameworks have so far been developed primarily at the national level. A comparative overview of these competency frameworks from Canada, the USA, the United Kingdom, and Australia can be found in Thistlethwaite et al. 2014. The first competency framework was developed in the United Kingdom with the aim of creating an integrated and patient-centered approach to modernizing the education of future health professions. The content includes knowledge in practice, ethical practice, interprofessional collaboration, and reflection on learning processes. The Canadian Interprofessional Health Collaborative (CIHC) subsequently published its own national competency framework for IPC in 2010. Based on a systematic review of interprofessional competencies, these were grouped into six competency areas: interprofessional communication, patient-centered care, role clarity, team functioning, collaborative team leadership, and interprofessional conflict resolution. The competency frameworks of the USA (values & ethics, roles & responsibilities, interprofessional communication, teamwork & team-based care) and Australia (communication, team functioning, role clarity, conflict resolution, reflection) were published in 2011.

In addition to the countries mentioned, Germany (National Model Curriculum for Interprofessional Collaboration and Communication in Medicine from 2015) also has uniprofessional approaches from medicine that define interprofessional competencies and provide guidance on how to teach them in medical education with other professions. The four interprofessional competency areas—mutual respect and shared values, the role of health professions, communication in teams, and acting as a member of a team—are to be acquired in joint learning modules between two or more professions. The respective formulations and sub-competencies can be found in the NKLM (National Competence-Based Learning Objectives Catalogue for Medicine). At a higher level, the following competencies are defined for these four areas. Graduates ...

- work together with different health professions on the basis of mutual respect and shared values
- can explain their own role and the role of other health professions for the health of the population and for patient care. They can apply this knowledge in health promotion and prevention, cure, rehabilitation, and palliative care
- communicate appropriately as a member of a team with representatives of different health professions in order to optimize collaboration and quality of care
- can act successfully as a member of a team with the aim of optimally shaping health promotion, prevention, cure, rehabilitation, and palliative care (nklm.de Section VIII.3).

A model more strongly oriented toward IPP and adaptable was developed by the European Interprofessional Practice and Education Network (EIPEN). The model comprises five central building blocks: planning and managing, referring and transferring, dealing with problems and opportunities, consulting and collaborating, as well as reflecting and evaluating. The associated competencies are formulated so that they can be adapted to specific contexts. In addition, there is an assessment sheet that contains behavioral indicators for IPC. This can be used at different points in time to identify and make visible the development of competencies—from not yet present/acquired to fully acquired/present.

The research group led by Vaseghi investigated competencies for IPC in practice in a review. The competencies from 17 studies were clustered into six areas: transparency of tasks and responsibilities, patient-centered care, interprofessional communication, participative leadership, conflict resolution, and teamwork. Patient-centered care and interprofessional communication have been identified as key competencies for practice, enabling various healthcare professionals to exchange knowledge, ideas, and values regarding patients (Vaseghi et al. 2022). The competency of participative leadership creates an appropriate working environment in which interprofessional relationships and information exchange are enabled. The resolution of emerging disagreements or conflicts is achieved through conflict resolution competencies. The competency for establishing transparency also helps to develop an understanding of one's own tasks as well as those of others and to obtain the necessary knowledge and skills for task completion.

It should be noted that, both for education and for practice, competencies can be broadly divided into the areas of communication, values, role, leadership, and cooperation. These are also the framework conditions that can have a supportive or hindering effect on collaboration.

33.3 Facilitating and Hindering Conditions for Interprofessional Collaboration

Uncoordinated IPC based on poor communication and information exchange can have a negative impact on health services and patient care. However, according to a Cochrane Review, there is currently no clear evidence regarding the effects of coordinated measures based on a shared knowledge base (Reeves et al. 2017). Nevertheless, there are indications that IPC leads to improvements in care processes and patient health outcomes.

Individual studies in various settings with diverse populations implement and evaluate specific measures. Doornebosch et al. (2022) identified facilitating and hindering factors of IPC for the care of multimorbid individuals in long-term inpatient care and geriatric rehabilitation as part of a systematic review. The influencing factors can be grouped into three main themes: team performance, organizational framework conditions, and information exchange.

With regard to team performance, the relationships among team members themselves as well as with patients and their relatives, and the presence of a shared vision or common goals, are important. Advantages arise from equal status and knowledge of the tasks, roles, and responsibilities of team members. Further supportive factors include trust, respect, and appreciation within the team, as well as a sense of belonging. Conversely, boundaries, tensions, status inequalities, lack of mutual knowledge, stereotypes, negative behaviors, and attitudes act as hindrances. The team climate and internal team culture can also have a facilitating or hindering effect on IPC and the team, and further influence participants' attitudes regarding job satisfaction, engagement, and well-being (Doornebosch et al. 2022).

Organizational framework conditions can either support or prevent collaboration. Accordingly, the organization should provide enabling conditions to allow for interprofessional collaboration, i.e., provide appropriate resources and enable joint work processes. Formal structures such as the composition of teams and departments, power structures and their distribution, as well as accessibilities and responsibilities, can also influence collaboration. Perceived and structurally established hierarchies can have a hindering effect.

Only effective communication ensures that necessary information is shared and available. This communication is based on a common language, prioritization, feedback, and openness to address even critical issues. Lack of or ineffective communication can hinder IPC and result in information not being passed on and remaining in content/profession-specific language.

Facilitating and hindering factors are two sides of the same coin. Depending on how individual factors are handled, they can have a positive or negative effect. Organizations should strive to increase the facilitating factors for IPC. The factors mentioned are interdependent. Organizations, teams, and individuals are in reciprocal relationships with each other and can strengthen IPC. At its core, the influencing framework conditions can be summarized into three pillars: individual factors, team factors, and organizational factors (Wei et al. 2022). The two foundations for interprofessional collaboration are illustrated in the following Fig. 33.1.

With regard to team factors, this contribution concludes with notes for large interprofessional teams, which are less frequently focused on in the literature.

33.4 Interprofessional Practice in Large Teams

Care and education experts recommend interprofessional collaboration among health professions to meet the demands of practice and to increase the effectiveness and efficiency of care. However, the larger an interprofessional team becomes, the more likely (partly disciplinary) subgroups are to form, which are temporarily cohesive to varying degrees. A key factor in this cohesion is the coherence in terms of discipline-specific and interprofessional goals in patient care.

With regard to interprofessional action, it is particularly the case that global goals such as improving quality of life, autonomy, and participation, etc., in the care of chronically ill people are pursued in parallel by various professions. At the same time, each

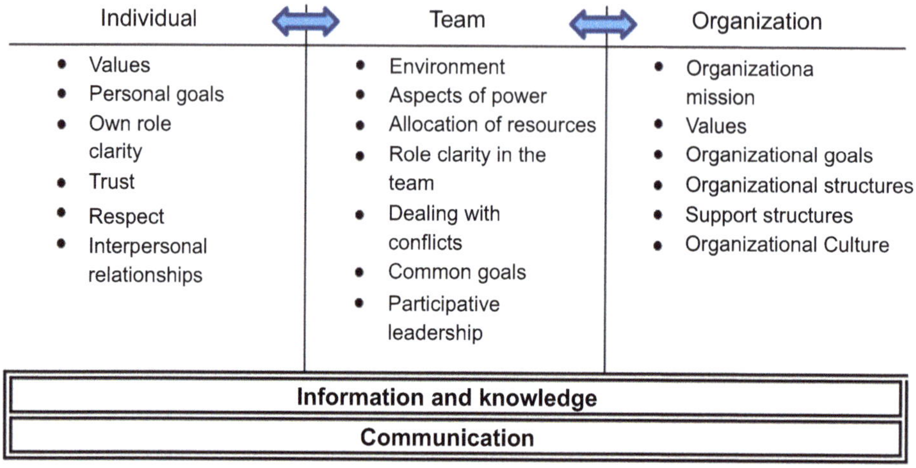

Fig. 33.1 Influencing factors of IPC, extended presentation according to Wei et al. 2022, p. 11

profession pursues specific goals that make the realization of global goals possible in the first place. Achieving global goals through coherence requires interprofessional action, which can be optimized through competencies for interprofessional collaboration. On the one hand, interdisciplinary competencies and authorities that emphasize shared values and contribute to the definition of one's own and other professions' roles are necessary to promote and enable specificity. Especially IPP requires mutual trust, respect, and appreciation, and may need to break free from traditional or hierarchical structures and mindsets. Participative leadership in patient care also means that all health professions are (actively) involved in decision-making and that an open discussion culture with room for innovation, conflict resolution, and teamwork is fostered. On the other hand, transparent tasks and responsibilities combined with adequate communication can convey the specific goals of one's own profession and create awareness of the goals of other professions. In addition, this can communicate profession-specific approaches for patient-centered care.

By comparing and, if necessary, adapting all profession-specific goals, coherence can be created that enables the realization of the global goals of patients and the identification of all involved professions. As an example, activating-therapeutic care based on the postulate of help for self-help can be cited. To achieve the global goal of maximum autonomy, it is the specific goals of nursing (increasing self-care), occupational therapy (targeted action planning and implementation), physiotherapy (improving mobility and endurance), and speech therapy (safe food intake), etc., which, through coherent collaboration, enable the autonomy of patients in terms of independent living.

References

D'Amour D, Ferrada-Videla M, San Martin Rodriguez L, Beaulieu MD (2005) The conceptual basis for interprofessional collaboration: core concepts and theoretical frameworks. J Interprof Care 19(Suppl 1):116–131

Doornebosch AJ, Smaling HJA, Achterberg WP (2022) Interprofessional collaboration in long-term care and rehabilitation: a systematic review. J Am Med Dir Assoc 23(5):764–777.e2

Guraya SY, Barr H (2018) The effectiveness of interprofessional education in healthcare: a systematic review and meta-analysis. Kaohsiung J Med Sci 34(3):160–165

Kaap-Fröhlich S, Ulrich G, Wershofen B, Ahles J, Behrend R, Handgraaf M, Herinek D, MItzkat A, Oberhauser H, Scherer T, Schlicker A, Straub C, Waury Eichler R, Wesselborg B, Witti M, Huber M, Bode SF (2022) Position paper of the GMA committee interprofessional education in the health professions—Current status and outlook. GMS J Med Educ 39(2):Doc17

Reeves S, Pelone F, Harrison R, Goldman J, Gurein M (2017) Interprofessional collaboration to improve professional practice and healthcare outcomes. Cochrane Database Syst Rev 6(6):CD000072

Thistlethwaite JE, Forman D, Matthews L, Rogers G, Steketee C, Yassine T (2014) Competencies and frameworks in interprofessional education: a comparative analysis. Acad Med 89(6):869–875

Vaseghi F, Yarmohammadian MH, Raeisi A (2022) Interprofessional collaboration competencies in the health system: a systematic review. Iran J Nurs Midwifery Res 27(6):496–504

Walkenhorst U, Mahler C, Aistleithner R, Hahn EG, Kaap-Fröhlich S, Karstens S, Reiber K, Stock-Schröer B, Sottas B (2015) Positionspapier GMA-Ausschuss—„Interprofessionelle Ausbildung in den Gesundheitsberufen". GMS Z Med Ausbild 32(2):Doc22

Wei H, Horns P, Sears SF, Huang K, Smith CM, Wie TL (2022) A systematic meta-review of systematic reviews about interprofessional collaboration: facilitators, barriers, and outcomes. J Interprof Care 36(5):735–749

World Health Organization (2010) Framework for action on interprofessional education and collaborative practice. https://www.who.int/publications/i/item/framework-for-action-on-interprofessional-education-collaborative-practice. Accessed 03.02.2023

Knowledge Management in Multiprofessional Care Processes

34

Daniela Schmitz and Jan-Hendrik Ortloff

Contents

34.1 Knowledge, Knowledge Management, and Knowledge Transfer

34.1.1 Forms of Knowledge

Not every piece of information needs to be stored within the framework of knowledge management or transmitted in a knowledge transfer process. The key distinction is

D. Schmitz (✉) · J.-H. Ortloff
Department of human medicine, Witten/Herdecke University, Witten, Germany
e-mail: Daniela.Schmitz@uni-wh.de

J.-H Ortloff
e-mail: Jan-Hendrik.Ortloff@uni-wh.de

D. Schmitz et al. (eds.), *Chronic Care—Science and Practice*,
https://doi.org/10.1007/978-3-662-72298-5_34

between data, information, and forms of knowledge. Data are signs and symbols, that is, individual elements of information. For example, the data sequence 31011961. These data become information when a context is assigned to them, meaning they are linked with additional information. In the example, the context becomes clear by inserting periods: 31.01.1961. By definition, information becomes knowledge when it is associated with personal meaning; in this example, it could be the birthday of a family member.

Knowledge is differentiated into explicit and implicit knowledge. Explicit knowledge is knowledge that can be clearly communicated as verbalized rules and factual knowledge. This form of knowledge can be easily put into words and thus readily shared with others (Wilkesmann and Wilkesmann 2009). For example, forum posts about common software problems, in which users write instructions for others to solve the problem and thus share their knowledge. Implicit knowledge, on the other hand, is less accessible and often difficult to articulate, as it consists of internalized knowledge gained from experience and routines. Figuratively speaking, it resides in the minds of employees and is not documented. In the context of knowledge transfer, this knowledge should, for example, be passed on from departing employees to their successors. An example would be the knowledge of a machine operator who can identify a problem and the part that needs repair by recognizing changes in the machine's operating sounds.

34.1.2 Approaches to Organizational Knowledge Management

The guiding question from an organizational perspective is: What does the organization know, how can its knowledge be identified, preserved, and distributed? The goal is a conscious and responsible approach to the resource of knowledge. Models of knowledge management originate from the business sciences, as knowledge functions here as a central competitive factor alongside the classic production factors of labor, land, and capital. Due to processes of globalization and digitalization, there is an exponential increase and volatility of knowledge, so an organization must constantly assess which knowledge needs to be stored and distributed. Probst et al. (2012) have identified areas of activity for this—so-called building blocks of knowledge management:

- Knowledge objectives: What do I want to know and for what purpose?
- Knowledge identification: What do I already know?
- Knowledge acquisition: What knowledge products and knowledge carriers are available?
- Knowledge development: How can I acquire the knowledge I need?
- Knowledge distribution: How can I share my knowledge?
- Knowledge utilization: How can I use my knowledge productively?
- Knowledge preservation: What techniques for selecting, storing, and updating are necessary?
- Knowledge evaluation: What is the quality of the knowledge to be collected? What standards are suitable for this?

All these activities can be understood as a cycle and are also interrelated. As a result of knowledge evaluation, it may be necessary to adjust the knowledge objectives.

34.1.3 Transfer of Knowledge

For knowledge to be transferred from one person to others, it is necessary to repeatedly consider the two forms—explicit and implicit knowledge—which has consequences for knowledge transfer. Nonaka and Takeuchi (2012) explain this using a knowledge spiral, the so-called SECI model (= Socialization, Externalization, Combination, Internalization), in which the acquisition of knowledge is described from the individual's perspective:

- **S**ocialization focuses on the transfer of implicit knowledge from one person, which is received as implicit knowledge by another person. This can be described as an exchange of experience, in which implicit knowledge is acquired through observation or imitation in practice and is taken up as implicit knowledge by another person.
- **E**xternalization describes the transfer and transformation of implicit into explicit knowledge. This is a common goal of knowledge transfer, so that, for example, the implicit knowledge of departing employees becomes explicit and thus permanently available to the organization. In this process, implicit knowledge is articulated in the form of metaphors or analogies. Through reflection and interpretation of the knowledge, gaps between the figurative representation and the verbal expression are filled. This is the key to knowledge creation, as new explicit knowledge is developed from implicit knowledge in this way.
- **C**ombination encompasses knowledge transfer processes in which explicit knowledge is further developed into new explicit knowledge by adding or linking information.
- **I**nternalization represents the transformation of explicit into implicit knowledge. The experiences of others are internalized through learning by doing, grasped at their core, and transferred into an individual, implicit mental model.

Since knowledge is always tied to a person and can only be transmitted through processes of communication and interaction, the knowledge conveyed in a knowledge transfer is never exactly the same knowledge that the receiving person constructs for themselves. This is based on the epistemological position of constructivism, which holds that knowledge is an individual construction of reality. Therefore, knowledge can only be transferred through processes within the framework of an interaction model and ultimately represents a knowledge transformation. The knowledge provider can also change their knowledge during the interaction (Renzl 2003). In the interaction, both knowledge transfer partners negotiate a shared understanding of the knowledge. This rules out outdated notions of a package model, in which knowledge, packaged as a parcel, is logistically distributed from one person to the next.

34.2 Relevance of Knowledge Transfer in Multiprofessional Care

Knowledge transfer serves a dual function in the multiprofessional care of people with chronic diseases. On the one hand, it occurs within the team, involving the sharing and development of knowledge, and on the other hand, the person receiving care always acts as a third knowledge transfer partner. In interprofessional collaboration, each discipline possesses profession-specific knowledge as well as areas of knowledge that overlap with other professions. Thus, they can also be understood as knowledge-based professions (Kurtz 2003), which, through the exchange of knowledge, arrive at shared interpretations of problems. On this basis, joint problem-solving takes place by and for individuals, which also considers the knowledge of those being cared for and involves them in an exchange of knowledge relevant to them.

For cross-professional knowledge transfers, the focus is ultimately also on knowledge cooperation. This includes the willingness and extent to which one contributes their own knowledge to multiprofessional work processes (keyword: knowledge is power). Ideally, the professional groups involved pursue the common goal of mutually supporting each other with their own knowledge, even if no individual benefit is apparent (Moser 2002). Lived knowledge cooperation arises reciprocally between employees and the organization. Therefore, the employees involved must have the opportunity to contribute their competencies (see Contribution 32), to experience themselves as competent, to develop motivation for performance, and to perceive themselves as effective. The organization must actively manage knowledge, provide temporal and financial frameworks for knowledge transfers, and promote a positive image of reciprocity. One's own willingness to share knowledge must be appropriately recognized and reciprocated so that knowledge cooperation is worthwhile. Individual and organizational factors flow into collective factors within the framework of knowledge cooperation, which is based on mutual trust, includes qualitative communication, and is founded on a collective expectation of effectiveness, in which all employees assume that mutual knowledge exchange is worthwhile in order to provide good care together.

Overall, two areas must be addressed for knowledge management and knowledge transfer in healthcare: on the one hand, from the operational perspective of managers, to enable and organize knowledge processes, and on the other hand, from the perspective of the actors, to make the required knowledge available at the patient's bedside at the right time (Giehoff 2008). In terms of content, meetings with the multiprofessional team and with patients should be distinguished from each other, as they pursue different objectives. While the former focus on the team itself, the frequently held meetings with and about patients in particular require a formally and substantively coordinated timeframe. Especially in nursing, knowledge transfer is addressed as a practical issue for imparting knowledge during training (Schaeffer 2006). The introduction of knowledge management and knowledge transfer stands and falls with the managers and the culture they embody in dealing with knowledge, as well as the promotion of a sense of togetherness.

34.3 Methods for Implementing Knowledge Transfer

There are various options for the concrete implementation of knowledge transfer methods between a knowledge-giving and a knowledge-receiving person (Pleskina 2002). Methods of direct verbalization of the experience to be transferred include, for example, analogies, in which understanding is established pictorially through something familiar, such as *this unit works like a vacuum cleaner*, or metaphors, using images from everyday life, such as the image of a bridge.

Methods of indirect verbalization of the implicit knowledge to be transferred include, for example, after-action reviews or active observations followed by feedback. The former is characterized by implementation and reflection following a training session. This involves taking stock of what was planned, how it was implemented, and where the differences lie, in order to identify missing knowledge components. In active observation, the knowledge-receiving person observes the knowledge-giving person for extended periods to identify the behaviors central to implicit knowledge.

Other methods involve creating experiential situations in which experiential knowledge is made explicit and reflected upon. This can be achieved through interviews or the formulation of lessons learned. In interviews, explicit questions about procedures, thoughts, and underlying concepts can make behavior and actions conscious, making the associated implicit knowledge reproducible. Lessons learned are often documented in projects, capturing relevant experiences for future projects. The aim is to record critical experiences and identify issues that need to be considered in the future. Alternatively, situations can be created in which typical cases are presented, thereby demonstrating implicit knowledge.

For longer-term knowledge transfers, so-called socialization methods are suitable, such as job rotation, communities of practice, or mentoring models. In job rotation, work content and workplace are regularly changed to stimulate the acquisition of new knowledge and the expansion of existing knowledge. Communities of practice are voluntary, informal discussion groups that come together due to a shared activity and a common interest in exchange. For example, current issues can be addressed through the exchange of implicit knowledge during an informal, shared lunch. Mentoring models include, for example, coaching or mentoring, in which mentors are available as contacts for professional and organizational issues for a knowledge-receiving person, in order to support knowledge-building processes.

34.4 Prerequisites and Obstacles for Implementing Knowledge Transfer

The successful implementation of knowledge transfer depends on several factors, which lie in the knowledge to be transferred itself, the people involved, and the framework conditions. The quality of the knowledge to be transferred must be carefully considered in the methodological design of the knowledge transfer, as, for example, knowledge components that are more experience-based require more time and more experiential situations with personal interactions (von Krogh and Kröne 1998).

From the perspective of the knowledge-giving and knowledge-receiving person, previous experiences with knowledge transfer initially influence the upcoming transfer. Furthermore, motivation, openness, and existing skills are central. On the part of the knowledge-giving person, barriers include a lack of motivation to share knowledge, a lack of common language, a poor relationship with the knowledge-receiving person, as well as possible generational conflicts or negatively shaped generational images. Barriers for the knowledge-receiving person can include a lack of motivation to accept and adopt the knowledge to be transferred, a lack of trust in the transfer partner, or limitations in the person's perception and processing abilities. Ultimately, there must be a trusting relationship between the transfer partners, in which mistakes are dealt with openly and knowledge is shared openly. If the organization provides incentives for knowledge transfer, these can have a positive effect (von Krogh and Kröne 1998).

The framework conditions for successful knowledge transfer primarily include sufficient time, space, and autonomy to carry it out. The organization must therefore create appropriate structures and provide resources. The organizational culture must also have a positive view of collaboration and knowledge sharing, in which knowledge is not interpreted as power and thus withheld. Organizational structures can also be decisive, such as which interaction and communication styles are maintained, what hierarchies, adaptability, and transparency exist in the organization, and how well information flows function. Ultimately, the role of managers and their leadership style is also crucial, that is, the value and attitude they have toward knowledge transfer and thus the support they provide.

34.5 Documentation as a Concrete Application Field for Knowledge Management

Documentation in healthcare encompasses all information communicated by the involved disciplines. In addition to professional findings, all actions performed must be documented in order to serve as proof of service. This results in a flood of documentation entries and a time-consuming process for the involved actors, as the information must be collected, selected, and formulated as concretely as possible to clearly present the relationships between diagnostics, therapy, and the current status. In particular, chronic diseases and multimorbidity require extensive documentation, as treatment is provided over a longer period, by multiple professions, and across interfaces. Using the building blocks of knowledge management, knowledge can be focused, acquired, identified, evaluated, distributed, preserved, and utilized through documentation. Documentation also includes a communicative intent. Resource-oriented documentation can explain current measures, while described deficits can justify the necessity of future treatments.

On a formal level, it is advisable to be aware of the intended recipients of the documentation. These may include internal professionals from one's own profession, department, or institution, as well as external parties, such as payers, authorized relatives, and the patients themselves. Thus, it is often, but not always, a professional report using technical terminology that should be employed eloquently. In addition, accessibility is another formal prerequisite for successful knowledge transfer. Only if all involved professions have barrier-free access to the required information can knowledge transfer occur on an equal footing.

According to quality management principles, documentation is carried out in writing, but often simultaneously across multiple channels in digital, printed, and handwritten form. Due to the volume of information (explicit knowledge), this can lead to duplicate information, information gaps, as well as contradictory statements. These should be avoided as much as possible for efficient documentation, as duplicate information and contradictory statements consume unnecessary resources in an already comprehensive process, and information gaps must be discovered during the treatment process. In addition to patient case discussions, digital documentation in particular can provide a low-threshold opportunity for the transfer of explicit knowledge, provided it is adequately organized.

Multiprofessional documentation can be understood as knowledge transfer based on the SECI model, in which information from one professional (knowledge provider) is made accessible to other knowledge recipients. During the onboarding of new employees, for example, implicit knowledge can be passed on by adopting routines regarding the formal and substantive design. The way in which (and how extensively), where, and when documentation is carried out is therefore also the result of *socialization*.

The course of illness and the current care status of patients should be determined as objectively as possible. Nevertheless, interactions, contextual factors, and objectives can be interpreted through experience (implicit knowledge). Through documentation, this implicit knowledge can become explicit knowledge by making implicit knowledge conscious and recording it as relevant information. This form of *externalization* determines what knowledge is passed on. Precise documentation with structured reading aids can facilitate the process of externalization and enable inferences. Consequently, it is important, especially in multiprofessional documentation, to coordinate the focus and responsibility for content.

From the perspective of the recipients, it is also helpful if comparative values between diagnostic findings and the progress or final report are evident, and if the documentation makes clear how conclusions were reached, which prior information or comparative values the treating professionals received (external medical history) or collected themselves (self-reported medical history). This enables recipients to generate new knowledge through *combination*. When the information is accessible to the involved actors, they can transform explicit knowledge into implicit knowledge through *internalization* and apply it to their treatment of the patient.

The bio-psycho-social model and the International Classification of Functioning, Disability and Health can be used as structuring foundations for assessing health status, in order to also address social aspects and individual environmental factors. However, since these provide only limited guidance for a person-centered and holistic approach, it is advisable to design multiprofessional documentation collaboratively and not hierarchically. Documentation that is simultaneously adapted to the patient situation must address both the impact of chronic diseases and the work-related resources of the professionals.

The goal of multiprofessional knowledge transfer can therefore, among other things, be an optimized documentation process that is efficiently designed and whose actors are appropriately trained.

References

Giehoff C (2008) Wissensmanagement in der Pflege. Shaker, Aachen.

Krogh von G, Kröne M (1998) Der Wissenstransfer in Unternehmen: Phasen des Wissenstransfers und wichtige Einflussfaktoren. Die Unternehmung 52(5/6):235–252

Kurtz T (2003) Professionen und Wissensberufe. Sind alle Professionen Wissensberufe, sind alle Wissensberufe Professionen? ARBEIT 12(1):5–16

Moser KS (2002) Wissenskooperation: Die Grundlage der Wissensmanagement-Praxis. In: Wehner T (Hrsg) Wissensmanagement – Praxis: Einführung, Handlungsfelder und Fallbeispiele. vdf Hochschulverlag, S 97–113

Nonaka I, Takeuchi H (2012) Die Organisation des Wissens. Wie japanische Unternehmen eine brachliegende Ressource nutzbar machen, 2. edn. Campus, Frankfurt am Main

Pleskina S (2002) Explikation von Wissen. Mehrung von Erfahrungswissen in Unternehmen. Emporias, Unterföhring

Probst G, Raub S, Romhardt K (2012) Wissen managen. Wie Unternehmen ihre wertvollste Ressource optimal nutzen. 7. edn. Gabler, Wiesbaden

Renzl B (2003) Wissensbasierte Interaktion. Selbst-evolvierende Wissensströme in Unternehmen. Dt. Univ.-Verl, Wiesbaden

Schaeffer D (2006) Wissenstransfer in der Pflege. Ein Problemaufriss. In: Schaeffer D (Eds) Wissenstransfer in der Pflege. Ergebnisse eines Expertenworkshops. Institut für Pflegewissenschaft an der Universität Bielefeld (IPW), Bielefeld, pp 1–14

Wilkesmann U, Wilkesmann M (2009) Wissensmanagement. In: Gessler M (Hrsg) Handlungsfelder des Bildungsmanagements. Ein Handbuch. Waxmann, pp 157–182

Setting-Specific Process Planning and Organizational Development

35

Manfred Fiedler

Contents

35.1 On the Necessity of Organizational Development

Healthcare provision is a complex matter. The reason for various interventions is often an acute or chronic illness. Different institutions and professions are involved in care simultaneously, as well as upstream and downstream. Care frequently takes place in different care settings; even when services can be described as such, process flows vary depending on the characteristics of the individuals affected. For example, in a CT scan, the duration varies due to the complexity of positioning the person, depending on mobility limitations, body weight, or cognitive impairment. Classic pathways *to achieving health* are therefore abandoned in organizational development (OD) and process planning.

M. Fiedler (✉)
Department of human medicine, Witten/Herdecke University, Witten, Germany
e-mail: manfred.fiedler@uni-wh.de

D. Schmitz et al. (eds.), *Chronic Care—Science and Practice*,
https://doi.org/10.1007/978-3-662-72298-5_35

35.2 Peculiarities of the Organization of Healthcare Institutions

In healthcare institutions, the professional responsibility of the healthcare professional takes precedence over the organizational responsibility of the enterprise. The relationship between the professional and those affected involves a special knowledge of the subject, content, and impact of professional health actions. We therefore speak of inverted organization. The professional responsibility for concrete actions with and for those affected can only be very limitedly restricted by managers at *higher* hierarchical levels. This has consequences for the organizational development of healthcare institutions. In hospitals, for example, the management is traditionally structured by profession into a directorate consisting of nursing, medicine, and administration. Care facilities are also generally managed by professional discipline.

However, the tasks of these professional leaders are not those of classic line managers. In hospital management, they represent the professional standpoint. In the professional line organization, their role is even more diffuse. Especially at the middle management level, ambiguities may arise, as their task is to implement global operational requirements in practice. Studies on nursing ward and area managers show that, on the one hand, they feel they belong to the nursing team, but at the same time, as managers, they function as part of the more practice-removed management levels.

Medical directors, in turn, have a moderator function in the line, since professional responsibility fundamentally lies with the respective department heads. The medical department head, due to their role in medical specialist training, is both the professional superior to the residents and, at the same time, in a mentoring position as a professional role model. With respect to specialists, the role is much more diffuse, as they cannot delegate their professional responsibility in medical practice to the department head.

In hospitals, professional structuring dominated, as siloing, with parallel, rigid hierarchies that made professional collaboration on the horizontal level more difficult, but also represented traditional understandings of hierarchy within the silos.

The performance requirements of recent years have been characterized by increasing complexity. This affects intra- and interprofessional collaboration as well as intra- and interinstitutional collaboration, which in turn impacts organizational structure and processes, and thus leadership tasks. Leadership roles therefore differ by profession, despite similar leadership positions in the line.

35.3 Principles of Organizational Development

The aforementioned challenge is the subject of OD as "a long-term effort to improve problem-solving and renewal processes in an organization, primarily through more effective and collaborative management of organizational culture" (French and Bell 1990) using social science methods. The focus is on addressing current and future challenges facing the organization in terms of organizational, social, and economic environmental factors. The understanding presented here is that of participative OD, as action in action (own translation, French and Bell 1990), as change directly within the field of action. In contrast, there are hierarchical structures in which change processes are initiated and implemented as top-down directives. Here, hierarchy is understood as a differentiation of rank based on the (threatened) potential for negative and positive sanctions (Kühl 1998).

Hierarchies are reflected in the organizational structure as a static structure, while processes in the operational structure represent the dynamic structure of a business.

The classic form of organizational structure is the line organization, in which the hierarchical structure follows a pyramid shape (see also Fig. 35.1), which branches out more and more hierarchically and functionally from the top management at the apex.

In the matrix organization, the line is partially abandoned. Internal professional relationships are the essential structural organizing principle. This means that the internal organization of a department is oriented toward the internal professional relationships within the company. On the one hand, this is intended to strengthen the internal service character, and on the other, to enable problem-solving in the form of a decentralized project organization.

Decentralization of responsibility, in the form of streamlining hierarchical levels (lean management), can be particularly well achieved with the matrix organization. Lean management is intended to facilitate adaptation to technological innovation, changes in performance, and new performance structures by having solutions developed decentrally by and with the affected work teams, while at the same time enabling decisions to be made more appropriately and quickly. In this moment, structure is combined with methodological procedure.

Closely linked to the lean organization is the concept of the Continuous Improvement Process (CIP). CIP is often explained using the Deming Cycle (Plan-Do-Study-Act, PDSA), which the American engineer Deming first introduced in Japan in the 1950s as a development cycle (Moen and Norman 2009). Originally developed for product development, the cycle has become a fundamental concept in quality management. Following this understanding, the concept of semi-autonomous work groups was developed, initially in Japan, in which team members in a given area work autonomously to improve their own work processes within basic guidelines for the performance process.

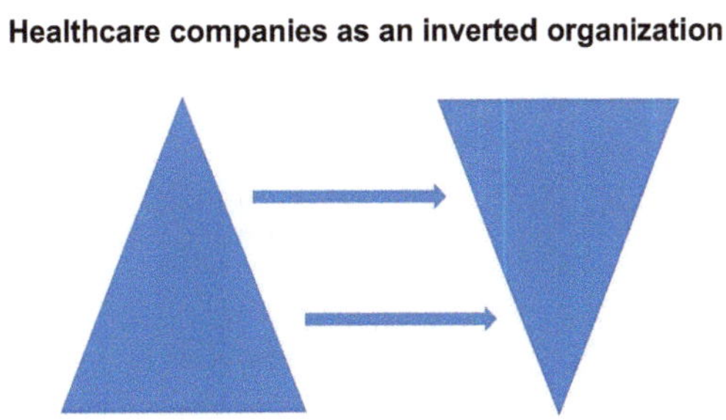

Fig. 35.1 Reversal of hierarchy in healthcare organizations. (Own illustration)

A special organizational structure is the fractal organization, in which the classic line is abandoned. The operational areas organize themselves, company relationships and thus collaboration are organized in networks, and communication is direct and de-hierarchized. Other principles include self-similarity, i.e., the fractal areas structure themselves according to similar principles, as well as a continuous development dynamic required by the network relationships (Probst 1991).

Decentralized structures, especially in organizations with high professional responsibility, have strengths in terms of the appropriateness, sustainability, and dynamism of change processes. However, there are also limits and contradictions. These result from the multidimensionality of OD processes (see Fig. 35.2).

Overall strategies and decentralized processes must be *harmonized*. Especially when OD is organized decentrally but hierarchical decision-making paths still exist,

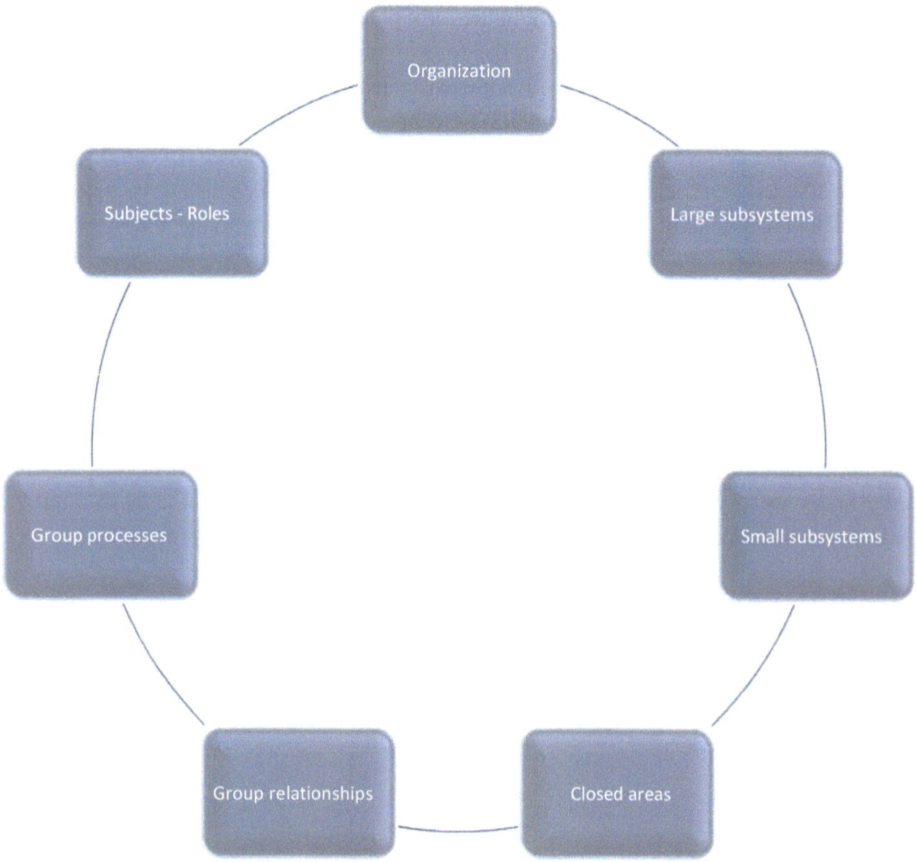

Fig. 35.2 Levels of organizational development. (Own illustration based on Hill et al. (1989))

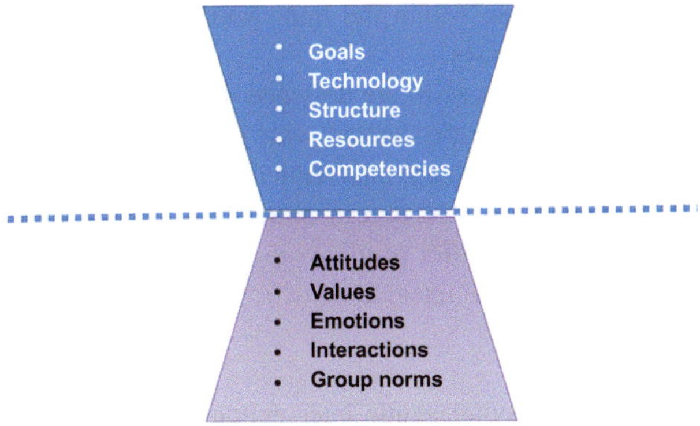

Fig. 35.3 The visible and the hidden in an organization (French and Bell 1990, p. 33, own illustration)

decentralized solutions can be blocked and the dynamics of decentralized processes can be counteracted.

Finally, every organization has visible and hidden characteristics (see Fig. 35.3). For example, in decentralized teams, conflicts can arise when weaker team members slow down the team's dynamics. Also, fractal organizations within the network of relationships do not always pursue the same interests. The understanding of self-organization in a radiology team may differ from that of a surgical team, and there is a risk that interface problems remain statically unresolved. Professional attitudes and norms can also cause decentralized processes to become hierarchical again, leading to the existence of *final decision-makers* on the one hand and the loss of team dynamics on the other.

OD processes therefore always require supplementary OD structures that, on the one hand, bring developments together and, on the other, moderate processes within teams and between teams and departments. What is needed is access to knowledge, i.e., the organization of knowledge as well as information and transparency about the company's development processes, in the form of an adapted, decentralized controlling system, internal communications management, internal or externally organized organizational consulting, and an established company-wide knowledge management system.

35.4 The Importance of OE in Healthcare Institutions

A large proportion of healthcare services are complex interventions. This means that individual interventions, sometimes referred to as singular interventions, are provided in conjunction with other services, both temporally and procedurally interconnected. They are also mutually dependent and influence each other. Typically, several professional groups are involved (Robert Koch Institute 2012). This coherence requires, on the one hand, professional situational decision-making responsibility based on occupational expertise, and at the same time, within the framework of a multiprofessional setting, mutually coordinated care processes.

The way in which service processes are designed depends on the care setting. In the home setting, we are predominantly dealing with individual workstations, which are initially organized as monoprofessional interventions. In institutional care, on the other hand, we generally find multiprofessional team structures.

The conditions of the setting differ primarily due to the complexity of the interventions and the degree of institutional integration.

Three examples illustrate this:

- Home treatment is a psychotherapeutic intervention in the home environment. It is organized for each patient by a multiprofessional team consisting of physicians, specialist nurses, and therapists. Singular interventions are often carried out monoprofessionally or in small teams. In addition to regularly scheduled interventions, crisis interventions also take place, which in individual cases may be conducted digitally. The exchange of information about the implementation of interventions and case discussions must be organized within the team.
- Home-based long-term care is usually provided by a primary nurse in coordination with the affected individuals and their relatives. The patients are generally under outpatient medical care, which typically involves ongoing and, in individual cases, acute pharmacotherapy (see contribution 24), especially for multimorbid patients as a polypharmaceutical arrangement. Therapeutic interventions are also provided on a case-by-case basis. The primary nurse is usually familiar with the nursing and home situation of the patients. Other nurses who are temporarily involved should be appropriately informed. Coordination within the nursing service team regarding assignments, the development of the patients' situation, critical situations, and professional requirements in care and nursing processes must be discussed within the team. However, information from the medical and therapeutic care arrangement is not necessarily available. In individual cases, treatment care may be provided on medical prescription, for example, to ensure safe medication administration.
- A general ward in an acute care hospital is also a predominantly nurse-led setting. Medical care is provided by ward physicians, who generally do not have specialist qualifications. The admission, transfer, and discharge of patients are daily occurrences and must be organized both routinely and on a case-by-case basis. Patients must be coordinated and, if necessary, accompanied with regard to non-nursing diagnostic, medical, and therapeutic interventions. Daily care, especially medication administration, food intake, or nursing activation, must be tailored to each patient. Due to continuous shift operations and the unplanned admission and discharge of patients, systematic coordination and assessment within the nursing team are necessary. These nursing handovers and coordination processes are supplemented by medical rounds for the patients.

These roughly outlined examples illustrate the requirements for OD processes. Even where there are initially less complex, monoprofessional processes, there are relevant connections to interventions from other service processes, which, however, are not routinely available. At the same time, the examples show that OE in healthcare can only be designed as a participatory process.

References

French WL, Bell CH (1990) Organisationsentwicklung: Sozialwissenschaftliche Strategien zur Organisationsveränderung, 3. edn. Bern-Stuttgart, UTB für Wissenschaft Uni-Taschenbücher, Bd 486. Haupt

Hill W, Fehlbaum R, Ulrich P (1989) Organisationslehre: Ziele, Instrumente und Bedingungen der Organisation sozialer Systeme, 4., durchges. Aufl. UTB für Wissenschaft Uni-Taschenbücher Betriebswirtschaft, Bd 259. Haupt

Kühl S (1998) Wenn die Affen den Zoo regieren: Die Tücken der flachen Hierarchien, 5., akt. u. erw. Neuaufl. Campus

Moen R, Norman C (2009) Evolution of the PDCA Cycle [In Proceedings of the 7th ANQ Congress, Tokyo]. https://rauterberg.employee.id.tue.nl/lecturenotes/DG000%20DRP-R/references/Moen-Norman-2009.pdf. Zugegriffen am 08.09.2023

Probst GJB (Hrsg) (1991) Vernetztes Denken: Ganzheitliches Führen in der Praxis, 2., erw. Aufl. Gabler

Robert Koch-Institut (2012) Beiträge zur Gesundheitsberichterstattung des Bundes. Evaluation komplexer Interventionsprogramme in der Prävention: Lernende Systeme, lehrreiche Systeme. Robert-Koch-Inst

Concepts of Digitalization from the Perspective of the Organization

36

Wolfgang Deiters and Sven Meister

Contents

W. Deiters (✉)
Hochschule Bochum, Fachbereich Gesundheitswesen, Bochum, Germany
e-mail: wolfgang.deiters@hs-bochum.de

W. Deiters · S. Meister
Abteilung Gesundheitswesen, Fraunhofer-Institut für Software- und Systemtechnik ISST, Dortmund, Germany

S. Meister
Lehrstuhlinhaber für Gesundheitsinformatik, Fakultät für Gesundheit/Department Humanmedizin, Universität Witten/Herdecke, Witten, Germany

D. Schmitz et al. (eds.), *Chronic Care—Science and Practice*,
https://doi.org/10.1007/978-3-662-72298-5_36

36.1 Digitalization in Organizations

One of the leading terms in this article is digitalization, a widely used but often vaguely defined concept. The English language offers the terms *digitization* and *digitalization* to provide greater distinction, allowing us to differentiate between the conversion of analog data and information into zeros and ones and a process of transformation or change. In the following, digitalization will be used in the sense of digital transformation. Within this definition, we will examine the perspective of organizations in the context of chronic care processes.

From the perspective of healthcare organizations, digitalization is now, on the one hand, a voluntary option to support internal processes and offer additional services. On the other hand, digitalization is increasingly becoming a legal requirement. Laws such as the Hospital Future Act (Krankenhauszukunftsgesetz, KHZG), the Digital Care and Nursing Modernization Act (Digitale Versorgung und Pflege Modernisierungs Gesetz, DVPMG), or the Health Data Use Act (Gesundheitsdatennutzungsgesetz, GDNG) sometimes specify deadlines for the implementation of individual digital processes. Both aspects lead to a constant transformation of existing work and care processes within organizations, which inevitably also affects the people involved in these processes. This change must be addressed and structured. We will address this necessity in Chap. 2 of this article.

Chronic care involves multiprofessional collaboration among the professional groups involved, both within a single care organization and across organizational boundaries. Care thus takes place across both spatial and temporal boundaries. The latter means that subprocesses in the provision of care may occur in parallel or asynchronously. Ideally, all actors always have access to the right information at the right time and place for the purpose of care, for example, the medication plan. Digitalization now makes it possible to distribute information differently. This *differently* is often associated with speed, clarity, quality, cost-effectiveness, and other attributes. However, evidence for this exists—if at all—only for a few specific subprocesses, which is why we will critically examine this in the course of Chap. 3.

Finally, we ask ourselves to what extent today's healthcare in Germany can be understood as a managed process. Sometimes referred to as the patient journey, we look at both the intra- and inter-organizational segments of care and the impact of digitalization. In this context, terms such as case management, navigation functions, or health kiosks arise. It seems evident that the existing management principles in Germany are rather limited.

Thus, examining digitalization concepts from the perspective of organizations paints a multidimensional picture of people, technology, care, and processes. Bringing these dimensions together requires strategic components within organizations.

36.2 Healthcare Organizations as Expert Organizations:Ð The 'Human Factor' in Times of Digital Transformation

Addressing chronic care usually requires the involvement of a multitude of care endpoints with a multiprofessional character. Healthcare institutions have recognized digitalization as a suitable means to address universal challenges such as increasing service complexity, cost and reform pressures, and the shortage of qualified professionals. Digitalization is mostly associated with the introduction of technology. The discussion then centers on the type of technology to be used and the extent of its application. Technology is intended to support processes—processes in which people continue to play a significant role. This chapter examines the *human factor* and its roles within the framework of digital transformation.

Rasche and Braun von Reinersdorff (Rasche and Braun von Reinersdorff 2016) define expert organizations as knowledge- and competence-intensive service organizations whose value creation is primarily based on the recruitment, refinement, and utilization of highly specialized human capital. Experts are thus characterized by being highly qualified, often holding leadership or coordinating roles, possessing a high degree of autonomy, and dealing with complex services or products. Expert organizations provide a suitable environment for the individual development of knowledge toward greater specialization, but not for integrated, interprofessional learning processes across the boundaries of one's own profession and subsystem (Schmerfeld and Schmerfeld 2000).

Both the intra- and inter-organizational perspectives of healthcare institutions as expert organizations inevitably lead to the requirement and ability to work beyond one's own profession. However, to optimally utilize expert knowledge (see contribution 34) and contribute to the best possible treatment of patients, continuous cooperation among the various medical disciplines is necessary. The *willingness* is the motivational aspect—"Why am I doing this?"—and the *ability* addresses the "How," which, in the context of this article, is deliberately answered in a one-dimensional way with digitalization.

Digitalization inevitably leads to change, and such change should be guided and managed—requiring change management. The absence of this, as is the case in most healthcare institutions, has a significant impact on people's behavior. There are numerous behavioral effects, such as openness to and acceptance of change. Common portrayals regarding digitalization include: artificial intelligence or humans, or robots or healthcare professions. This competitive framing is a reality but does not foster acceptance. People must be part of the change process in order to experience a high degree of self-determination. The self-determination theory by (Deci and Ryan 2012) describes the interplay of autonomy, competence, and social relatedness as key pillars for high motivation and well-being.

The current approach to implementing digitalization in organizations relegates people to supporting roles on their own stage. The lack of participatory design prevents the development of collaborative, cooperative, or coexistent human-technology interaction, as well as potential positive effects such as greater needs orientation in healthcare.

Self-determination theory already emphasizes the high importance of competencies. Over- or under-challenging can lead to reduced acceptance of changing processes. A survey commissioned by the European Parliament in 2016 already found that many healthcare professionals had received no or only insufficient further training in the field of *digital health* (Dalati et al. 2016). The Federal Ministry of Health (BMG) emphasizes the need for digital and data competencies in relation to the digitalization strategy for health and care presented in 2023 (Federal Ministry of Health 2023).

The education system responds sluggishly in the areas of initial and continuing education. The new National Competence-Based Learning Objectives Catalogue for Medicine (NKLM 2.0) specifies mandatory digital competencies for future medical studies—implementation ongoing. The *TIGER International Framework for Recommendations of Core Competencies in Health Informatics 2.0* (Hübner et al. 2019) provides a broad perspective on the necessary competencies of various actors and roles in healthcare. Looking at the continuing education offerings of the German Medical Association, initial links to the topic of digitalization can be seen. Further activities are mostly project-based, such as the BMG-funded project *Digi-Manager:in* for the further training of medical assistants in the field of digitalization in outpatient care.

However, focusing on educational policy actors does not absolve healthcare organizations of their responsibility. *Learning on the job*, that is, building knowledge within the context of employment, is a fundamental component of continuous knowledge acquisition. This requires framework conditions such as financial support and the release of employees from their duties.

36.3 Digitalization in Different Healthcare Organizations

Digital technologies promise numerous possibilities, including ensuring the quality of care through data access, data quality, and data readability, saving valuable time by facilitating documentation, and reducing repetitive tasks through automation (Sætra and Fosch-Villaronga 2021). This chapter is dedicated to intra-organizational digitalization and examines the status quo in various healthcare organizations.

36.3.1 Digital Maturity: Measuring the Status Quo of Digitalization

Various approaches from the industrial sector, such as models describing Industry 4.0, can provide guidance for the structured assessment of digital maturity, the identification of corporate objectives, and the bridging of existing gaps. The measurement of the digitalization status quo is carried out across industries using so-called maturity models. These often have their origins in software development, specifically in the Capability Maturity Model (CMM). Healthcare institutions also use maturity models, including for benchmarking, self-assessment, change management, or organizational learning. The World Health Assembly points to the benefits of maturity assessments in identifying areas in need of improvement. It therefore calls on member states to evaluate the use of digital technologies.

In the field of inpatient care, particularly for hospitals, several maturity models have recently been developed. The most widely used international maturity model in this context is the Electronic Medical Record Adoption Model (EMRAM) by the Healthcare Information and Management Systems Society (HIMMS). This also includes the HIMSS

Outpatient Electronic Medical Record Adoption Model (O-EMRAM), an adaptation of the classic EMRAM for outpatient healthcare facilities.

It is important to note critically that the majority of models for measuring digital maturity focus on technology and do not sufficiently take the human factor into account (Burmann and Meister 2021; Neunaber and Meister 2023). In particular, aspects such as motivation, acceptance, and competence are not captured and can negatively impact the achievable effect of digitalization within organizations.

36.3.2 Hospital

A multitude of surveys have shown that German hospitals lag significantly behind in terms of digitalization, both in European and international comparison. One reason often cited is that engaging with digitalization requires appropriate financial resources. With the Hospital Future Act (KHZG) of 2020, funding for projects was made possible along eleven funding criteria (eligible focus areas). The defined funding criteria, the short-term deadlines, and initial experience reports already make it clear: The *human factor* is at risk of being pushed into the background.

On this subject, the authors, together with the Hospital Association of North Rhine-Westphalia (KGNW), conducted a survey among hospital management (n = 184 out of N = 354) regarding the current state of digital development, the challenges and obstacles to further digitalization, and the general sentiment regarding the associated transformation (Fischer et al. 2019). The results showed that management, IT, medical technology, or a steering committee were the main drivers of digitalization initiatives, with the final decision resting with management. Employee involvement in the process usually took place through training. Digital penetration was highest in patient billing at 74%—work on the wards lagged far behind at 47%. Most hospitals were still far from being paperless.

However, people are the essential asset in this system, both in their role as active subjects (service providers) and as treated objects. To digitally transform a single hospital or a hospital group, it is essential to create transparency about the initial state, as well as to know the relevant organizational and analytical levels and their stages of development for this process. The short development cycles of digital innovations can lead to an overload of the *human factor* if structured change management is lacking.

Creating this structure, in turn, means first assessing the status quo. With DigitalRadar, another instrument for evaluating the digitalization status of hospitals has been developed. This tool, initiated as part of the KHZG, aims to direct funds from the hospital future fund financed by this law, to highlight development, and to identify the needs of individual hospitals (in the context of distributing funding from the fund). In 2022, the first results were presented, showing an average score of 33/100 points (Hesser 2022)—indicating significant room for improvement. Unfortunately, this instrument also lacks an explicit measurement of the *human factor*.

36.3.3 Medical Practice

A look back at 1994 in the National Health System (NHS) raises the question of what effect paperless documentation could have in general medical care (Purves 1996). Even then, it was noted that, with sufficient process support, the elimination of paper could lead to significant efficiency and effectiveness gains. Several decades later, we now see that this insight has only been partially realized.

The work of general practitioners is now increasingly shaped by digitalization. The possibilities for using digitalization in general practices and primary care facilities are diverse. Application examples range from simplifying administrative processes and online appointment scheduling to the direct use of telemedicine applications in patient treatment. While digitally connected medical history forms are used in the waiting room, decision support systems assist with diagnosis, and telemedicine applications support treatment. Patients can be issued e-prescriptions, resulting in fewer doctor visits. Administrative processes in a general practice, such as inventory management or staff scheduling, can also be digitally supported. The use of digital solutions can contribute to high-quality healthcare, for example by improving patient safety.

In contrast to the hospitals described above, medical practices have a significantly different organizational and operational structure. The structures and team sizes are smaller, and practice owners often take on roles in strategy development, business management, and digitalization—in addition to providing medical care. This multiple burden usually leaves little room for adequately addressing non-medical areas of responsibility. Running a healthcare facility requires additional staff beyond the physicians, with medical assistants being particularly important. The success of a medical practice depends on these staff members and their satisfaction. This, in turn, means that processes must be aligned not only with the needs of patients and practice owners but also with those of the employees. The PraxisBarometer Digitalisierung 2021 (Albrecht et al. 2022) notes that private practitioners are open to digitalization, but the practical suitability of the available applications is usually lacking. High error rates are met with an unfavorable cost-benefit ratio.

Can digital maturity be adequately measured in this structure? Unlike hospitals, maturity models for this area are still very much in development. Thus, for now, it is necessary to look beyond one's own field and consider the target vision from the citizens' perspective. A prominent example from Europe is the implementation of the strategy in the National Health Service (NHS) with its goal of *GP at hand* (general practitioner always available). The smartphone or desktop PC serves as the access point to primary care, supported by artificial intelligence and patient management along care pathways.

36.3.4 Care Facility

When considering the field of care, it becomes apparent that the degree of digitalization is significantly less pronounced than in the medical sector. First of all, the majority of care is provided by non-professional caregivers (often family members). For this portion of care, there is virtually no technological support, apart from a few app offerings that assist with communication and coordination among caregivers.

In the area of professional care, the topic of support through technology/digitalization has only recently gained momentum. This is mainly because care is largely understood as relationship work, where the personal attention of the caregiver to the person being cared for is paramount. Emotional support, social interaction, and physical care are considered the core aspects of caregiving activities. Any form of technology that intervenes in this relationship (that comes between the caregiver and the person being cared for) has often been perceived as a destruction of the fundamental principles of care and was initially vehemently rejected—the human factor is seen as central.

Digitalization in care therefore initially took place almost exclusively in the area of care documentation. Both in outpatient and inpatient care, legal requirements for documenting caregiving activities have been repeatedly tightened, leading to frequent complaints that the time required for such documentation comes at the expense of the time available for actual caregiving. Against this background, digital systems that make it possible to limit or make documentation more efficient are viewed positively, as they free up time for actual care. In distinguishing between inpatient and outpatient care, documentation systems were first introduced in the inpatient sector, with the outpatient sector following after some delay. In the meantime, digital care documentation is now widespread in outpatient care as well; many care services are moving towards documenting not only in the central care office but also using mobile devices at the point of care in the living environment of the person being cared for.

In the wake of a shortage of skilled workers in the care sector—which became even more publicly apparent during the COVID-19 pandemic—there is a growing recognition that digital applications can be a building block in combating the so-called care crisis. The range of solutions considered extends from ambient assisted living systems (sensor-based systems that can detect and report needs for assistance and provide data analyses for assessing care requirements), to specialized technologies for specific care groups (such as dementia clients), and even robotic systems that can assist with lifting or repositioning, delivery and collection services, or monitoring (such as fluid intake logs/dehydration). However, for all these technologies, while they are used in individual projects or facilities, they are not yet in widespread use. This also applies to the group of digital care applications (DiPAs), for which a legal basis was established in 2022, modeled after the concept of digital health applications (DiGAs). However, for regular funding through care insurance funds, a DiPA directory must first be established by the Federal Institute for Drugs and Medical Devices (BfArM); work on this is currently underway. In summary, it should be noted that, apart from the area of digital care documentation, there is still no broad experience regarding the effects of these technologies—particularly with respect to how they impact the *human factor* in care.

36.3.5 Therapeutic Facility

Similar to the field of care, digitalization in many therapeutic healthcare facilities often does not take place as part of a strategic plan. Connection to the telematics infrastructure is often not available or is still in its infancy. As a result, therapeutic practices are frequently not integrated into digital, cross-sectoral medical care structures.

Of course, digitalization has nevertheless found its way into this area. IT systems exist for performance verification, i.e., for treatment documentation and billing of services rendered. Therapeutic facilities use digital applications for staff scheduling or for presenting a customer presence (web presence). This digitalization of administrative processes contributes to more efficient practice management, helps optimize workflows, and ensures quality. Thus, it provides a small contribution to addressing the shortage of skilled workers by freeing up time for the core therapeutic business and work with patients.

In addition, there are digital solutions in all therapeutic disciplines to support the respective therapeutic service (e.g., in speech therapy, apps to support therapy for aphasia; in physiotherapy, digital tools to promote mobilization or treat balance disorders, gait support, etc.). These digital applications can, in some cases, be highly innovative AI-supported or robotic systems (such as exoskeletons for gait support in (neuro)rehabilitation for patients after stroke or with paraplegia). However, these are often (sometimes highly specialized) standalone systems, whose interoperable interaction—even within the facility—leaves room for improvement, let alone broader networking.

Thus, digitalization in therapeutic facilities usually also takes place as an isolated solution. From the organizational perspective, this means at most support for the intra-organizational perspective, while the cross-organizational and multiprofessional view is virtually not supported.

36.4 The Strength of the Individual Organization Lies in its Interaction with the Entirety of Healthcare Organizations

Looking at digitalization concepts from an organizational perspective, it becomes apparent that the various efforts toward digitalization primarily focus on individual sectors or single organizations. This reflects the deeply rooted segmentation in the German healthcare system between medical, therapeutic, and nursing care, as well as between the outpatient and inpatient sectors. An intersectoral and, above all, interprofessional perspective is often still underdeveloped and not the norm.

Although the explicit goal of the telematics infrastructure, which was launched as early as 2004, was and is to support intersectoral communication and thus improved collaboration through digital solutions, issues related to data protection, technological implementation, and especially concerns from various interest groups (medical associations, health insurance funds, pharmacists' associations, etc.) have led to significant delays in the system. In addition to the introduction of appropriate authentication systems for patients and physicians (EGK, HBA), the first administrative service (VSSD) was implemented in 2015. It was not until 2019, based on the Appointment Service and Supply Act (TSVG), and in 2020, based on the Patient Data Protection Act (PDSG), that the electronic patient record (ePA) was introduced as the first medical service. However, to this day, it has not achieved significant relevance in medical care. The ePA offers great potential, especially in chronic care, as it enables access to the care history. This project also reveals the highly segmented perspective of the German healthcare system. The original concept of the telematics infrastructure only provided access to this system for medical personnel. It was only since 2021/22 that professional IDs for non-chambered health professions (initially nursing, midwifery, physiotherapists, with others to follow) have been issued, thus enabling these groups to participate in the system.

While the discussion around the telematics infrastructure takes a technical view of networking and interoperable data exchange between different organizations, it is also necessary to consider the various health professions and, in particular, their cooperation in medical and nursing care situations. Interprofessional collaboration among different health professions is considered highly important (Behrend et al. 2020). Especially when considering the increasing number of multimorbid and aging patients, collaboration among physicians, nurses, therapists, nutritionists, etc., becomes essential, as only together can they develop a holistic picture of a person in need of care and implement comprehensive care through cooperative, task-sharing collaboration. However, this holistic picture often fails to emerge due to inadequate collaboration—a collaboration for which suitable joint learning concepts still need to be developed (Behrend et al. 2020). There are many examples of this, such as when a person in need of care is transferred back to their facility after a hospital stay for medical treatment, and it is not known there that a change in medication has increased the risk of falls.

Adequate intersectoral collaboration across organizational boundaries and interprofessional collaboration across different occupational groups therefore often remains in need of improvement. In this context, the potential of digitalization in terms of designing new, interprofessional work processes (digitalization) across various professions for the creation of efficient and effective care structures often goes untapped. This discussion also shows that viewing digitalization solely from the perspective of a single organization is too limited; it is precisely the cross-organizational and cross-professional perspective that reveals great potential for digitalization to coordinate and cooperate among various health professionals in the sense of holistic, innovative care structures.

A similar picture emerges from the perspective of those affected. Often, they move through the system for treatment of their condition, being referred from general practitioners to specialists to therapists and back again. This creates patient journeys that, on the one hand, are not efficient from a system perspective and, from the patient's point of view, often seem aimless and not conducive to a rapid cure of their condition. Since there is no digital support for the patient journey (such as through an electronic patient record), it is neither transparent nor assessable.

In addition to the demand for transparency in patient journeys through digital solutions, this also leads to calls for new professional roles and organizations. Navigator concepts are needed that are capable of reading, analyzing/optimizing patient journeys and, on this basis, advising patients and competently guiding them through the healthcare system. This includes advice on the medical situation as well as on physical activity or nutrition. Health navigators connect prevention, diagnosis, and cure, and as advisors, they are a valuable tool for patient empowerment and for strengthening patient compliance in an optimized patient journey.

Navigator concepts can be implemented in various professional roles (such as community health nurses, advisors in neighborhood management, case managers) and can be installed in different organizational settings. In this regard, the concept of the health kiosk is particularly interesting: neighborhood-based counseling and referral services that are currently under political discussion and implementation. Located in socially disadvantaged areas, they offer low-threshold counseling, often for particularly vulnerable groups. They facilitate access to medical treatment, prevention, and health promotion services and can support the coordination of services, especially at the interface between health and social issues. Health kiosks as a new organizational form or navigator concepts as a component of new health professions can build interorganizational bridges in care. However, this can only work with the help of digital solutions in integrated data repositories. With these organizations and professional roles, today's systemic focus can be redirected to the focus on patients, thus strengthening the human factor in a digitally supported patient journey.

36.5 Outlook

People work together in expert organizations along processes and are increasingly supported by digital innovations. The target vision must be a multiperspective approach, as shown in Fig. 36.1.

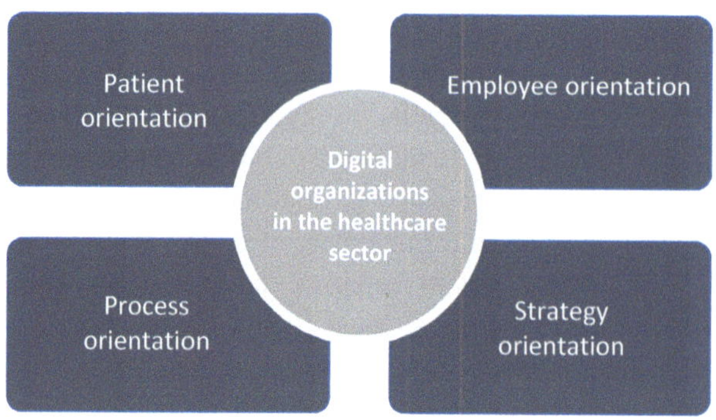

Fig. 36.1 Target vision of digitalization. (Own illustration)

Digitalization is not an end in itself and therefore requires a focus on patients, employees, processes, and strategy. The *human factor* (patients and employees) is prominent, as is human-to-human interaction. People act together with other people along processes—sometimes mediated by digitalization (e.g., digital nursing records, video consultations, etc.) and sometimes in an analog way. Processes should be developed in line with strategic goals (care objectives, corporate goals, etc.). In this context, a process that was previously analog is not always a good digital process.

The introduction of digital innovations into processes usually promotes the generation of data, which in turn can be used for research, care, or company-specific strategic decisions. This availability of data is also accompanied by the discourse on the use of artificial intelligence methods. Here again, the human factor is in focus, as the narrative is *human or AI*. This confrontational depiction must in the future be replaced by opportunities for cooperation or collaboration in order to unlock the potential of digitalization for organizations.

More stringent cooperation and collaboration are also needed interorganizationally. The diversity and frequency of interactions with healthcare institutions in the context of chronic care necessitate a high degree of collaboration. Digitalization can overcome information gaps between organizations. Within a single organization, for example through asynchronous communication, the information status regarding care can be kept transparent. Both people and technology will undergo changes in this process, which must be strategically managed. Management means that a target vision must be formulated, resources provided, and the necessary competencies developed. This form of change requires the participation of all stakeholders, as it affects us all.

References

Albrecht M, Sander M, Otten M (2022) PraxisBarometer Digitalisierung 2021: Stand und Perspektiven der Digitalisierung in der vertragsärztlichen und -psychotherapeutischen Versorgung. https://www.kbv.de/media/sp/IGES_PraxisBaroDigit2021_Kurzbericht.pdf. Accessed 10.02.2024

Behrend R, Maaz A, Sepke M, Peters H (2020) Interprofessionelle Teams in der Versorgung. In: Jacobs K, Kuhlmey A, Greß S, Klauber J, Schwinger A (Eds) Pflege-Report 2019. Springer, Berlin/Heidelberg/Deutschland pp 201–209

Bundesministerium für Gesundheit (2023) Gemeinsam Digital: Digitalisierungsstrategie für das Gesundheitswesen und die Pflege. https://www.bundesgesundheitsministerium.de/fileadmin/Dateien/3_Downloads/D/Digitalisierungsstrategie/BMG_Broschuere_Digitalisierungsstrategie_bf.pdf. Accessed 01.04.2023

Burmann A, Meister S (2021) Practical application of maturity models in healthcare: findings from multiple digitalization case studies, proceedings of the 14th international joint conference on biomedical engineering systems and technologies. SCITEPRESS – Science and Technology Publications, Scitepress/Setúbal/Portugal, pp 100–110

Dalati F, Lenglet G, Steen L, Giedrojc M, Filipe J, Florindi F, Gohlar M, Lim R, Mao X, Pastore M, Schmidt M, Vandamme T (2016) Digital skills for health professionals. https://www.healthparliament.eu/wp-content/uploads/2017/09/Digital-skills-for-health-professionals.pdf. Accessed 22.01.2023

Deci EL, Ryan RM (2012) Self-Determination Theory. In: van Lange PAM (Hrsg) Handbook of theories of social psychology. Sage, London/United Kingdom, pp 416–437

Fischer B, Burmann A, Brinkkötter N, Meister S (2019) Das Digitale Krankenhaus. www.das-digitale-krankenhaus.nrw. Accessed 24.05.2023

Hesser A (2022) Erste Ergebnisse des Digitalradar: „Solide" Digitalisierung in den Kliniken. kma 27:26–29

Hübner U, Thye J, Shaw T, Elias B, Egbert N, Saranto K, Babitsch B, Procter P, Ball MJ (2019) Towards the TIGER international framework for recommendations of core competencies in health. Informatics 2.0: extending the scope and the roles. Stud Health Technol Informat 264:1218–1222

Neunaber T, Meister S (2023) Digital maturity and its measurement of general practitioners: a scoping review. IJERPH 20:4377

Purves IN (1996) The paperless general practice. BMJ (Clinical research ed.) 312:1112–1113

Rasche C, Braun von Reinersdorff A (2016) Krankenhäuser als Expertenorganisationen. In: Pfannstiel AM, Rasche C, Mehlich H (Hrsg) Dienstleistungsmanagement im Krankenhaus. Springer Fachmedien, Wiesbaden, pp 1–23

Sætra HS, Fosch-Villaronga E (2021) Healthcare digitalisation and the changing nature of work and society. Healthcare 9:1007

Schmerfeld K, Schmerfeld J (2000) Interprofessionelle Kooperation im Krankenhaus 1. Problembeschreibungen. Jahrb Krit Med 33:94–109

Normality and Equality in Self-Determined Living with Chronic Diseases

37

Helen Güther and Manfred Fiedler

Contents

37.1 Normality and (In)Equality

The desire to be *normal* is deeply rooted in us as social beings. It conveys a sense of belonging and the idea of an ideal way of life. As such, the notion of what is *normal* shapes our everyday perception, thinking, speaking, and actions. At the same time, the normality we orient ourselves by is so familiar to us that we usually do not question it,

H. Güther (✉)
Fakultät für Gesundheit, Department für Humanmedizin, Universität Witten/Herdecke, Witten, Germany
e-mail: helen.guether@uni-wh.de

M. Fiedler
Department of human medicine, Witten/Herdecke University, Witten, Germany
e-mail: manfred.fiedler@uni-wh.de

D. Schmitz et al. (eds.), *Chronic Care—Science and Practice*,
https://doi.org/10.1007/978-3-662-72298-5_37

but rather take it for granted. Yet, there is no such thing as *the* normal. Rather, normality is a construct shaped by historical and sociocultural factors, and is therefore variable and subject to change (normalism), which has gained increasing significance in the understanding of social order processes with the development of larger nation-states since the 18th century.

The literary scholar and discourse theorist Jürgen Link (1997) conceptually bases his studies on *normalism* on the statistical measure of the normal distribution, which is defined by a central normal spectrum and, at its edges, by boundary values (normality or tolerance limits). The distribution curve is mathematically continuous, i.e., the boundary between normal and abnormal is fluid. Historically, two ideal-typical concepts can be distinguished for Western industrial societies: protonormalism and flexible normalism. *Protonormalism* is characterized by narrowly defined boundaries of normality and a rigid delimitation of what is normal, resulting in authoritarian to violent exclusion and sanctioning of all those declared abnormal (examples include earlier closed psychiatric institutions and the euthanasia laws of the Nazi regime). Only in modern postwar industrial societies does the understanding of normality shift toward *flexible normalism*, with a broader spectrum of characteristics and behaviors accepted as normal. What is judged abnormal or degenerate in protonormalism is, in the understanding of flexible normalism, a tolerable otherness that is included within the spectrum of the normal. In flexible normalism, the notion of normality is changeable over time, resulting in a multitude of normalities (Link 1997). Nevertheless, it must be noted that the experiences of people with chronic illnesses and disabilities, despite the predominance of flexible normalism in Western societies today, (still) paint a picture of sometimes severe exclusion. Unequal health, social, economic, demographic, geographic, and other conditions that lead to health and social inequality must be critically examined.

37.1.1 Chronic Illness as Deviation from the Norm (Experiences of Discrimination)

First and foremost, people with disabilities, people with (severe) mental, behavioral, and intellectual illnesses (depression, schizophrenia, dementias) are affected by stigmatization and, as a result, discrimination. The life situation of people with communicable infectious diseases, such as sexually transmitted diseases or HIV, is also highly burdened by experiences of exclusion. In contrast, people with more age-typical illnesses, such as diabetes mellitus or cardiovascular diseases, are less frequently affected. Barriers to access (e.g., to the labor market, to care facilities outside certain neighborhoods/districts), segregation (e.g., through institutionalization of those affected in psychiatric clinics or nursing homes), a physician-centered healthcare system, inadequate staffing and personnel development, as well as insufficient involvement of those affected (e.g., in decision-making and health services research), and financial disadvantage can be understood as *structural* discrimination. Demeaning and shame-inducing actions such as verbal belittlement (for example, using first names, baby talk, etc.) or even measures that deprive individuals of their liberty are to be regarded as *depersonalizing* discrimination. The spectrum of social disadvantage outlined here raises the question of *why* people affected by chronic illness and people with dementia, even in times of widespread flexible normalism, still find themselves at and moving along the boundaries of what is considered normal.

37.2 Social Construction of Normality and Deviation

Link's concept of normalism provides insight into the fundamental understanding of normality in societies. However, the structural and functional influences on a society that cause diversity in line with flexible normalism or, conversely, homogeneity in the sense of protonormalism, are not yet fully explained. Therefore, the following questions need to be explored in more depth: What mechanisms promote abnormality at the interpersonal level (Sect. 37.2.1)? How is normality produced at the societal level (Sect. 37.2.2)? How does (social and health) inequality arise (Sect. 37.2.3)?

37.2.1 Stigmatization—Between Social and Personal Identity (Erving Goffman)

Discrimination, as a factual exclusion and disadvantage, goes hand in hand with stigmatization. 1963 Goffman published his work "Stigma," which was not only widely received but also became the starting point for a broad scientific discourse on the social phenomenon of stigmatization. Stigma (Latin = tattoo, brand, marking of a person) is understood as a negative deviation that is attributed to the person. In reality, however, stigmas are never naturally given, but are always dependent on interpretation and are ascribed to a person (*labeling*). Through this, individuals are socially devalued (discrediting) and excluded (discrimination). In the context of illness, stigmatization occurs especially when it is assumed that the affected person is to blame for their flaw, or when there is a mental impairment (perceived as behavioral abnormality, see contribution 21). Stigmatization begins where a person's identity deviates from normative and stereotypical expectations, i.e., simplified, socially established, or even personal value judgments about individuals (or groups). At the center of Goffman's analyses is therefore the *identity* of those affected, which is determined by characteristics of their body, their behavior, their cognitive abilities, or simply their belonging to a group, such as people with chronic illness. Goffman distinguishes three aspects of identity that every person possesses:

1. The public *social identity* (social identity), which on the one hand expresses social status, but can also include external characteristics such as attributed abilities and

traits. It is changeable, as both prestige and negative, attributed characteristics (stigmas) can be projected onto it. As such, it can and must be managed by those affected.
2. The *personal identity* (personal identity), which encompasses the uniqueness of the person and especially biographical characteristics that are inextricably linked to the individual.
3. The *ego-identity*, as a self-reflective, self-constructed identity that engages with and organizes both personal and social identity.

Social and personal identity exist in a field of tension, especially when personal identity includes characteristics that are discreditable (*discreditable secrets*), i.e., that are or can become the subject of stigmatization.

To manage this tension, those affected, from the perspective of ego-identity, employ various techniques (*stigma management*). These include, in particular, concealing discreditable characteristics (*covering*), avoiding stigmatized and stigmatizing groups, people, and situations (*distancing*), targeted information control—deciding who is given access to which information—and finally, the staging of a public identity (*professional presentation*).

For example, people with discreditable characteristics such as chronic illness or disability distinguish between the group of normals, to whom they do not feel they belong and from whom they withhold information or present an expected social identity, and their *own group*, such as the chronically ill, within which they reveal more or different information about themselves. Goffman illustrates his considerations using the example of a woman with dwarfism: She must adapt her social identity to the expectations of the supposedly normal, non-disabled group due to the hardly concealable characteristic of short stature. To do so, she stages the role of a clown imposed upon her and denies her personal identity. Within the safety of her own group, where the socially dominant expectation of a certain body size loses significance, she can express and experience her personal identity—her need for equal recognition—freely and un*im*peded. The own group consists not only of people directly affected by chronic illness or disability, but also of close friends, relatives, partners, as well as trusted caregivers and health professionals, up to entire professional groups (such as nursing, psychiatry, and therapeutic education professions). Belonging to an own group, for example close family members, can result in the same stigma—either covertly or openly—being attributed to them as to the affected person. While those not directly affected in the own group play an important role as advocates and mediators for the primarily stigmatized person, this connection can also lead to them becoming secondarily stigmatized (*courtesy stigma*) and experiencing corresponding discrimination.

However, the problem with stigma management is not only that those affected must move as if between two worlds (the world of the normal and that of the abnormal). Attention must also be paid to the socialization process through which the actual identity (*actual social identity*) of those affected is adapted to a normative, stereotypical, social expectation (*virtual social identity*). By conforming to the social expectations placed upon them, they involuntarily orient themselves toward a normality imposed on them, which they begin to internalize (*normification*). Goffman's reference to *normification* thus points to a socially constructed normality that shapes and frames the life situation of people with chronic limitations and their own group—although Goffman himself did not reflect on the broader social context of norms. Therefore, considerations of Foucault's concept of power and Bourdieu's theory of habitus are relevant at this point.

37.2.2 Disciplining the Body (Michel Foucault)

Unlike Goffman, who traces the process of stigmatization at the social micro-level through everyday interactions, Foucault (2016) reconstructs the emergence of social functions and structures, and thus hierarchies, as the exercise of power. The starting point is also the *body*, but less as an expression of information and bearer of subjective identity (or stigma), and more in its social functionality as an object of (conditioning) subjected to structural, institutionalized power. Foucault demonstrates that the body and the behaviors exercised upon it, beyond its biological functionality, are primarily treated as a socially disciplined and controlled object (body discipline). This *disciplining* secures social hierarchies and is guided by prevailing norms. At the same time, it limits individuality and deviant behavior. Foucault highlights social body techniques that serve to control human diversity through the regulation of the body. Key features by which the disciplining of the body can be traced are *space* (partitioning), *function* (coding), *activity* (developments, actions), and *time* over the course of life. Thus, the behaviors of children and also the sick, in contrast to (healthy) adults, can be tolerated as temporary and situational deviations from the norm. They are granted—temporarily—a higher degree of individuality. Parallels to Parsons' sick role, in which those affected are freed from social norms and functions for the duration of their illness, are evident. In the case of permanent deviation from the norm, such as that caused by a chronic illness, however, the body is understood as dysfunctional and loses its value within the prevailing social order, since those affected have no chance of returning to a norm-compliant bodily structure. Thus, the chronically ill person loses their function and place in society. Foucault points out that the disciplining of the (chronically ill) body is the result of a genealogical developmental process: With the triumph of scientifically based medicine in the 18th century, the meaning of illness changed. The medical gaze took shape and, since then, has determined, based on empirically measurable symptoms and diagnosable deviations, what counts as health (the normal) and what counts as illness (the abnormal) (*medicalization*). Therapeutic intervention sets the path for returning from illness and abnormality to health or normality. In order to exclude the abnormal, in a medicalized society, this can, in extreme cases, lead to institutional exclusion (for example, from the company) or to spatial confinement and exclusion (institutionalization) in, for example, closed psychiatric hospitals (referred to by Goffman as *total institution*) of people diagnosed as ill. Power is to be understood as an abstract form of domination, in which social significance is expressed and measured through space and time. Thus, the forms of expression extend beyond the actual human body and also include a virtual, spatial corporeality: The higher the hierarchical position, the more significant the social function, the greater the virtual body, i.e., the space (body structure) granted to the individual. Conversely, the *institutional techniques of domination* are intended to stabilize social hierarchies in the form of disciplining through surveillance (control) and punishment, and to enforce norm-compliant behavior within the body structure attained or assigned to the individual. Unlike in archaic societies, where physical violence was used, in modern societies the most important concept for punishing deviation from the norm is *panopticism*—the seamless and efficient surveillance of the many by the few in *partitioned space*. The surveillants remain hidden from the view of those being surveilled. Surveillance as such is therefore anonymous, yet it is always present and possible. Power thus becomes automated and at the same time de-individualized. In the panoptic disciplinary society, anyone can be both the surveilled and the surveillant, and this at every level, whether in the family, in public institutions such as hospitals, schools, in the company, or at the workplace. Even though he repeatedly analyzes historically, Foucault emphasizes the detachment from a personally named ruler, the subtlety of the mechanisms, and thus the reference to modern societies. In this way, he highlights the persistence of what we, following Goffman, can consider normification, because this is based, on the one hand, on social hierarchies and structures that operate as an automatism in all areas of life. At the same time, the interplay between the idea and the experience of control and sanction means that the individual must always fear the loss of their position and thus must strive for norm-compliant behavior. Foucault does not use the terms stigma or discrimination. But the panoptic mechanisms to which a person with a potentially discreditable characteristic in their living space (body space) is exposed can, with regard to the limitation of individuality, be fundamentally analyzed as an interplay of public, personal, and self-identity.

37.2.3 Habitus and Social Inequality (Pierre Bourdieu)

The disciplined virtual and biological corporeality observed by Foucault also proves to be power-stabilizing in that it can lead to the internalization of a social position, which then becomes incorporated as *habitus*. For the biological body is not merely a passive object of stigmatization and disciplining. It also reproduces social structures within and through itself and thus—albeit unconsciously—actively contributes to an existing social order. Pierre Bourdieu demonstrates this in his theory of habitus, developed in the 1960s and 1970s on the basis of biographical studies. According to Bourdieu (2021), *habitus* is a *structured* and at the same time *structuring structure* that unconsciously shapes both the patterns of action and perception of a person. It embodies an *attitude*. At times, Bourdieu also refers to habitus as a *lifestyle*, which, with regard to health and illness, reveals interesting connections to the concept of the social determinants of health (see Section 16). Thus, the fact of where we live, with whom we live, and the geographical and social space that shapes us, has a direct impact on the development of our habitus. At the same time, the habitus, in the way we move, dress, and behave, always involuntarily reveals information about our origins and biographical development and, in turn, shapes our living environment. Through the sociality thus expressed, we position ourselves in the social space and are positioned within it. Bourdieu illustrates the social positioning of individuals in a two-dimensional social space consisting of class or stratum affiliation (vertical axis) and capital accumulated over the life course (horizontal axis). In terms of class affiliation, Bourdieu distinguishes rather broadly between dominant, middle, and subordinate classes; in terms of capital, he differentiates between *economic capital* (money or assets directly convertible into money) as well as *cultural* and *social capital* (Bourdieu 2015, 2021). Social capital consists of existing or created social networks and social relationships. Cultural capital is differentiated into embodied (education), objectified (acquired cultural goods), and institutionalized (titles, awards) forms. Thus, habitus is on the one hand an expression of the hierarchical social order, and at the same time, through it, we internalize and stabilize social power structures and positions. Due to this interaction, a change or even a break out of a social position (unreflectively) is hardly possible, since we do not consciously experience de facto inequality and disadvantage as such, because they have become self-evident to us.

Bourdieu therefore also understands this mechanism as *symbolic violence* (Bourdieu 2005). Applied to the situation of people with chronic illnesses, symbolic violence is evident wherever social status within one's own class is weakened, for example by persistently high medical or care expenses, restriction of cultural capital (such as in the case of a dementia illness), and loss of social capital through the erosion of existing networks, e.g., due to limited mobility, without any resistance being raised against it. Unlike with Goffman, lack of demands, gratitude, or silence on the part of the stigmatized are not to be understood as conscious stigma management in order to secure a favorable social position in society despite deviation from a norm. Rather, those affected unconsciously practice a habitualized self-deprecation, which makes them appear invisible and unimportant, with the consequence that they are accorded only a low social status (cf. Section 37.1.1). From the perspective of symbolic violence, the concept of courtesy stigma described by Goffman also takes on a much more central significance. Thus, the question arises as to whether entire occupational groups and professional disciplines in the context of chronic care are also subject to the symbolic violence of self-deprecation, as can be seen in the developments of deprofessionalization of non-medical health professions. The normification described by Goffman is then not only to be understood as the subtle power of a socially dominant norm such as the biomedical interpretation (Foucault), to which one is indeed powerless but can consciously criticize. With Bourdieu, it is both internalized and embodied, and thus (almost) invisible.

37.3 Promoting Equality through Self-Determination

Against the backdrop of the three major sociological theories of stigma, power, and habitus, the final question to be addressed is how equality in self-determined living with chronic illnesses can be made possible.

37.3.1 Cultural Change

In a medicalized society as described by Foucault, the chronically ill person is reduced to their body. This body is then declared a deviation from the norm of health, rendered abnormal, and disciplined both through the shaping of its virtual corporeality (e.g., through segregation and institutionalization) and its biological corporeality (e.g., through efforts to medically and technically (re)establish a state of health defined as normal). Framed in Link's terminology, this one-sided societal orientation leads to protonormalistic structures, which, under the pressure of Goffman's normification, cause self-stigmatization. To counteract this, stigma management must be shifted from the level of individual action to the societal level (*Cultural Change*). In other words, the burden of the problem must be reversed onto the socio-cultural level in order to structurally establish a flexible normalism, as Link suggests. The World Health Organization has coined the concept of *Health Equity* to ensure equal health opportunities. This is described as "the absence of unfair, avoidable or remediable differences among groups of people, whether those groups are defined socially, economically, demographically, or geographically or by other dimensions of inequality (e.g. sex, gender, ethnicity, disability, or sexual orientation)" (WHO 2022). The challenge of implementing health equity, in light of Foucault's theory of power, lies in moving beyond the biomedical interpretive framework. Thus, health policy instruments such as outreach, low-threshold, and broadly culturally appropriate services, patient education, or the initiation of health-promoting cities must always be critically reflected upon with regard to the risk of even further-reaching encroachment of medical interpretive frameworks and power influences on the lifeworld of the so-called *affected*, in order not to implement the existing biomedical protonormalism even more powerfully instead of making it more flexible. For the implementation of a flexibly normalistic health policy and socio-cultural framework, people with chronic illnesses must be able to participate equally and not be reduced to a medical diagnosis, so that they can help shape this framework in the sense of political participation and plurality (see contributions 29 and 51).

37.3.2 Habitus Sensitivity

In addition to changing societal framework conditions, there is also a need for a response at the level of immediate interaction in order to counteract the symbolic violence that both shapes and manifests societal conditions. To realize and stabilize a flexible normalism through lived practice, the empowerment of those affected is therefore of central importance at the interaction level (e.g., through self-help groups). The experience of one's own competence despite and with a chronic illness fosters a positive self-image and strengthens ego identity. In this way, negative self-images can ideally be countered, contrary to biomedical pressure to conform, and one's own sense of control—i.e., the competence for self-determination as well as the conviction of being able to manage one's own affairs—can be promoted, thereby positively developing one's own habitus. People with chronic illnesses, in particular, should be regarded as experts regarding their own life situations. In recent decades, the concept of *Shared-Decision-Making* has become established as a model for joint decision-making in health therapies. This refers not only to the legal respect for the patient's will. Especially for people who find it difficult to articulate their will and needs, such as those in critical life situations or with cognitive impairments, it is not just a one-time clarification, but requires an ongoing, safeguarded process. Since chronic illnesses do not represent a temporary disruption of social position, special attention must be paid in the care of chronically ill people to the development of profession-specific cultural competence, which addresses questions of body perception, as well as the emotional and social needs of chronically ill people in their illness-influenced lifeworld. This forms the basis for multiprofessional, culturally sensitive services and should be established as a component of interprofessional cooperation. According to Bourdieu, it is the opportunity—perhaps even the duty—especially of professionals to become aware of their own habitus (habitus sensitivity), in order to develop a reflective practice. This can then help to question one's own familiar protonormalistic, i.e., biomedical, normative concepts and to learn from new experiences, which in turn begin to shape a self-determined lifestyle or habitus and, through this, a flexible normalism.

References

Bourdieu P (2005) Die männliche Herrschaft. Suhrkamp, Frankfurt am Main

Bourdieu P (2015) Die verborgenen Mechanismen der Macht. VSA, Hamburg

Bourdieu P (2021) Die feinen Unterschiede. Kritik der gesellschaftlichen Urteilskraft, 28. edn. Suhrkamp, Frankfurt am Main

Foucault M (2016) Die Hauptwerke, 4. Aufl. Suhrkamp, Frankfurt am Main

Goffman E (1963) Stigma. Notes of management on spoiled Identity. Touchstone, New York

Link J (1997) Versuch über den Normalismus. Wie Normalität produziert wird. Westdeutscher Verlag, Wiesbaden

World Health Organisation (WHO) (2022) Health equity. https://www.who.int/health-topics/health-equity#tab=tab_1. Accessed 04.22.2022

Chronic Illness—A Family Affair 38

Christiane Knecht

Contents

38.1 Family/Families Today

With the "pluralization of familial and non-familial life forms" (Peuckert 2019, p. 18), the traditional family constellation of father, mother, and child(ren) is losing its preeminence. Characteristics such as lifelong marriage, child(ren), a shared household in which the woman assumes responsibility for care work and the man takes on the role of breadwinner, define the societal image of a *normal family*. Alternative family and life forms, such as same-sex partnerships, single parents, blended families, or spouses who live in a long-distance relationship in two separate households, complement the picture of family/families today (Nave-Herz 2019; Peuckert 2019). In contrast, narrowly defined concepts of family may even exclude such modern familial and non-familial arrangements (Nave-Herz 2019). Referring to all these previously described family and life forms, three attributes can be identified that Nave-Herz (2019, p. 16) describes as constitutive features

C. Knecht (✉)
FH Münster, Fachbereich Gesundheit, Münster, Germany
e-mail: knecht@fh-muenster.de

D. Schmitz et al. (eds.), *Chronic Care—Science and Practice*,
https://doi.org/10.1007/978-3-662-72298-5_38

of family: (1) "reproductive and socialization function," (2) "cooperation and solidarity," and (3) "differentiation of generations." Jurczyk (2014, p. 66) also emphasizes the aspect of care and describes family as a system of care-related generational and gender relationships in which care work is naturally assumed. Through these private and semi-public care services, the family simultaneously makes an indispensable contribution to society (Jurczyk 2014). Bertram (2002) highlights further developments that allow statements to be made about cohabitation and relationships within families. Due to the aging of society, it is now possible, for example, for older family members to witness the weddings of grandchildren or the growing up of great-grandchildren. Even if families of origin and their members do not live in the same place, relationships within families persist and can be maintained. From both developments, Bertram (2002, p. 517) derives the concept of "multi-local multigenerational families." At the same time, this means that heterogeneous lifestyles interact in families at various locations, requiring coordination and negotiation work, especially with regard to maintaining emotional and social connectedness, in order to make family practically livable in everyday life (Schier 2009). While the deinstitutionalization thesis predicts the decline of the classic family, other authors point to the transformation evident in family cultures with modern forms of solidarity that "extend beyond spatial distances and kinship boundaries" (see, e.g., Peuckert 1991; Lüscher 1989; Lüscher and Schultheis 1993, cited in Backes 1998, pp. 6–7). Jurczyk (2014) therefore asks how doing family, or the active creation of family, can be practically realized so that families can even assume care responsibilities under today's conditions?

38.2 Living in a Family with Chronic Illness

The characteristics described above apply not only to healthy families, but also when one or more members of a family are affected by chronic illness. While there is a lack of valid data regarding chronic diseases, in 2021, 2.55 million—more than half of the nearly 5 million people in need of care in Germany—were cared for predominantly by their families alone, while another 1.05 million were supported by care and support services (Federal Statistical Office (Destatis) 2022). This trend, which has remained stable for years according to the biennial care statistics, emphatically demonstrates the solidarity in Germany regarding the assumption of caregiving responsibilities within families. However, it is not only care work that is taken on as a matter of course; rather, health itself is shaped both positively and negatively within families (Büscher and Schnepp 2011). Chronic illness is thus a family matter that affects not only the life of the person concerned, but indeed the entire family structure, its individual members, and their relationships with one another (Grypdonck 2005). Conversely, this can mean that changes affecting one member can in turn influence the chronic illness and family dynamics. The significance of chronic illness and family coping strategies can therefore only be understood in this context. Apart from a few state-specific initiatives, such as the model project "Familiale Pflege," which became part of standard care in 2019 (Lebeda et al.

2017), the family perspective—with its experiences, biography, family roles, actions, and dynamics—is only here and there and rarely systematically considered in professional nursing care in Germany.

The focus in social legislation is, by its nature, also directed at the affected individuals. However, family care begins before other (professional) assistance is involved and does not end when such assistance is provided (Schnepp 2002). Caring families are therefore often "silent service providers" (Schnepp 2006, p. 69), and there is a risk of their instrumentalization. Especially when care within families is not understood as a shared family project but rather takes place in a dyad, where one primary caregiver assumes the caregiving tasks alone, the burden on this person can be enormous. The discourse on the burden of family caregivers has been extensively described in meta-analyses by Pinquart and Sörensen (2003, 2006, 2007, 2011). The experience of burden ranges, for example, from physical and psychological to social effects. Caring families are confronted with social rejection and isolation. Roles and relationships within the family change. Life and daily routines are arranged around the chronic illness. It is difficult to assess the duration of care relationships, and care periods are now significantly longer due to increasing life expectancy.

That caregiving responsibility involves varying time commitments, that the experience of burden can differ, and that family caregivers are not a homogeneous group is also shown by the ZIPA study by Bohnet-Joschko (2020). While previous findings label family caregivers as a risk group, family care does not necessarily have to be associated with burden. Family care, in the sense of "doing family," can also be understood as a shared developmental task that brings new meaning. Schnepp (2006) therefore recommends identifying burdens, assessing them carefully, understanding and explaining how they arise, and how families deal with them. Only from this understanding can support for families succeed. Corbin and Strauss (1991) studied couples in which one partner is affected by a chronic illness and the other is healthy. The authors make it clear that coping strategies are directed at the life disrupted by the illness, not at the chronic illness itself, using the concept of "work" and its three lines of work (illness, everyday life, and biography), which interact with the illness trajectory curve. After the manifestation of the illness, acute phases alternate with crises, normalization phases, and downward developments, with these phases occurring less in health care institutions and more at home, shaped by those affected themselves, their families, and professional care. Care thus takes place in a triangular relationship. Twigg and Atkin (1994) describe four roles of family caregivers, from which different role assignments and expectations of professional care regarding informal helpers result:

1. Carer as resource: The focus is on the person affected. Informal helpers are seen as a resource, while professional care is substituted.
2. Carer as co-worker: The focus is on both the person affected and the informal helpers, with the goal of connecting both support systems.

3. Carer as co-client: The focus is on the informal helpers, who are considered a second target group for professional care.
4. Superseded carer: The focus is on promoting the independence of the person affected and reducing dependence on the caregiving family, while maintaining the relationship.

The perspectives of caregiving families and professional care differ significantly, and their cooperative relationships must be negotiated (Büscher 2007).

38.3 Family-Centeredness—Perspectives for Germany

The experiences and perspectives of relatives form the starting point for family care of people with chronic illnesses. It is therefore important to recognize the significance of caregiving families and not to diminish or instrumentalize them. A prerequisite for this is a definition of family that includes today's diverse forms of living and is useful for clinical nursing care. Wright and Leahey (2005, p. 60) therefore propose a broad definition: "The family is who they say they are." While other countries are more advanced in establishing family-centered care, Germany still has some catching up to do. Professional nurses must be trained in family-centered care and acquire competencies to systematically support families willing to take on caregiving responsibilities. What professional nurses can do is to care together with the family. It is the small interventions that are perceived as helpful and can provide short-term relief, such as developing respect for the uniqueness of the family, sharing information, involving the family in care at the level they are comfortable with, communicating openly, and entering into a care-family partnership. In the spirit of *think family*, caregiving families should therefore be considered important target groups.

References

Backes GM (1998) Individualisierung und Pluralisierung der Lebensverhältnisse: Familie und Alter im Kontext der Modernisierung. Z Familienforsch 10(2):5–29

Bertram H (2002) Die multilokale Mehrgenerationenfamilie. Von der neolokalen Gattenfamilie zur multilokalen Mehrgenerationenfamilie. Berl J Soziol 12(4):517–529

Bohnet-Joschko S (Hrsg) (2020) Zielgruppenspezifische Unterstützungsangebote für pflegende Angehörige. Transferbericht, Witten

Büscher A (2007) Negotiating helpful action. A substantive theory on the relationship between formal and informal care. Doctoral dissertation, University of Tampere. https://trepo.tuni.fi/bitstream/handle/10024/67689/978-951-44-6843-8.pdf;sequence=1. Accessed 06.02.2024

Büscher A, Schnepp W (2011) Die Bedeutung von Familien in der pflegerischen Versorgung. In: Schaeffer D, Wingenfeld K (Eds) Handbuch Pflegewissenschaft. Juventa Verlag, Weinheim, pp 469–487

Corbin JM, Strauss A (1991) A nursing model for chronic illness management based upon the trajectory framework. Sch Inq Nurs Pract 5(3):155–174

Grypdonck M (2005) Ein Modell zur Pflege chronisch Kranker. In: Seidl E, Walter I (Hrsg) Chronisch kranke Menschen in ihrem Alltag. Das Modell von Mieke Grypdonck bezogen auf Patientinnen nach Nierentransplantation. Pflegewissenschaft heute, vol 8, pp 15–60. Verlag Wilhelm Maudrich, Wien/München/Bern

Jurczyk K (2014) Familie als Herstellungsleistung. Hintergründe und Konturen einer neuen Perspektive auf Familie. In: Jurczyk K, Lange A, Thiessen B (Eds) Doing Family. Warum Familienleben heute nicht mehr selbstverständlich ist. Beltz Juventa, Weinheim/Basel, pp 50–70

Lebeda D, Waterböhr J-W, Gröning K (2017) Die praktische Konzeption und die Instrumente im Modellprojekt „Familiale Pflege unter den Bedingungen der G-DRG". Bielefeld University, Studienbrief

Nave-Herz R (2019) Familienformen in Deutschland. In: Nave-Herz R (Eds) Familie heute. Wandel der Familienstrukturen und Folgen für die Erziehung. wbg academic, Darmstadt, pp 14–30

Peuckert R (2019) Pluralisierung der Lebensformen. In: Peuckert R (Eds) Familienformen im sozialen Wandel. Springer VS, Wiesbaden, pp 133–145

Pinquart M, Sörensen S (2003) Differences between caregivers and noncaregivers in psychological health and physical health: a meta-analysis. Psychol Aging 18(2):250–267

Pinquart M, Sörensen S (2006) Gender differences in caregiver stressors, social resources, and health: an updated meta-analysis. J Gerontol B Psychol Sci Soc Sci 61(1):33–45

Pinquart M, Sörensen S (2007) Correlates of physical health of informal caregivers: a meta-analysis. J Gerontol B Psychol Sci Soc Sci 62(2):126–137

Pinquart M, Sörensen S (2011) Spouses, adult children, and children-in-law as caregivers of older adults: a meta-analytic comparison. Psychol Aging 26(1):1–14

Schier M (2009) Räumliche Entgrenzung von Arbeit und Familie: Die Herstellung von Familie unter Bedingungen von Multilokalität. Informationen zur Raumentwicklung 1/2: 55–66. https://nbn-resolving.org/urn:nbn:de:0168-ssoar-65363-7. Accessed 06.02.2024

Schnepp W (2002) Einleitung. In: Schnepp W (Hrsg) Angehörige pflegen. Huber, Bern, pp 6–12

Schnepp W (2006) Im Angesicht des Anderen: „Schützen müssen". Antrittsvorlesung am Lehrstuhl für familienorientierte und gemeindenahe Pflege, Institut für Pflegewissenschaft, Universität Witten/Herdecke. Pflege & Gesellschaft 11(1):61–76

Statistisches Bundesamt (Destatis) (2022) Pflegestatistik 2021. https://www.destatis.de/DE/Themen/Gesellschaft-Umwelt/Gesundheit/Pflege/_inhalt.html. Accessed 21.09.2023

Twigg J, Atkin K (1994) Carers perceived. Policy and practice in informal care. Open University Press, Maidenhead

Wright LM, Leahey M (2005) Nurses and families: a guide to family assessment and intervention. F.A. Davis, Philadelphia

Self-Determined Living at Home: Diversity of Living Arrangements

39

Kirstin Schütz

Contents

39.1 Self-Determined Living at Home

The care of chronically ill and often elderly people takes place in various institutional contexts. Different ongoing physical, mental, or emotional limitations generally require long-term support, or result in a need for care. In particular, the appropriate form of housing can be crucial in providing those affected with independence and the highest possible quality of life. It is important to involve the individuals themselves in the decision-making process or, better yet, to empower them to make their own choices.

K. Schütz (✉)
Witten, Germany
e-mail: Kirstin.Schuetz@uni-wh.de

D. Schmitz et al. (eds.), *Chronic Care—Science and Practice*,
https://doi.org/10.1007/978-3-662-72298-5_39

39.2 Negotiating the Care Arrangement

With regard to the institutional context, or rather the space in which care is provided, there can be a wide variety of care settings. When focusing on the living situation, the main types to mention are inpatient and outpatient settings, which (see contribution 30) in turn form the basis for the design of care and are considered complex care arrangements that go far beyond mere care arrangements. The complexity of a care arrangement in particular requires the ongoing negotiation of care goals as part of care planning. The actors involved in this process should primarily be the individuals affected themselves, their relatives, as well as professionals from health and non-health professions. Multiprofessional collaboration is therefore advantageous. Even though the care goals are generally prevention, rehabilitation, maintenance of function, quality of life, and *end of life care*, the individual actors often interpret their implementation very differently from their own perspectives. Therefore, this negotiation should always include a comparison of perspectives that places the ideas and wishes of those affected at the center and takes their self-determination into account. Especially for people with dementia, relatives and close contacts should ask early on how the person wishes to be cared for and which form of housing is preferred. It is therefore advisable to gain an overview of the variety of housing options together with the person affected and to keep the framework conditions of each type of housing in mind. Both inpatient and outpatient facilities, such as shared apartments, often offer interested parties the opportunity to visit the premises or try living there temporarily. The participation of those affected also relieves relatives when it comes to making later decisions regarding care and living arrangements. Professional support and advice from a housing advice center, a senior citizens' office, a care support center, or Alzheimer societies can generally be accessed free of charge. Open questions about financing or options for support to remain in one's familiar environment can thus be clarified.

39.3 Diversity of Housing Forms

There is a variety of common housing forms, which are divided into fully inpatient, partially inpatient, and outpatient settings.

The fully inpatient housing forms, that is, the classic

- nursing homes or residential care homes for the elderly
- senior residences

are distinct from the wide range of partially inpatient options

- assisted living/service living (services can be booked as needed)
- day care, night care
- short-term care, respite care

and outpatient housing settings. These include:

- (dementia) shared apartments (self-organized or provider-organized)
- multi-generational houses
- one's own apartment (support from relatives and/or nursing service)
- living with relatives.

39.4 Living Conditions Are Crucial for Quality of Life

As early as 2015, the Care Report *Care between Home and Institution* (Teti 2015) addressed the importance of housing in old age. The quality of housing is a decisive factor in terms of health, well-being, quality of life, and autonomy. In particular, older and ill people have a much smaller radius of activity, which is focused on the home environment, as the majority of this group is not or no longer employed. Everyday life mainly takes place in the immediate living area, and people spend more than three-quarters of the day at home. Thus, the living environment is of great importance for people with chronic illnesses.

Both the objective living conditions and the subjective experience of living have an impact on life satisfaction and independence. At the same time, the spatial and social living conditions form the basis for mobility and social participation. In other words, optimized living conditions offer opportunities and preserve resources by promoting independence and thus enabling, for example, self-care. Deficient living conditions, on the other hand, restrict independence and pose risks, such as increased risk of falls and accidents due to insufficient accessibility. Social consequences such as isolation and loneliness are also possible, which can promote mental illnesses such as depression and anxiety. In addition, unfavorable living conditions have a negative impact on the risk of needing care and can lead to an increased need for assistance and care services, for example by preventing self-care in the home environment. Thus, quality of life in all its facets is a fundamental factor in the choice of housing options for people with chronic illnesses.

39.5 Numbers Under Scrutiny

According to the Federal Statistical Office, about in Germany 4.96 million people were in need of care as defined by SGB XI in 2021. Compared to 2011 (2.5 million), the numbers have almost doubled. In particular, since the expansion of the definition of need for care as part of the Second Care Strengthening Act (2017), the numbers have risen sharply. A stronger emphasis on dementia-related illnesses is reflected here. Looking ahead, the number of people in need of care will continue to rise, with projections for 2050 estimating 6.5 million. The number of people over 80 is also increasing. While 5.7 million were recorded for 2020, statisticians expect almost 10 million people over 80 by 2050.

Of these nearly five million people currently in need of care, 16% are cared for in fully inpatient settings. The majority, 84%, live at home or in an environment referred to as home care. Based on the number of people cared for at home, relatives provide about 70% of the care and support alone. Thus, the group of caregiving relatives, that is, informal caregivers, is very large, and care without these people is hardly conceivable (Brandt 2022; Janson 2022).

39.6 Rethinking Domesticity

Rüsing (2020) advocates for a new perspective on the figures from the Federal Statistical Office and simultaneously raises the question of whether people truly want to live the way they currently do. This means questioning whether the health policy mandate of *outpatient before inpatient care*, which is derived from the guiding principle of the new Nursing Strengthening Act, actually takes into account the population's preferences regarding life in old age.

In his critical analysis, Rüsing refers to the results of the representative study by Spangenberg (2013), which examined images and aspirations of aging. People between the ages of 14 and 97 were surveyed. Specifically, the group aged 45 to 97 was asked to indicate how and, above all, where they would like to live in old age if they required care. 66% of respondents wish to remain in their own home and, if necessary, would like to use an outpatient care service. 20% can imagine living in a so-called new housing concept, such as assisted living, living in a shared apartment, or in a multigenerational house. According to the study, only 5% of respondents would choose to move into a traditional nursing home.

These results were partly to be expected, but also surprising in one crucial aspect. While the number of people who can imagine living in an institutional facility amounts to only 5%, there is, surprisingly, only one other place that is equally unpopular: living with one's own relatives. Only 5% of respondents wish to live with their children or other family members. Rüsing emphasizes that most people, in the event they require care, want to remain in their own home, but do not want to move into the home of their relatives. Both living situations are referred to as domesticity, but are nevertheless perceived completely differently by those surveyed.

Especially in the context of the living situation of people in need of care, the term domesticity is used in a wide variety of contexts. Rüsing finds this usage diffuse and misleading. He calls for a rethinking here, as it is interesting that the Federal Statistical Office classifies everything as domesticity that is not institutional. This also includes any form of living in a private household, which does not necessarily have to be one's own. For those affected, however, domesticity generally means the apartment or living environment in which they have always lived, that is, their own home, and not being cared for in the domestic environment of relatives.

Thus, one's own perspective on living in domesticity is completely different from what is represented by the figures of the Federal Statistical Office. Likewise, the mandate of outpatient before inpatient care does not align with the wishes of those surveyed if outpatient or domestic is used to describe everything that is not institutional. Rüsing sees urgent need for action here, as these official figures are frequently used by policymakers and the media. The concept of domesticity must be redefined to ensure the self-determination of those affected.

39.7 Demographic Change—Pathways to New Forms of Living

In summary, it can be stated that the success of self-determined living in a residential environment chosen as freely as possible is subject to conditions that can be either supportive or obstructive. Whether this environment must be defined as domesticity remains open. What is crucial is the possibility for those affected to participate in decision-making. The initially obstructive conditions are shaped by the shortage of skilled workers and the often inadequate care situation that accompanies it, which, due to demographic change and the associated increase in the need for care, will continue to intensify and place a burden on the healthcare system. At the same time, new perspectives on life in old age are emerging, as the coming generation—the so-called baby boomers—brings a different level of acceptance toward alternative forms of living, such as shared apartments, multigenerational houses, or service-oriented housing. This shift in perspective enables a focus on the supportive conditions for living with a chronic illness. The participation of those affected, which is already anchored at the health policy level through legal provisions (for example, through the Housing and Participation Act or the requirements for participation in SGB IX), should be routinely implemented in the future. This can be achieved through multiprofessional collaboration in the design of care arrangements. Comprehensive and early information about the variety of options for self-determined living should always be available to those affected and their relatives. Politics and society should continue and expand the existing structures of neighborhood work and district development, and ensure a barrier-free and livable environment that offers safety and quality of life for people with limitations, even in old age.

References

Brandt M (2022) Fast 5 Millionen Pflegebedürftige. https://de-statista-com.uni-wh.idm.oclc.org/infografik/7593/anzahl-der-pflegebeduerftigen-in-deutschland/. Accessed 31.05.2023

Janson M (2022) Pflegerepublik Deutschland. https://de-statista-com.uni-wh.idm.oclc.org/infografik/26535/anzahl-der-pflegebeduerftigen-und-ueber-80-jaehrigen-in-deutschland/. Accessed 31.05.2023

Rüsing D (2020) „Häuslichkeit“ ist nicht immer „zu Hause“! https://www.dzla.de/zu-hause-ist-nicht-gleich-zu-hause/. Accessed 02.05.2023

Spangenberg L, Glaesmer H, Brähler E, Kersting A, Strauß B (2013) Nachdenken über das Wohnen im Alter. Z Gerontol Geriatr 46:251–259. https://doi.org/10.1007/s00391-012-0363-x

Teti A (2015) Wohnen im Alter: Versorgungsformen in der Pflege. In: Jacobs K, Kuhlmey A, Greß S, Schwinger A (Hrsg) Pflege-Report 2015: Pflege zwischen Heim und Häuslichkeit. Schattauer, Stuttgart, pp 15–26

Household-Related Services for Self-Determined Living

40

Ulrike Pfannes and Pirjo Susanne Schack

Contents

U. Pfannes (✉)
HAW Hamburg, Department Ökotrophologie, Professorin für Verpflegungs- und Versorgungsmanagement, Hamburg, Germany
e-mail: ulrike.pfannes@haw-hamburg.de

P. S. Schack
FH Münster, Fachbereich Oecotrophologie-Facility Management,
Professorin für Haushalts- und Dienstleistungsmanagement, Münster, Germany
e-mail: schack@fh-muenster.de

D. Schmitz et al. (eds.), *Chronic Care—Science and Practice*,
https://doi.org/10.1007/978-3-662-72298-5_40

40.1 Background

As a result of chronic illnesses, there may be a need for support in everyday care, often long before there is an "official" need for care as defined by the long-term care insurance (PflegeVG). This article, from the perspective of home economics/family and consumer science, aims to highlight the importance of everyday domestic care for quality of life.

40.2 The Importance of Household-Related Services

Household work and HRS are of great importance for a good life, both on an individual and societal level:

- On an individual level, it is about the security of being cared for, personal well-being, quality of life, and relief from everyday tasks, possibly also for relatives.
- On a societal level, it concerns aspects of prevention and financing: for example, delaying the onset of the need for nursing and moving into a residentitial care facility for the elderly.

HRS can also be seen as complementary services, among others, to care and create a reliable foundation for everyday life (Maier-Gräwe 2013). Not infrequently, the scope of domestic tasks significantly exceeds the amount of nursing care required (Heinemann-Knoch et al. 2006).

▶ **Definition of Household-Related Services** *Household-related services (HRS) are person- and/or object-related services that are necessary for people in need of assistance to cope with everyday life in their private homes: They serve to provide relief, support, participation, and self-determination. HRS are usually provided by non-household members for a fee.* (Pfannes and Schack 2014, p. 20)

40.3 Characteristics of Household Work and the Possibilities and Limits of Outsourcing

Living and private household management serve not only to meet basic needs, but also to foster the culture of living together and personal development (Schweitzer 1991). In this sense, household work affects many aspects of quality of life and creates well-being. Household work is both labor and care, and it is essential for life.

40.3.1 Work in the Household: Management and Practical Work

Household work can be divided into household management and practical work. Household management is a prerequisite for the execution of tasks. Both the ability to manage a household and to carry out tasks can be impaired by illness. If pracitical work is outsourced, household management remains with the person managing the household. If this is not possible (e.g., in the case of dementia), it must be transferred to another authorized person, such as family members or a legal caregiver. Figure 40.1 illustrates this situation.

40.3.2 Organizational Principles in Households and Barriers to the Use of Household-Related Services

A typical feature of private households is that they have their own organizational principles. When HRS are outsourced, it is expected that things will be done the way one does them oneself. Communication can be challenging, as this individual household style is often practiced unconsciously as a habitus (see article 37) (Deeken 2009).

The privacy, individuality, and emotionality of household work are reasons for typical barriers to using HRS. Major barriers include allowing strangers into one's home and affordability. Therefore, professional services are usually only used when support options from the immediate environment (e.g., family) are lacking.

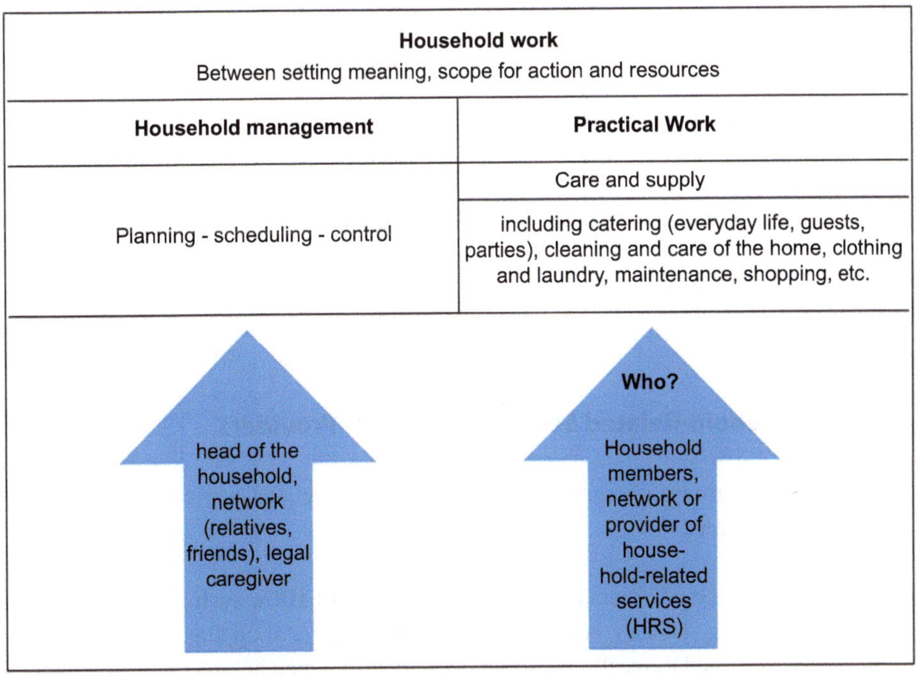

Fig. 40.1 Household work – between management and practical work. (Pfannes and Schack 2014a, p. 19)

40.3.3 Requirements for Household-Related Services

From these characteristics of the private household, requirements for the provision of professional HRS can be derived:

- Recognize and respect barriers regarding privacy, individuality, emotionality, affordability, and feelings of shame when in need of help
- Adapt to individual lifestyles, organizational principles, and standards of expectation
- Take into account the importance of care and relationship aspects
- Coordinate with relatives and, if necessary, other professional groups
- Be aware that commissioning HRS is a household management task and must be carried out by the chronically ill person themselves or by an authorized person.

40.4 Participation and Self-Determination through Domestic Care

Domestic care enables people in need of assistance to carry out everyday tasks as independently as possible (dgh 2012). It is a joint, meaningful activity that ensures self-care and maintains and promotes abilities and skills. In principle, it can refer to both household management and pracical work. The degree of involvement of the assisted individuals can be structured in a differentiated way (Feulner and Pfannes 2014). Thus, domestic care differs from concepts of *occupational therapy* and *activation* (Schmidt and Döble 2010), which are generally not linked to supply.

40.5 The Market for Household-Related Services

Market aspects of HRS concern the types of providers, private households as employers, and financing.

40.5.1 Household-Related Services—Types of Providers

There are various groups of legal providers of household-related services, who generally offer operational tasks:

- Household service providers offer a broad spectrum of HRS, such as room cleaning, window cleaning, laundry care, (child and senior) care, shopping, accompaniment, and services related to meals. These services are also aimed at target groups without a need for assistance.
- Nursing services additionally offer HRS for people in need of help and care, often financed through long-term care insurance.

- Companies specializing in cleaning also provide cleaning services for private households.
- Facility service organisations offer, for example,, cleaning services, winter services, and gardening services.

HRS are usually offered by small businesses. The most frequently requested service is apartment cleaning, supplemented as needed by laundry, ironing, shopping, cooking, etc. (BMFSFJ 2012).

Legal providers of HRS compete intensively with illegal providers. The share of undeclared work among domestic helpers in Germany is estimated at 88% (Enste 2019). Both, providers and clients benefit from undeclared work, as both sides see short-term financial advantages. The objective risks of undeclared work are often ignored by both parties: for households, for example, liability for work accidents; for domestic helpers, the (long-term) lack of social security, such as in the case of illness or protection against dismissal (Pfannes and Schack 2014). It can be assumed that without political measures (e.g., through voucher systems, tax benefits, subsidies), legalizing the market for household-related services will be difficult to achieve (Prognos 2012).

Another challenge is the shortage of (qualified) personnel for HRS. The Competence Center for Professionalization and Quality Assurance of Household-Related Services (PQHD) has, among other things, developed qualification concepts (Hochschule Fulda 2021).

40.5.2 Households as Employers or as Clients of a Service Company

The household can either act as an employer itself (e.g., mini-job) or commission a service company. In HRS, relatives are often the clients who also check the results. However, the everyday requirements of the commissioning relatives can (significantly) differ from those of the chronically ill, which can lead to contradictory orders or work instructions for the service providers.

HRS almost always have, in addition to the aspect of domestic work, a communication and relationship aspect, even if this is not explicitly agreed upon as a service. Chronically ill individuals may simply want to have a conversation. In such cases, this caregiving service may come into conflict with the operational work.

40.5.3 Financing of Household-Related Services

When it comes to financing, it should be noted that HRS generally involve regular demand, which often increases over time. Even at low hourly rates, this results in monthly costs that those affected often cannot afford.

Legally provided HRS can be deducted from taxes up to a maximum amount. In the case of acute, severe illness of the person managing the household, a domestic helper can be financed by the health insurance for up to four weeks if there is no other person in the household who can, for example, care for children or dependents. For those in need of care from care level 1, the relief amount of €125 per month can be used to access HRS from certified providers. Commissioning and utilizing such financial support options is part of household management.

40.6 Quality in Household-Related Services

For HRS, customers consistently see quality—alongside price—as a key factor. They particularly name the following as quality characteristics: reliability, trustworthiness, continuity, empathy, flexibility, and professional competence (Prognos 2012). Standards and qualification are used by HRS providers as instruments to ensure the desired quality.

The following institutions have published professional guidelines for household-related services, which are available for free download:

- BMWi – Federal Ministry for Economic Affairs (BMWI 2015)
- DIN – German Institute for Standardization (DIN 2015 and DIN 2018)
- KoHW – Competence Center for Home Economics, Bavaria (KoHW 2020)
- Innovation and Competence Center for Home Economics Baden-Württemberg (Innovations- und Kompetenzzentrum 2021a, b)
- Consumer organisation also provide information on commissioning HRS (Verbraucherzentrale o.J. n.d.).

For qualification activities, the reference framework "Modular (Partial) Qualification for Household-Related Services and Home Economics" can be used (PQHD and dgh 2020).

40.7 Care Arrangements

Arrangements that ensure everyday care and enable self-determination and participation are central to quality of life. It is not the optimization of individual services that is relevant, but rather the combination into a tailored, coordinated, and practical mix of assistance that is decisive.

Figure 40.2 illustrates that with increasing need for assistance, a continuum emerges in which the (barrier-free) living environment, everyday care with HRS and other services, etc., interlock. This is supplemented by local infrastructure and opportunities for participation as well as information and counseling services. The family network usually plays a key role in this.

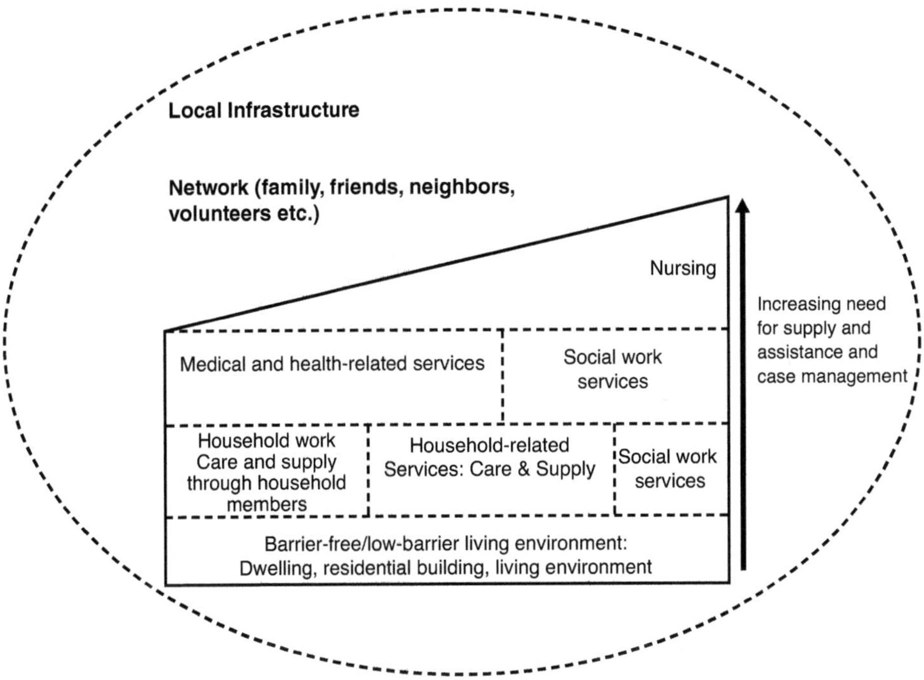

Fig. 40.2 Care arrangements for chronically ill people: a continuum of various support services. (Adapted from Pfannes and Schack 2014, p. 94)

40.8 Interprofessional Approaches to Collaboration

Household management is care work, which means that household-related professions are part of the SAHGE professions (SA: Social Work, H: Household Management/ household-related services, G: Health Professions, Nursing Professions, E: Educational Professions) (Gutachten Sachverständigenkommission 2017). The professional characteristics and attitudes of these fields can form a common foundation for collaboration (DHWiR 2021).

With regard to the interfaces between nursing and everyday domestic care, the AEDL care model (Activities and Existential Experiences of Life) can be referenced. Maier-Ruppert (1996) has provided a detailed explanation of how domestic care can be linked to the AEDL model.

In addition, the resource-oriented approach, as used in pedagogy and social work, is also applied in household-related services and domestic care (Feulner and Simpfendörfer 2006).

Furthermore, biographical work is also an approach in the field of domestic care to gain a better understanding of people's concerns (dgh 2009).

Based on these approaches, points of connection for interprofessional collaboration and mutual appreciation can be developed. The boundaries between domestic care, assistance and nursing in private households are fluid. Networking and interprofessional collaboration among the various professional groups are in the interest of people with chronic illnesses.

40.9 Conclusion and Final Considerations

Household-related services play a central role in enabling people with chronic illnesses to live self-determined lives: Reliable everyday domestic care—as part of a comprehensive care arrangement—is an important foundation for quality of life. The use of household-related services currently faces a number of structural challenges (e.g., market situation, financing, recognition).

Home economics/Family and consumer science make a central contribution to the transdisciplinarity of chronic care with their expertise in everyday life.

References

BMFSFJ – Bundesministerium für Familien, Senioren, Frauen und Jugend (2012) Anbieter haushaltsnaher Dienstleistungen in Deutschland – Angebotsbedingungen, Strukturen, Perspektiven, Berlin. https://www.bmfsfj.de/resource/blob/93264/1a03566d76745fa7cb4e02ff97a212d9/anbieter-haushaltsnaher-dienstleistungen-in-deutschland-data.pdf. Accessed 17.05.2023

BMWi – Bundesministerium für Wirtschaft und Energie (Hrsg) (2015) Qualitätssicherung für haushaltsnahe Dienstleistungen – Checkliste für Anbieter. Eine Arbeitshilfe für Anbieter haushaltsnaher Dienstleistungen. https://www.bmwk.de/Redaktion/DE/Downloads/P-R/qualitaetssicherung-fuer-haushaltsnahe-dienstleistungen-checkliste-fuer-anbieter.pdf?__blob=publicationFile&v=5. Accessed 17.05.2023

Deeken (2009) Eigenerstellung oder Fremdvergabe von Versorgungsdienstleistungen im Alter. Baltmannsweiler

dgh – Deutsche Gesellschaft für Hauswirtschaft e. V. (Eds) (2009) Biografiearbeit in der bewohnerorientierten Hauswirtschaft. https://www.dghev.de/fileadmin/user_upload/HW_Biografie_Fragebogen.pdf. Accessed 17.05.2023

dgh – Deutsche Gesellschaft für Hauswirtschaft e. V. (Eds) (2012) Den Alltag leben! Hauswirtschaftliche Betreuung. Ein innovativer Weg für soziale Einrichtungen und Dienste, dgh, Osnabrück

DHWiR – Deutscher Hauswirtschaftsrat e. V. (Eds) (2021) Arbeitspapier – Beschreibung der gemeinsamen Merkmale und Haltungen der Professionen der SAHGE-Berufe. https://www.dghev.de/fileadmin/user_upload/News/21-10-29Arbeitspapier_SAHGE.pdf. Zugegriffen am 17.05.2023

DIN SPEC 77003 (2015) Information, Beratung und Vermittlung von Personen- und haushaltsnahen Dienstleistungen, Berlin

DIN SPEC 77004 (2018) Personen- und haushaltsbezogene Dienstleistungen – Dienstleistungserbringung, Berlin

Enste D (2019) Haushaltshilfe: Keine Entlastung in Sicht. Institut der deutschen Wirtschaft (Eds), IW-Kurzbericht Nr. 42, Juli 2019

Feulner M, Pfannes U (2014) Hauswirtschaftliche Betreuung – ein partizipatives Konzept für nachhaltiges Handeln. In: Hauswirtschaft und Wissenschaft (HuW) 1/2014, pp 7–19. https://www.dghev.de/fileadmin/user_upload/HuW_2014_Heft_1_Feulner_Artikel.pdf. Accessed 17.05.2023

Feulner M, Simpfendörfer D (2006) Soziale Dienste – den Alltag bewältigen. Handwerk und Technik, Hamburg

Heinemann-Knoch M, Knoch T, Korte E (2006) Invested time in private care: estimated by people in need of help and care and their private caregivers. Z Gerontol Geriatr 39:413–417

Hochschule Fulda (Eds) (2021) Wahrnehmung haushaltsnaher Dienstleistungen. https://www.hs-fulda.de/fileadmin/user_upload/FB_Oe/PQHD/Bericht_Studie_Haushaltsnahe_Dienstleistungen_Endf_22.12.21.pdf. Accessed 17.05.2023

Innovations- und Kompetenzzentrum Hauswirtschaft Baden-Württemberg (Eds) (2021a) Qualitätsstandards für haushaltsnahe Dienstleistungen – Perspektive der Nutzenden, Stuttgart. https://jimdo-storage.global.ssl.fastly.net/file/2a388222-7d45-4603-bd33-9929b0836ba5/Qualit%C3%A4tsstandards%20f%C3%BCr%20hnDL%20in%20BW_Kundinnen_01.21.pdf. Accessed 17.05.2023

Innovations- und Kompetenzzentrum Hauswirtschaft Baden-Württemberg (2021b) Qualitätsstandards für haushaltsnahe Dienstleistungen – Perspektive Anbieter, Stuttgart. https://jimdo-storage.global.ssl.fastly.net/file/43634449-2bf0-4969-a57b-9b1cd6955838/Qualit%C3%A4tsstandards%20f%C3%BCr%20hnDL%20in%20BW_Anbieter_01.21.pdf. Accessed 17.05.2023

KoHW – Kompetenzzentrum Hauswirtschaft (Eds) (2020) Qualitätsmanagement-Handbuch – Vorlage nach DIN SPEC. https://www.stmelf.bayern.de/mam/cms01/berufsbildung/dateien/qm-handbuch_nach_din-spec_haushaltsnahe_dienstleistungen.pdf. Accessed 17.05.2023

Maier-Gräwe U (2013) Wertschöpfungspotentiale haushaltsnaher Dienstleistungen. In: Justus-Liebig-Universität Gießen: Cooking, Caring, Cleaning. Zukunftsperspektiven haushaltsnaher Dienstleistungen in Deutschland. Tagungsdokumentation 17.09.2013. Gießen, pp 11–28

Pfannes U, Schack P (2014a) Metastudie haushaltsbezogene Dienstleistungen, im Rahmen des Projektes des vzbv: „Gutes Leben im Alter – Verbraucherpolitische Aspekte des demografischen Wandels am Beispiel Wohnen, Haushaltsnahe Dienstleistungen und Pflege", Berlin, 9/2014. https://www.vzbv.de/sites/default/files/downloads/Metastudie-Haushaltsbezogene_Dienstleistungen-vzbv_2014.pdf. Accessed 08.06.2023

PQHD (Kompetenzzentrum „Professionalisierung und Qualitätssicherung haushaltsnaher Dienstleistungen"), dgh (Deutsche Gesellschaft für Hauswirtschaft) (2020) Referenzrahmen Modulare (Teil-)Qualifizierung für haushaltsnahe Dienstleistungen und Hauswirtschaft. https://www.hs-fulda.de/fileadmin/user_upload/FB_Oe/PQHD/Referenzrahmen_Modulare__Teil_Qualifizierung_fuer_haushaltsnahe_Dienstleistungen_und_Hauswirtschaft_1.pdf. Accessed 17.08.2023

Prognos (2012) Dynamisierung des Marktes haushaltsnaher Dienstleistungen. Endbericht. Basel, Berlin. https://docplayer.org/8468211-Dynamisierung-des-marktes-haushaltsnaher-dienstleistungen.html. Accessed 06.06.2023

Sachverständigenkommission zum Zweiten Gleichstellungsbericht der Bundesregierung (Hrsg) (2017) Erwerbs- und Sorgearbeit gemeinsam neu gestalten – Gutachten für den Zweiten Gleichstellungsbericht der Bundesregierung. https://www.gleichstellungsbericht.de/gutachten-2gleichstellungsbericht.pdf. Accessed 17.05.2023

Schmidt S, Döble M (2010) Demenzbegleiter – Leitfaden für zusätzliche Betreuungskräfte in der Pflege. Springer, Heidelberg

Schweitzer R v (1991) Einführung in die Wirtschaftslehre des Haushalts. UTB, Stuttgart
Verbraucherzentrale (Hrsg) (o.J.) Haushaltshilfen – so bekommen Sie Hilfe bei Krankheit oder Pflegefall. https://www.verbraucherzentrale.de/wissen/gesundheit-pflege/pflegeantrag-und-leistungen/haushaltshilfen-so-bekommen-sie-hilfe-bei-krankheit-oder-pflegefall-42718. Accessed 17.05.2023

Further Reading

BAGSO – Bundesarbeitsgemeinschaft der Senioren-Organisationen e. V. (Hrsg) (2017) Mittagstisch-Angebote für ältere Menschen erfolgreich organisieren IN FORM Leitfaden-Mittagstisch, Bonn. https://im-alter-in-form.de/fileadmin/user_upload/6_Weiterbildung/Materialien/Mittagstisch/Broschuere-Mittagstisch_neu_Klo__ckner_kl.pdf. Accessed 17.05.2023
Bundesfinanzminsterium (o.J.) Steuerermäßigung bei Aufwendungen für haushaltsnahe Beschäftigungsverhältnisse und für die Inanspruchnahme haushaltsnaher Dienstleistungen. https://www.bundesfinanzministerium.de/Content/DE/Downloads/BMF_Schreiben/Steuerarten/Einkommensteuer/2021-09-01-steuerermaessigung-bei-aufwendungen-fuer-haushaltsnahe-beschaeftigungsverhaeltnisse-und-fuer-die-inanspruchnahme-haushaltsnaher-dienstleistungen.html. Accessed 08.06.2023
DGE – Deutsche Gesellschaft für Ernährung e. V. (Eds) (2012) 12. Ernährungsbericht, Bonn
Feulner M, Pfannes U (2012) Betreuung und Versorgung – zwei Säulen der Hauswirtschaft für die Weiterentwicklung von sozialen Einrichtungen und Diensten. In: Hauswirtschaft und Wissenschaft (HuW), 2/2012, pp 93–104. https://www.dghev.de/fileadmin/user_upload/HuW_2012_Heft_2_Feulner_Artikel_Version_2.pdf. Accessed 17.05.2023
Feulner M, Pfannes U, Schukraft U, Sobotka M (2012) Freiburg & Osnabrück. https://www.dghev.de/fileadmin/user_upload/dgh_Den_Alltag_leben_2012.pdf. Accessed 17.05.2023
ILO (International Labor Organisation) (Hrsg) (2011) Übereinkommen über menschenwürdige Arbeit für Hausangestellte, ILO-Konvention 189, Genf
Kaufmann JC (1999) Mit Leib und Seele – Theorie der Haushaltstätigkeit. UVK, Konstanz
Maier-Ruppert, Inge (1996): Das Pflegemodell der AEDL und hauswirtschaftliche Leistungen in der stationären Altenhilfe, in: Hauswirtschaft und Wissenschaft Heft 9, pp 17–23
Pfannes U (2014) Hilfreiche Hände – Hauswirtschaftliche Betreuung. In: Hauswirtschaft und Management, Nachlieferung 1/2014. Raabe, Stuttgart
Pfannes U (2016) Haushaltsnahe Dienstleistungen gefragt: Die Hilfen bei der eigenständigen Lebensführung sollen ausgebaut werden. In: Blätter der Wohlfahrtspflege 1/2016, pp 19–22. https://www.nomos-elibrary.de/10.5771/0340-8574-2016-1-19.pdf?download_full_pdf=1. Accessed 17.05.2023
Pfannes U, Schack P (2014b) Gutes Leben im Alter – der Beitrag haushaltsbezogener Dienstleistungen zur Lebensqualität (Teil I). In: Hauswirtschaft und Wissenschaft (HuW) 4/2014, pp 195–202
Pfannes U, Schack P (2015) Gutes Leben im Alter – der Beitrag haushaltsbezogener Dienstleistungen zur Lebensqualität (Teil II). In: Hauswirtschaft und Wissenschaft (HuW) 1/2015, S 9–19. https://www.dghev.de/fileadmin/user_upload/HuW_2015_Heft_1_Pfannes_Artikel.pdf. Accessed 17.05.2023
Thiele-Wittig M (1993) Schnittstellen der privaten Haushalte zu Institutionen. Zunehmende Außenbeziehungen der Haushalte im Wandel der Daseinsbewältigung. In: Grabe, Sylvia (Hrsg) Der private Haushalt im wissenschaftlichen Diskurs. Campus, Frankfurt am Main, pp 371–388

Weinkopf C, Hieming B (2007) Instrumente der Arbeitsmarktpolitik und haushaltsnahe Dienstleistungen, IAQ-Expertise im Auftrag des BMFSFJ, Gelsenkirchen. https://www.bmfsfj.de/resource/blob/76406/2cc6aa4ff5916edbf08e59df2dbf8bc6/instrumente-arbeitsmarktpolitik-data.pdf. Accessed 07.06.2023

Part IV

System Level Chronic Care: Framework Conditions, Health Care Economics, Community and Public Health Care, Digital Health as a Societal Innovation

41 Fundamentals of Social Law in Health Care

Manfred Fiedler

Contents

41.1 Social Law and Social Equality

Following Graser, we understand social law as law that generates equality (Graser 2010). To work with this concept, it is necessary to define equality and inequality. Usually, reference is made to equal or unequal income or wealth. This means that questions of distribution policy are initially at the forefront, which are then translated into social law. Thus, it is about economic participation. With regard to the phenomena of health and illness, participation has further aspects that make social law a specific health social law, such as the living situation of individuals or social groups (see Contribution 44). The opportunity

M. Fiedler (✉)
Department of human medicine, Witten/Herdecke University, Witten, Germany
e-mail: manfred.fiedler@uni-wh.de

D. Schmitz et al. (eds.), *Chronic Care—Science and Practice*,
https://doi.org/10.1007/978-3-662-72298-5_41

for health and illness is shaped by equal opportunity, such as non-discriminatory access to health services, and equal treatment as legal equality. In the context of social law, the aim is to enable equal and needs-based access to services in the event of illness. Since chronic illnesses in particular can lead to restrictions in participation, it is also about participating in societal institutions in terms of well-being, as people without these limitations or illnesses do. Health social law, as the legal implementation of health policy principles, is an instrument for defining and ensuring access to health services, especially with regard to the care of people with chronic illnesses.

41.2 On the Principle of the Social State

Even though Germany is defined as a social state with regard to the Grundgesetz, this is only defined in very general terms in the Basic Law itself. In Article 12 of the Grundgesetz (GG), Germany is defined as a democratic and social state. There are no further elaborations on the social state mandate. In Germany, it is up to the legislature to provide specifics. This gives special significance to the political consensus expressed in social law. Constitutionally, the prohibition of discrimination (Art. 3 GG), the respect for and protection of human dignity (Art. 1 GG), and the equivalence of living conditions (Art. 72 GG) can be understood as principles that flank the principle of the social state.

The German definition of the social state, and thus also of the principle of the social state, is primarily the result of a historical development in social law, which concretizes the social state through social law regulations. This includes, in particular, Bismarck's social reform at the end of the 19th century, which was unique worldwide at the time, the formulation of social insurance in the Reich Insurance Code (RVO) of 1911, its consolidation and expansion after the Second World War, and the consolidation of social security law in the form of the Social Code Books. Of particular importance is the separation into social insurance, as a public-law security system, largely mandatory for employees, separated from the core public budget, to protect against major social risks such as unemployment, old-age poverty, illness, and occupational accidents, as well as the state's direct responsibility for supporting people in special life situations.

A special feature is the social self-administration in social insurance as a form of social self-determination of the insured. The safeguarding of special social benefits is largely left to municipal self-administration, such as regulations on inclusion and the promotion of participation for people with disabilities.

Contradictory concepts such as solidarity and Subordination of the state (subsidiarity) accompany the development of social law. The question is when and where the state should intervene in solidarity, how far the area of individual self-responsibility extends, and how this self-help of individuals can be legally defined (see Contribution 44). The principle of solidarity underlying social insurance, the solidarity principle, involves the mutual obligation to provide support in the event of damage, whereby, unlike in classic mutual insurance, the risk community is understood in a comprehensive social sense, thus in principle including all employees.

41.3 Social Law and Social Justice

The subject of social policy, and thus of social law, is the principle of social justice (Ebert 2015). A corresponding term in the field of health is health justice or health equity. These terms, too, are not clearly defined as ethical orientations of social security. The simplest definition is that the legal constitution itself contains social justice, that the principle of legally enforceable rights itself guarantees justice. This definition avoids a substantive definition.

Another principle, which stems more from an economically liberal understanding, is the principle of merit-based justice. Equality and inequality are thus contradictory concepts, whereby inequality is regarded as a natural order in which everyone is rewarded according to their individual productivity. The market economy order implies that, through market-based remuneration of market participants, distributive justice arises automatically. The market develops a just order naturally through the so-called invisible hand.

In contrast stands the principle of utility. Just is what is useful. The utilitarianism of the 19th century saw this in the maximization of the benefit of the many, if not all. This means that social benefits are meaningful and just if, without diminishing the benefit of individuals, they increase the benefit of all, the overall social benefit. The social order of a society must be oriented toward this goal of justice for the many. Since benefit is not defined solely in economic terms, the specifics remain abstract and subject to political debate.

Another principle of justice is found in the German constitution through the prohibition of discrimination, or better, equal opportunity as a standard of justice. Everyone should have equal opportunities for self-fulfillment. In the health care system, this corresponds to the context of health equality, the principle that every person, regardless of their personal background, has the same opportunities to achieve health and must not be arbitrarily excluded from them. The differences between people are not yet taken into account with this ideal of equality.

The principle of health equity (Braveman et al. 2018) differs as a more far-reaching principle of justice, which accepts that people are unequal and bring different abilities as well as non-economic starting conditions, such as education, lifestyles, living environment conditions, etc., as access to health services. It is about the person-specific appropriateness of service provision and access.

For the law, this means that it is not sufficient and just if it merely enables everyone to have formally equal access, but only when it takes into account the differences inherent in the person and thus enables a relatively understood equality of access to services. This means, for example, that a person with mobility impairments is enabled to access health services in the same way as someone without such impairments, for instance through mobility-promoting measures.

Given the diversity of understandings, social justice is an unspecific ethical norm that can be defined in terms of non-discrimination, but must be critically reflected upon in the contradiction between the social state and market economy principles and the respective resulting ethical principles. Merit-based justice and equivalence of performance, for example, are consistent with market economy principles. The equity concept stands in contrast to this. Since social law is the result of social policy negotiation, the different principles are also inherently reflected in health social law.

41.4 Concepts of Social Security

Concepts of social security justify the necessity of a social security system. In other words, they form the basis for measures in social policy and social law.

The following section presents two fundamental concepts that guide social policy and social law measures.

First, we start from the understanding of social inequality as economic inequality. In this context, social policy has the task and goal of leveling economic inequality through appropriate redistribution measures. At this point, we are referring to the change from the primary distribution created by market-based allocation to the leveled secondary distribution. This means that the income generated by the original market or societal distribution without state intervention is redistributed to compensate for economic inequalities.

The reduction to purely economic inequality is expanded by other concepts. For example, we understand living conditions to encompass all circumstances that significantly influence a person's social situation (Leßmann 2015). In this sense, it is not only income that is distributed, but also living conditions, which may include, for example, questions of family constellations, social environment, and housing situation. All these conditions influence an individual's social situation and can, accordingly, lead to exclusion from participation in society and its institutions. From this perspective, social law should not only focus on the redistribution of income, but also on leveling living conditions, thereby fundamentally promoting opportunities for participation. As a general concept, the constitutional principle of ensuring equivalent living conditions can be invoked. The Indian economist Sen (Sen 2002) has described the limited perspective of income equality, even when taking into account people's particular situations, as an insufficient concept. He points out that people with physical, mental, and other impairments must spend more financial resources to cope with their situation and individually compensate for disadvantages. They would still be disadvantaged even with income equality.

41.5 Fundamental Principles of Social Law

The manner in which social benefits are granted follows certain principles that are relevant in different areas of social security law (Bauer 1992).

1. The causality principle refers to the causation of a damage event. In order to assert a claim to benefits, there must be a justified causal connection in the sense of a case context that gives rise to entitlement. An example is the law on occupational diseases,

where the claim to benefits from the statutory accident insurance provider is based on proof of causation by the occupational activity performed.

2. The equivalence principle means that benefits are granted in relation to the amount of insurance contributions or prior payments made by the individual, as well as with regard to the insured risk and the scope of coverage. An example of this is income replacement benefits, such as in pension insurance, which are granted under social law in proportion to the amount and duration of pension insurance contributions, and supplemented by non-monetary benefits such as child-rearing or caregiving. The equivalence principle is also constitutive for private health insurance.
3. According to the finality principle, benefits are granted unconditionally with regard to the desired benefit outcome or objective. The finality principle is particularly important in accident insurance, where, for example, the granting of benefits after a workplace accident is aimed at restoring the status quo ante as far as possible, in terms of comprehensive medical, occupational, and social rehabilitation.
4. The welfare principle involves protection without prior contributions in the form of insurance payments. Entitlement to benefits arises due to social need. Welfare is not only provided in cases of economic hardship, but whenever another form of protection is not individually possible.
5. Finally, a distinction should be made between object and subject subsidies. In object subsidies, facilities or institutions are directly funded from public or parafiscal budgets, for example by maintaining or establishing the service-providing entity. An example is investment financing for hospitals. Financial support for social housing construction is also an object subsidy. In subject subsidies, the focus is on relieving the individual financially, often based on need. An example is housing allowance for low-income individuals or households. While object subsidies reduce the cost of accessing services and simultaneously increase the socially appropriate supply, subject subsidies leave the supply unchanged but increase potential demand at market prices. In cases of supply shortages, object subsidies are therefore generally more suitable.

41.6 Protection Against the Risk of Illness in Germany

The risk of illness in Germany is regulated in several codes of law. The foundation of German social law is the Social Code (Sozialgesetzbuch-SGB), which is divided into twelve books. For healthcare provision in case of illness, SGB V, Statutory Health Insurance (GKV), SGB VII, Statutory Accident Insurance (GUV), and SGB XI, Social Long-Term Care Insurance, are particularly relevant (see Fig. 41.1). SGB IX, concerning rehabilitation and disability law, as well as SGB XII, social assistance, are also significant. From a legal-historical perspective, the SGB is relatively recent. SGB V dates from 1989, SGB XI from 1995. The three major branches of social insurance—pension, accident, and health insurance—were previously regulated in the RVO. Especially for people

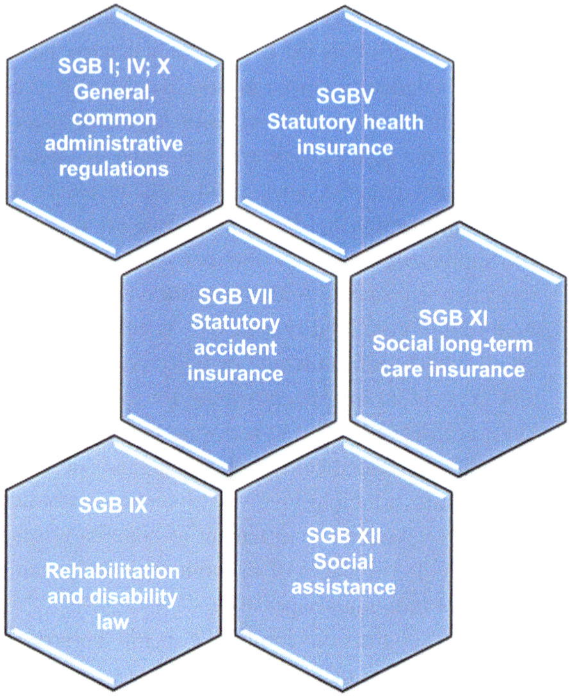

Fig. 41.1 Social Codes relevant to health social law. (Own illustration)

with special social security needs, other legal regulations applied, such as the Federal Social Assistance Act or the Employment Promotion Act. Rehabilitation law, which in terms of entitlements refers to various social benefit providers, was more or less implicitly summarized in the so-called Rehabilitation Harmonization Act.

In social law, we distinguish between the insured, who are the beneficiaries in case of illness, the payers, also called benefit providers, and the service providers, also referred to as providers of benefits.

The payers are those who ensure a benefit by securing its provision for the insured both financially and in terms of content and organization.

On the other side are the service providers, who are factually and substantively responsible for delivering the benefits. Since 1933, uniquely on an international scale, the responsibility for ensuring outpatient medical care has been assigned to the Associations of Statutory Health Insurance Physicians, which, as professional self-governing member organizations of contract physicians, are responsible for and organize comprehensive care for the insured. For hospital care, this responsibility lies with the federal states in the form of hospital planning. With regard to ensuring long-term care, there are formal planning responsibilities, but these are practically not implemented and, in reality, amount to a recognition procedure by the long-term care funds as payers of long-term care insurance.

Overall, the relationship between payers and service providers in the major service areas of statutory health insurance and long-term care insurance is based on a partially association-based, otherwise bilateral negotiation model. Association-level negotiations include, for example, the overall remuneration budget or the general financial guidelines for service remuneration, as well as specifications for billable services. Bilaterally, the billable services of the facilities, the remuneration rates (service prices), and the service volumes are negotiated.

In Germany, protection against the risk of illness is generally organized as an insurance benefit. The insurance-based nature means that health services in Germany are financed by contributions, with employers formally paying half of the contribution (parity financing). The principle of the individual financial capacity of the insured is achieved by levying the contribution rate on earned income, regardless of the risk of illness, social status, or individual risk behavior.

The co-insurance of family members represents another constitutive principle of statutory health insurance. This means that non-working spouses and children up to the age limit of 25 are entitled to benefits as co-insured persons.

Another principle is that of compulsory insurance and the compulsory insurance threshold. Employees are required to be members of a statutory health insurance fund. Above the compulsory insurance threshold, which is adjusted annually, this becomes a general obligation to take out health insurance, either as a voluntary member of a public health insurance fund or with a private health insurance provider. This allows the self-employed, civil servants, and employees with high incomes to secure themselves outside the social law institutions, which essentially violates the principle of equality in German social law.

Another principle is the contribution assessment ceiling. Health insurance contributions are levied proportionally to income. No contributions are levied on earned income above the contribution assessment ceiling. Here, the principle of solidarity reaches its legal limits.

As already mentioned, a constitutive principle of social insurance in Germany is social self-administration by the insured and employers, which determines the respective business policy. This principle also dates back to Bismarck's social legislation, which replaced the self-organization of the former workers' associations and, at the same time, restricted it through parity between employers and employees.

41.7 Benefit Law

Benefit law defines the services that can be billed within statutory health insurance and long-term care insurance. The basis is the so-called benefits catalog. This is generally developed in two ways. On the one hand, the associations (Federal Joint Committee (Gemeinsamer Bundesausschuss - GBA)) determine the approved services. The GBA is composed of representatives of the statutory health insurance funds and the service providers. Patient representatives are admitted in an advisory capacity. Through the self-administration of the respective health insurance funds, so-called voluntary benefits can also be determined. On the other hand, services are negotiated bilaterally between health insurance funds and service providers. In addition, the state/legislator can also set service requirements, for example in the form of a negative or positive list for billable pharmaceuticals.

In principle, we distinguish between cash benefits and benefits in kind. Benefits in kind are all services provided without financial contribution from the beneficiaries and are financed directly by the health insurance. Essentially, these are, minus any co-payments, all direct care services as well as physician-prescribed pharmaceuticals, i.e., material goods.

In contrast, cash benefits are those that are actually provided in monetary form, either as compensation, support, or as income replacement. For example, care allowance in long-term care insurance is a cash benefit, while professionally provided care is formally a benefit in kind.

In principle, benefits in statutory health insurance are provided according to the benefits-in-kind principle. In contrast, the reimbursement principle is an optional alternative, whereby the insured or affected person initially pays in advance and then receives reimbursement from the health insurance for eligible expenses. This has legal consequences. Under the benefits-in-kind principle, the direct contractual partner is the respective health insurance fund, and thus the service provider's claim is against the health insurance fund. This changes under the reimbursement principle. Patients become the contractual partner of the service providers, and invoices are issued to them. This alters legal clarity and certainty in billing disputes, especially if services are deemed non-billable in type or amount and the insurance does not wish to cover them fully or at all. Those affected may find themselves caught between the demands and the refusal of the health insurance. Reimbursement is a common principle in private health insurance. In statutory health insurance, it is little used because it is optional. Studies have so far failed to demonstrate the expected savings through better cost control. This makes it clear that the effort required to process payments (transaction costs) is significantly higher.

In addition to mandatory and voluntary benefits, service providers can bill patients for private services. This applies to dental services, special accommodations, treatment by chief physicians in hospitals, or listed individual health services (IGeL). These are higher-value services or services whose effectiveness has not yet been generally proven.

As already indicated, cash benefits are generally provided as compensation, income replacement, or as a subsidy. They can also be granted if insured persons are unable, for social and/or economic reasons, to provide certain services themselves. In such cases, these are granted as transfer payments according to individual need.

41.8 Care Requirements for Chronic Illness

In Germany, the treatment of chronic illness is secured for large parts of the population through statutory health insurance (Gesetzliche Krankenversicherung - GKV) in such a way that, despite co-payment regulations, economic overburdening should not occur. The legally established upper limit for maximum co-payments as a share of earned income is further reduced for people with chronic illnesses. Nevertheless, co-payments generally place a disproportionately high burden on chronically ill individuals.

The GKV is also a comprehensive insurance that finances necessary care services within the scope of its benefits catalog. The situation is different in the case of long-term care needs. With the introduction of long-term care insurance as a new branch of social insurance in 1995, no comprehensive insurance was created. This particularly affects inpatient care, where, due to personal contributions for care services and the need to finance accommodation and living expenses, a significant portion of those in need may face economic overload—even with an average retirement pension and after using up existing savings. In such cases, social welfare (assistance for care and basic security in old age) does apply, but since these are welfare benefits, there is recourse to direct relatives of the first and second degree.

The social law requirements for the care of chronically ill people relate to care over a long period, meaning continuous care that may vary over time, for example in the case of progressive diseases such as degenerative disorders or diseases with phases of acute episodes, such as epilepsy or multiple sclerosis. These disease-related requirements are legally separated from the support services provided due to the consequences of illness. With regard to care, acute treatment, prevention, rehabilitation, and social and family support services, those affected are confronted with a multiplicity of responsibilities under social law.

This multiplicity of responsibilities and the dominance of disease-related services, i.e., acute care, make it clear that chronic illness as such is not adequately represented in health social law.

This fragmentation under social law is also reflected on the side of service providers. This is especially true for people with multiple illnesses (multimorbidity). The professional care needs are distributed among a wide variety of service providers, who themselves have different legal relationships even within the GKV. This still applies to rehabilitation services, which are becoming increasingly important for chronically ill people. Prevention and health promotion also continue to play a subordinate role in social law, especially for risk groups.

The significance of this is demonstrated by a comprehensive dementia study (GBD 2019 Dementia Forecasting Collaborators 2022), according to which 40% of dementia cases can either be prevented, delayed in onset, or slowed in progression.

The number of people in need of care will increase, as will the number of chronically ill individuals, including those with multimorbidity. From a social law perspective, it is necessary to anticipate this development, particularly by integrating services that have so far been regulated under different responsibilities and financing systems into a unified legal framework that addresses the care needs of chronically ill people.

References

Bauer R (Eds) (1992) Lexikon des Sozial- und Gesundheitswesens. Oldenbourg, München

Braveman P, Arkin E, Tracy Orleans T, Proctor D, Acker J, Plough A (2018) What is health equity? Behav Sci Policy 4(1). https://journals.sagepub.com/doi/pdf/10.1177/237946151800400102

Ebert T (2015) Soziale Gerechtigkeit: Ideen, Geschichte, Kontroversen. Schriftenreihe/Bundeszentrale für Politische Bildung, Bd 1571, 2., erw. u. überarb. Aufl. Bonn, Bundeszentrale für Politische Bildung, Bonn

GBD 2019 Dementia Forecasting Collaborators (2022) Estimation of the global prevalence of dementia in 2019 and forecasted prevalence in 2050: an analysis for the Global Burden of Disease Study 2019. Lancet Public Health 7(2):e105–e125. https://doi.org/10.1016/S2468-2667(21)00249-8

Graser A (2010) Die Familie im Gefüge der Solidargemeinschaften: Ein Ansatz soziologisch orientierter Rechtsvergleichung: Ein Ansatz soziologisch orientierter Rechtsvergleichung. In: Becker U (Eds) Rechtsdogmatik und Rechtsvergleich im Sozialrecht I. Nomos Verlagsgesellschaft mbH & Co KG, pp 374–391. http://www.jstor.org/stable/j.ctv941wc7. Accessed 13.02.2024

Leßmann O (2015) Lebenslage, Capability Set – Spielraum bei neuen Konzepten von Ungleicheheit. In: Romahn H, Rehfeld D (Eds) Lebenslagen – Beiträge zur Gesellschaftspolitik: Jubiläumsschrift zum 50jährigen Bestehen des Instituts für beratende Sozial- und Wirtschaftswissenschaften – Gerhard-Weisser-Institut. Metropolis-Verlag, Marburg, pp 89–103

Sen A (2002) Ökonomie für den Menschen: Wege zu Gerechtigkeit und Solidarität in der Marktwirtschaft (C. Goldmann, Übers.) (Ungekürzte Ausg). dtv/Dt. Taschenbuch-Verl., München http://www.socialnet.de/rezensionen/isbn.php?isbn=978-3-423-36264-1

Legal Guardianship under the Guardianship Law

42

Kirsten Balcerzak and Manfred Fiedler

Contents

42.1 Guardianship Law

With the entry into force of the *Guardianship Act (BtG)* in 1992, guardianship and custodianship were replaced, and the associated deprivation of rights was substituted by a duty of care that respects individual rights. Guardianship law governs the legal care of adult persons who, due to a physical, mental, or psychological impairment or illness, are unable to manage their affairs wholly or partially on their own. It is strictly oriented to the individual needs of the person under care, takes into account their remaining abilities, and respects their right to self-determination. The aim is to foster a collaborative

K. Balcerzak (✉)
AWO Familienbildungsstätte, Schwerte, Germany

M. Fiedler
Department of human medicine, Witten/Herdecke University, Witten, Germany
e-mail: manfred.fiedler@uni-wh.de

D. Schmitz et al. (eds.), *Chronic Care—Science and Practice*,
https://doi.org/10.1007/978-3-662-72298-5_42

relationship between the guardian and the person under care on an equal footing. Guardianship only covers those areas in which the person in need of care requires support due to their impairment or illness, and these areas are reviewed and determined by the court. The goal of guardianship is to enable the person under care to lead a self-determined life (see Article 21). This means that guardians are fundamentally required to consider and comply with the wishes and will of the person under care. Exceptions are only made if fulfilling these wishes would cause significant harm to the person under care or would be unreasonable for the guardian.

Since its introduction, guardianship law has been amended several times. The provisions of the most recent reform of guardianship and custodianship law in 2021 (Federal Law Gazette Part I p. 882) have been in effect since January 1, 2023, and include an even more consistent focus on the self-determination rights of the person under care.

42.2 Requirements

According to § 1814 BGB, guardians can only be appointed if the person concerned has a need for support that is attributable to an illness or disability. The term illness includes both physical and mental illnesses, such as physically based diseases like neurodegenerative disorders (dementias) or consequences of illnesses (e.g., meningitis), as well as addiction disorders (e.g., due to alcohol, drug, or medication abuse), neuroses, and personality disorders. Both physical and intellectual disabilities, as well as congenital or acquired intellectual deficits resulting from early childhood brain damage, are encompassed by the term *disability*. Illness or disability alone is not sufficient grounds for the appointment of a guardian. In addition to the impairment, there must be a need for support that is causally related to the impairment. The person concerned has difficulty managing their affairs wholly or partially independently due to the illness or disability.

The appointment of a guardian can be requested by the person concerned, but also by relatives, physicians, or representatives of institutions such as hospitals, other facilities, or government agencies such as the competent guardianship court. The court examines whether the appointment is made against the free will of the person concerned. No guardian may be appointed against the will of the person concerned. Furthermore, the court checks whether the *principle of necessity* is fulfilled, as the appointment may only take place if the affairs of the person concerned cannot be managed by other already implemented means, such as a power of attorney. The principle of necessity refers to the actual need for guardianship, the scope of the guardian's responsibilities, the impact of the court's measure, and the duration of the guardianship. The areas of responsibility may include: health and personal welfare, legal and official matters, postal matters, right to determine place of residence, property and financial affairs, housing matters, accommodation and accommodation-related measures.

Guardians are tasked with managing the affairs of the person under care in their best interest. Furthermore, guardians may only be appointed for those areas in which guardianship is actually necessary (§ 1815 paragraph 1 BGB). The requirements of the guardianship court must be followed, and the person under care must always be informed about important decisions.

Guardianship may not be established for longer than necessary. It must be lifted or restricted if the requirements cease to exist. The duration of guardianship depends on the individual case and is limited to a maximum of seven years. After seven years, guardianship may be extended if it is still needed. An application to terminate guardianship can be submitted to the guardianship court at any time. The discontinuation of the need for guardianship must be substantiated in detail. In the event of the death of the person under care, guardianship ends automatically and the guardians are no longer authorized to make decisions (§ 1874 paragraph 2 BGB).

Through a *legally significant power of attorney*, affected individuals ensure that, in the event of incapacity to contract (§ 104 ff BGB), their interests are represented and safeguarded by the authorized persons. The authorized representatives can make decisions for the grantors of the power of attorney (similarly to guardians), negotiate with third parties, and enter into agreements that are in the interest of the grantors. The authorized representatives must adhere to the framework conditions set out in the power of attorney for the benefit of the person concerned. The grantors of the power of attorney must be of legal age. There are various types of power of attorney: general power of attorney (only this prevents the establishment of guardianship in the event of an emergency, e.g., coma), individual or partial power of attorney, and precautionary power of attorney.

42.3 Chronic Illnesses in Guardianship Law

Chronic illnesses play an important role in guardianship law, as they often lead to impairment of decision-making capacity and self-determination. In particular, in the case of neurodegenerative diseases such as dementia, legal guardianship may become necessary. The focus is especially on supporting the self-determination rights of the person concerned. Guardians are expected to assist in making decisions that are in the best interest of the person under care and take their personal needs into account. If free will is impaired by a non-temporary state of pathological disturbance of mental activity, the person is considered legally incapacitated according to § 104 BGB. Even if *legal incapacity* is present, the natural will of the person under care must be taken into account. This means that the person under care can still express understandable pain or needs such as hunger, thirst, etc., and request relief. This will should be appropriately implemented by those involved (physicians, nursing staff, and guardians).

42.4 Reservation of Consent

When it comes to influencing the legal capacity to act of affected persons, there is an important exception in guardianship law: the imposition of guardianship with a *reservation of consent* for specific areas of responsibility. This results in a restriction of the person's participation in legal transactions. The reservation of consent is ordered by the court if there is a significant risk that the person under care will harm themselves or their assets. This provides protection against reckless self-harm. The reservation of consent is a drastic measure and constitutes an intervention in the personal rights of the person under care, and can be equated with the former guardianship system. For this reason, the principle of necessity also applies here. In the case of guardianship with a reservation of consent, guardians may and must override the will of the person under care, as long as they act rationally and in the best interest of the person under care.

42.5 Medical Measures

Medical measures may only be carried out if patients have been thoroughly informed about the measures and any associated risks, and have given their consent. Only those who are capable of giving consent may do so. Guardians must therefore assess whether the person under their care is capable of giving consent. This involves determining whether the individual understands the nature, significance, and scope of the medical measure and is able to express their own will accordingly.

The capacity to give consent must be assessed individually in different treatment situations. If the person under care is not capable of giving consent, the guardians must receive sufficient medical information and decide whether to consent to the medical measure. Any existing advance directive must always be taken into account. If there is no advance directive, the guardians must determine the treatment preferences of the person under care or, if these are not known, their presumed will, and make a decision on this basis (§ 1827 paragraph 2 BGB). In doing so, physicians must inform the guardians about the medical measures in the same manner as they would inform competent patients, and must document this. Patients are also informed about the individual treatment steps according to their cognitive abilities. In certain cases, the consent of the guardians requires approval from the guardianship court. This is the case, for example, if there is a substantiated risk that the person under care could die or suffer serious health damage as a result of the measure (§ 1829 paragraph 1 and sentence 1 BGB). The risk of such harm must be concrete and imminent. Only hypothetical or unlikely risks do not require court approval. The approval process also serves to ensure that guardians are not left alone with such serious decisions.

42.6 Deprivation of Liberty Placement and Deprivation of Liberty Measures

Another important aspect in the context of guardianship law is the so-called deprivation of liberty placements and measures. *Deprivation of liberty measures* include, for example, mechanical devices, medications, or other interventions that deprive the person under care of their freedom for a period of time (§ 1831 paragraph 4 BGB). Such measures constitute a serious infringement of the fundamental rights of the affected person. Certain conditions must be met, which require approval by the guardianship court. This also applies if the person under care is already living in a closed facility with court approval.

Deprivation of liberty measures must be distinguished from interventions where the person under care would not be able to move about even without the measure, or where the measure does not prevent voluntary movement (e.g., a safety belt that prevents falling out of bed but can be opened independently by the person concerned). There is also no deprivation of liberty measure if the person under care agrees to the measure and possesses the corresponding capacity to consent. Only in the case of persons under care who lack capacity to consent do guardians decide on consent to the deprivation of liberty measure. According to § 1815 paragraph 2 number 2 BGB, this requires the express judicial assignment of the area of responsibility for decisions regarding deprivation of liberty measures (§ 1831 paragraph 4 BGB). Deprivation of liberty measures include, among others, bed rails, safety belts in bed or on a chair, restraints, locking the room or ward if it cannot be opened at the request of the person under care at any time, as well as medications administered primarily for sedation. It must also be examined in advance whether a less restrictive measure would be equally sufficient to avert the danger. Only then are deprivation of liberty measures considered.

For placement in a closed facility or ward, such as a hospital or nursing home, guardians also require, according to § 1815 paragraph 2 number 1 BGB, the express judicial assignment of the area of responsibility associated with deprivation of liberty placement (§ 1831 paragraph 1 BGB).

According to the requirements of § 1815 paragraph 1 BGB, *deprivation of liberty placement* is only permitted if, due to a mental illness or intellectual or psychological disability, there is a risk that the person under care will commit suicide or cause themselves significant health damage. This paragraph also applies if the person under care does not recognize the necessity of the placement and does not act in accordance with this insight, or if, without placement, the implementation of necessary medical treatment required to prevent health damage cannot be ensured.

Placement is only lawful with the approval of the guardianship court. An exception applies in cases of imminent danger that would be associated with delay. This is the case, for example, in acute suicidality. Approval must then be obtained without delay (§ 1831 paragraph 2 BGB). The placement is terminated by the guardians as soon as the conditions for it no longer exist. Termination of the placement does not require court approval; however, the guardians must notify the court of this without delay.

References

Bürgerliches Gesetzbuch (2023 & i. d. F.v. 2.1.2002 I 42, 2909; 2003, 738; zuletzt geändert durch Art. 1 G v. 14.3.2023 I Nr. 72). https://www.gesetze-im-internet.de/bgb/BJNR001950896.html#BJNR001950896BJNG000102377. Accessed 31.08.2023

Seichter J (2019) Einführung in das Betreuungsrecht: Ein Leitfaden Für Praktiker des Betreuungsrechts, Heilberufe und Angehörige Von Betreuten, 5. edn. Springer, Berlin/Heidelberg

Sorg W (2009) Geschichtliche Entwicklung des Betreuungsrechts. BGT – Betreuungsgerichtstag e. V. 7. Württembergischer Vormundschaftsgerichtstag Das Wohl des Betreuten. Wer bestimmt es? Wie? https://www.bgt-ev.de/fileadmin/Mediendatenbank/Tagungen/Württembergischer_BGT/07/AG4_Bericht2.pdf. Accessed 31.08.2023

Organizational Forms of the Health System

43

Manfred Fiedler

Contents

43.1 Organization of the Health System and Health Care

Internationally, health care at the macro level of the health system is organized very differently (Schölkopf 2017). This has an impact on care, especially for people with chronic illnesses. Both economic access (see Contribution 45), in terms of health equity, and needs-based access depend on the organization of the health system. The classic instruments of health policy (see Contribution 44) primarily concern the protection against the risk of illness as well as the assurance of care.

M. Fiedler (✉)
Department of human medicine, Witten/Herdecke University, Witten, Deutschland
e-mail: manfred.fiedler@uni-wh.de

D. Schmitz et al. (eds.), *Chronic Care—Science and Practice*,
https://doi.org/10.1007/978-3-662-72298-5_43

43.2 Protection Against the Risk of Illness

Basically, four types of financial protection can be distinguished: 1. Out-of-pocket, 2. Private insurance, 3. public or social insurance, and 4. tax funding or funding from the public budget.

1. **Out of Pocket**
   With *out-of-pocket* financing, health services are paid for from the current income of the individual concerned. This can also occur by liquidating savings. For people with low incomes and for small amounts, current income is typically used. Co-payments, i.e., a personal contribution by patients within the scope of a service otherwise covered by private or public health insurance, are also financed *out of pocket*. The burden of *out-of-pocket* financing particularly affects people with chronic illnesses and can negatively impact access to health services (Kočiš Krůtilová et al. 2021).
2. **Private Insurance**
   The insurance principle involves the *formation of a risk-sharing community* to protect against the uncertain occurrence of a risk event based on the principle of mutuality. In private insurance, this insured community is nowadays only formal in nature. It is therefore also referred to as 'individual insurance' today. The insurance premium is determined, in addition to the agreed scope of benefits, primarily by the individual risk of the insured. This may include pre-existing conditions, but also health risks arising from socioeconomic or sociobiographical characteristics, such as belonging to a social group or a particular high-risk occupational group.
   Since the risk of illness increases with age, the age at which insurance is taken out is also relevant for the amount of the insurance premium. With similar risk and similar entry age, we speak of an insured cohort.
   In principle, private insurance is based on the funded system, meaning that insurance premiums are saved and paid out in the event of a claim (in old age). Insurance premiums can change over time. They are calculated at the time the insurance contract is concluded based on the expected life expectancy, current claims experience, and the current scope of benefits. If these parameters for calculating the insurance premium change during the course of the insurance, for example due to higher life expectancy or a change in claims experience, the premium increases.
   Another principle is that of reimbursement of costs. In private insurance, patients remain, in principle, the debtors for the services received vis-à-vis the service provider. For example, they submit the invoice for a specialist treatment to the insurance company, which settles it, minus any agreed deductible. Especially for high-value invoices, such as those regularly incurred during hospital stays, private insurers are increasingly adopting the so-called benefits-in-kind principle. This means that the patient receives the service, in this case hospital treatment, not as a cash benefit but as

a benefit in kind. The insurance company thus becomes directly involved in the billing process.

An alternative to individual insurance is group insurance. In this form of insurance, not individuals but certain groups of people are insured, such as employees of a company as a (monetary) component of salary/wages. The insurance premium is usually charged as a uniform premium per insured person. The advantage for the insured person is that individual risk assessment is omitted. The disadvantage is that insurance coverage only exists as long as one is a member of the protection community. If a member leaves, for example due to termination of employment, insurance coverage usually ceases as well.

3. **Public or Social Insurance**

Like private insurance, social insurance is also based on membership. However, unlike private insurance, the insurance premium—or more accurately, the social insurance contribution—is not based on the principle of 'risk equivalence' but on the principle of ability to pay. It is therefore generally income-based. This means that the contribution/premium is determined by the income of the insured.

The model of competition among health insurance funds that exists in Germany is the result of historical health policy decisions and is not constitutive. This can be illustrated by looking at other branches of social insurance, such as the unified statutory pension insurance and unemployment insurance. A single social health insurance fund for everyone is therefore fundamentally conceivable and not incompatible with the principle of social insurance.

However, the in recent times discussed insurance premiums in the form of pe-capita-premiums, sometimes incorrectly referred to as per-capita-flatrates (Pfaff et al. 2003), or uniform contributions, however, represents a departure from the principle of income equivalence. This does not affect the provision of benefits. Depending on the amount of the uniform contribution, this would lead to financial overload for low-income individuals and would therefore require a needs-based compensation, which would then be paid from another public budget.

By contrast, the benefits-in-kind principle is constitutive. Since social insurance must insure a large number of people who have only a small disposable household income, these individuals would regularly reach the limits of their ability to pay if they had to make advance payments on a regular basis. In addition, since the insurance acts directly as a contracting party, insured persons are relieved of the need to check invoices for factual accuracy.

By contrast, the arguments for reimbursement of costs in social insurance are not convincing. The claim that the supposedly better information of the insured, leading to greater transparency of services, results in more accurate billing has not been substantiated by studies (Greß et al.2011): In fact, the transaction costs are higher, i.e., the effort required to carry out the billing process. Additional payment transactions arise, and both the patient and the health insurance fund must check the accuracy of invoices and the billability of services provided.

4. **Tax Funding**
   An internationally widespread form of protection against the risk of illness is tax funding. We speak of tax-funded health systems when health services necessary to meet needs are provided for all citizens of a country from public budgets. In contrast to other financing systems, access to health services is generally assured, since neither individual ability to pay nor, for example, membership in a health insurance fund is required to establish entitlement to benefits.
   In some cases, tax funding of health services is provided only for certain groups of people, such as those with low incomes or individuals who, due to a chronic impairment, are unable to earn sufficient income on their own.

In most cases, these systems exist side by side, for example when income replacement benefits in the event of illness are covered by insurance in otherwise tax-funded systems. Nevertheless, we refer to social insurance systems, as in Germany, when social insurance is the fundamental form of protection.

43.3 Ensuring the Provision of Care

In addition to the issue of safeguarding against the risk of illness, the public regulatory function is of great importance in all high-wage countries to ensure that the supply of healthcare services is adequate both quantitatively and qualitatively. The following provides a brief introduction to the main forms.

1. **Legislation**
   Through government legislation, the framework conditions for the organization and structures of the healthcare system are established. This sets out the basic structures and responsibilities. Legislation can also define (minimum) standards and determine procedures. The implementation of these national legal provisions can be delegated in various ways, for example to federal or state authorities. In Germany's federal system, for instance, state laws and implementing regulations of the federal states are used as instruments, which in turn can define processes, structures, and responsibilities at the state level and for municipalities.
2. **Associational Governance—Corporatism**
   The concept of associational governance is based on the (legal) delegation or commissioning of (interest) associations of professional healthcare actors to implement statutory requirements and regulations in healthcare practice. Corporatism is described as market-analogous governance or as an *equivalent to the market* (Czada 1994), as associational bi- or multilateral negotiation of, for example, prices or quality guide-

lines. In the absence of sufficient market-based solutions, it effectively replaces, *equivalently*, decentralized market negotiation processes.

Actors or their associations are also considered to possess greater professional and technical expertise than state actors. However, there is much to suggest that associational negotiation does not always lead to optimal outcomes. On the one hand, it always involves a negotiated compromise, which can also result in negotiation deadlock, as has led to statutory substitute actions in Germany. On the other hand, the parties involved are primarily concerned with advancing the interests of their members and thus are not initially focused on representing and actively shaping the overall societal interest in the healthcare system.

In addition to classic corporatism, medical and nursing professional associations develop guidelines and quality standards, which become recommendations or legally binding standards for healthcare procedures, as well as structural requirements for healthcare facilities such as care centers. These include, for example, minimum staffing standards in terms of qualitative and quantitative personnel allocation and the approval of medical, therapeutic, and nursing procedures.

3. **Mandate to Ensure Provision**

   By formulating the mandate to ensure provision, responsibility for parts/sectors of the healthcare system is transferred or defined (Schwartz 1995). This involves state authorization or commissioning. In Germany, the best-known form of this mandate is the provision of outpatient medical care by the Associations of Statutory Health Insurance Physicians (Kassenärztliche Vereinigungen, KV).

   A regular component of governance is needs-based planning, which is intended to ensure the regional availability and accessibility of general and specialized healthcare services.

   While the mandate to ensure provision can enable appropriate sectoral planning and service management tailored to regional requirements, the resulting sectoral structure can hinder the development of cross-sectoral care models and cross-sectoral interface management.

4. **Infrastructure Development**

   Healthcare facilities are considered part of the social and economically relevant infrastructure. Healthcare services are also counted as part of municipal public services or, internationally, as services of public interest. One instrument is the separation of investments from service remuneration. Instead of uniform, monistic financing through service remuneration, facilities are financed either dually through a separate financing mechanism or from an investment budget as part of regional investment planning.

43.4 Requirements for a Chronic Care-Oriented Organization of Care

Social security is intended to protect those who do not have sufficient financial and other resources and capabilities to insure themselves against the risk of illness. Chronic illness, on the one hand, reduces capabilities and, on the other, increases the need for health and health-related services. This ambivalence of chronic illness highlights the limitations of private insurance systems, in which chronic illnesses are penalized with a risk premium. At the same time, the complexity of care requirements necessitates innovative solutions that demand flexible law and open organization. This could be a publicly secured care system with a broadly understood corporatism in the sense of participatory involvement of self-help groups, health initiatives, and care networks.

References

Czada R (1994) Konjunkturen des Korporatismus: Zur Geschichte eines Paradigmenwechsels in der Verbändeforschung. Polit Vierteljahresschr 25:37–64

Greß S, Heberlein I, Heinemann S, Niebuhr (2011) Kostenerstattung in der Gesetzlichen Krankversicherung (pg-papers Nr. 1). https://fuldok.hs-fulda.de/opus4/frontdoor/deliver/index/docId/143/file/PgPapers_2011_01_Gress_et_al.pdf. Accessed 25 Sept 2023

Kočiš Krůtilová V, Bahnsen L, de Graeve D (2021) The out-of-pocket burden of chronic diseases: the cases of Belgian, Czech and German older adults. BMC Health Services Research 21(1):239. https://doi.org/10.1186/s12913-021-06259-w

Pfaff AB, Pfaff M, Kern AO, Langer B (2003) Auswirkungen verschiedener Modell-Varianten von Kopfpauschalen auf die Finanzierung von Krankenversicherungsleistungen in Deutschland. Projekt gefördert durch die Hans-Böckler-Stiftung. Augsburg. Inifes. https://www.sozialpolitik-aktuell.de/files/sozialpolitikaktuell/_Politikfelder/Gesundheitswesen/Dokumente/KOPFPA~2.PDF. Accessed 22 Sept 2023

Schölkopf M (2017) Das Gesundheitswesen im internationalen Vergleich: Gesundheitssystemvergleich, Länderberichte und europäische Gesundheitspolitik, 3., akt. erw. edn. Health Care Management. Berlin, Medizinisch Wissenschaftliche Verlagsgesellschaft. http://www.content-select.com/index.php?id=bib_view&ean=9783954663354

Schwartz FW (1995) Konjunkturen des Korporatismus: Zur Geschichte eines Paradigmenwechsels in der Verbändeforschung. Soz Fortschr 44(4):84–89

44 Health Policy Concepts for the Care of Chronically Ill People

Manfred Fiedler

Contents

44.1 Fundamentals of Health Policy

Health policy is understood as part of social policy in almost all high-income countries. Even in countries with a primarily market-oriented agenda, such as the USA, a large proportion of health expenditures (approx. 45%) is financed from public or parafiscal budgets. Despite this accepted public responsibility for health services, the respective national political agendas differ greatly.

The foundation of social policy concepts lies in the unequal distribution of economic resources within society and the partial redistribution of income to compensate for this. Gerhard Weisser's concept of life situations (1978) expanded this understanding. The concept of life situation has been incorporated into social policy in the form of the social indicators approach (Voges 2005). Social indicators are measurable, group-specific characteristics that can be used to describe life situations and scopes for action. One

M. Fiedler (✉)
Department of human medicine, Witten/Herdecke University, Witten, Deutschland
e-mail: manfred.fiedler@uni-wh.de

D. Schmitz et al. (eds.), *Chronic Care—Science and Practice*,
https://doi.org/10.1007/978-3-662-72298-5_44

such concept is the Socio-Economic Panel based at the German Institute for Economic Research.

A related, more person-centered concept is that of capabilities, developed by the economist Amartya Sen (2002). Capabilities are based on personal characteristics and resources and determine the ability to pursue and realize one's own goals. Those who, due to their social and economic situation, are unable to choose between different life options have correspondingly limited capabilities.

The aforementioned concepts highlight that focusing on multicausal, supportive or hindering factors for personal prospects and life chances is crucial. This forms the basis for another health and social policy concept, namely that of activating social policy. This refers to the much older principle of subsidiarity. According to Oswald von Breuning, the state should promote personal agency and self-determination (Möhring-Hesse 2015). Policy should enable such self-determined action. State-guaranteed institutions, such as healthcare provision, serve this purpose.

44.2 Policy for Securing the Risk of Illness: The Example of Germany

Regimes of health security have developed historically. As such, they imprint a kind of cultural stamp on healthcare provision and shape the system. The different types of risk protection for illness (see Contribution 41) are therefore not simply a toolbox from which policymakers can freely choose, but rather a form of national predisposition that forms the basis for political development.

For the Scandinavian countries, we speak of Nordic health policy; the US health system is interpreted as a system of private risk protection for illness, even though the share of public spending is high compared to European countries.

Health policy and reform policy are based on the reform of existing concepts and fundamental security regimes. Comparisons of health systems can reveal aspects of convergence, or system convergence, by adopting instruments that can be adapted to fit one's own regime.

German health security (see Contribution 41) is primarily based on statutory health insurance, which, from its inception, was supplemented by statutory accident insurance to cover the risk of occupational accidents and, since the 1920s, occupational diseases. Bismarck's social legislation emerged in the 1880s as a response to the growing labor movement and replaced the workers' mutual aid societies (Hansen et al. 1981), which were organized by trade unions. As part of the policy of *carrot and stick*, these were both an offer and an instrument of political control during a period when socialist parties were banned, since employers were also given equal representation in the social self-administration of the workers' health insurance funds. For this, they also had to contribute half of the contribution rate. It was not until 1911, with the Imperial Insurance Code, that the salaried employees' health insurance funds, whose self-administration was not based on parity, were established.

The development of German health policy can thus be divided into several phases. Up to the Nazi dictatorship, one can speak of the establishment phase, during which the foundations of today's structures were laid. The Nazi regime adopted these structures and made them part of its centralized social policy. For example, it established the mandate to ensure outpatient medical care by the Associations of Statutory Health Insurance Physicians, thereby ending fund-specific forms of care.

The restitution phase meant, in West Germany, the continuation and consolidation of the pre-war system, while in East Germany a fundamentally public health system was created, with public hospitals, polyclinics, outpatient clinics, and medical practices across the country. In West Germany, the 1960s and 1970s initially saw an expansion of social health security. With the Health Insurance Cost Containment Act of 1977 (Krankenversicherungskostendämpfungsgesetz - KVKG), the policy of cost containment emerged, introducing measures to limit expenditures and influence demand for health services, primarily through co-payments by those affected.

The unification of East and West Germany led to the dissolution of the previous outpatient care structures in East Germany and the adoption of the West German system of physician care based on individual practices. In this case, the merger was, at least in this respect, more of a takeover and integration.

The policy of cost containment did not achieve the desired success and was supplemented by market-oriented reforms with the Health Structure Act of 1992, particularly on the provider side and through the so-called competition among health insurance funds. At the same time, the increase in the need for long-term care was addressed by creating a new social insurance scheme in the form of statutory long-term care insurance.

Since the mid-2010s, even among supporters, there has been a sense of disillusionment regarding the effects of market-oriented reforms, and a shift—still unclear in its political direction—toward socio-economic adjustment of the instruments can be observed. The debates on binding staffing levels, the separation of nursing costs from the hospital case-based payment system, and the redesign of hospital financing make this evident.

44.3 Cost Containment and Market Regulation Policy

Over the past decades, so-called market regulation policy (Neubauer 1984) has emerged as a significant instrument of health policy. While in the 1980s the so-called cost containment policy dominated, aiming to control expenditures by increasing co-payments, this changed from the 1990s onward.

Based on the economically liberal perspective that publicly regulated and managed systems, including in healthcare, lead to inefficient and qualitatively inadequate outcomes, competitive structures were to be introduced in the healthcare sector as well.

Even the introduction of co-payments is based on the idea of economic behavior management. If access to and utilization of services is possible free of charge and without contribution, this, under the theoretical assumption of individual utility maximization, leads to overutilization (free-rider behavior, moral hazard). Co-payments are intended to influence this, so that only necessary services are used. In reality, this effect usually proved to be only short-term, as services were either brought forward or delayed, and the previous service volumes quickly returned. The so-called cost containment policy lost its priority and was replaced by market regulation policy.

As an ideal-typical principle, economic competition allocates resources much better than other distribution mechanisms can achieve. Accordingly, various concepts have emerged in recent years. This includes the so-called competition among health insurance funds. Those insured under statutory health insurance have the option to be insured with any statutory health insurance fund. Health insurance funds are intended to have an incentive, especially through a low contribution rate, to attract insured persons.

Another model is that of a unified insurance market based on the Dutch model, in which, under a general insurance mandate, the insured can freely choose between private and public insurers.

On the provider side as well, concepts for service design and financing have been developed to simulate market mechanisms. A good example is so-called administered prices, such as diagnosis-related groups (DRGs) in hospital financing. Generally, prices for services between customers and providers are supposed to be determined independently by the market without public intervention, which, through the automatic balancing of supply and demand, is expected to lead to optimal pricing from an economic perspective. In health systems, these theoretical possibilities for market-based price formation do not exist or are only possible to a limited extent, especially in light of social security objectives. Therefore, prices must be administered.

In the German healthcare system, the system of administered prices is based on a negotiation model at the association level (corporatism) (Kalvelage 1992) between the associations of health insurers and providers, the results of which are binding for their members. The externally set prices for hospital services are intended to force hospitals to operate more economically in order to avoid losses and generate profits, and also to increase transparency in the hospital sector.

Neither competition among health insurance funds, the unified insurance market in the Netherlands, nor hospital DRGs have been able to demonstrate the expected macroeconomic effects. The introduction of DRGs in hospitals has not led to a reduction in hospital care expenditures, nor have significant quality improvements been observed. Competition in health insurance, apart from the freedom of choice, has so far had no discernible effects on healthcare provision. In international comparison, systems with a more market-oriented health policy are neither superior economically nor in terms of system performance. However, evidence of disadvantages in care can be found in more privatized health markets, such as risk selection and the disadvantaging of risk groups like people with chronic illnesses.

44.4 Challenges

Demographic change is increasing the pressure on health policy not only in Germany. Health services, as predominantly personal services with a high proportion of personnel costs, can only be rationalized to a limited extent. At the same time, the labor market potential of health services is particularly high.

Demographic change has a dual and opposing effect. The demand for services is rising, while on the other hand, the labor market potential for education health professionals is tending to decline. Almost half of all primary care physicians in Germany are over 50 years old, as are nearly 40% of all nursing staff. We are seeing a widening gap between demand and supply. At the same time, the attachment of health professionals to their employers is decreasing, and especially in nursing professions, the willingness to leave the profession is increasing.

In contrast, the increasing number of chronically ill and multimorbid patients is leading to increasingly complex care requirements, which are met by a high degree of specialization, especially in specialist medical care.

What is needed, therefore, are care networks, cooperation in the healthcare sector, and thus a health policy that sets the framework for this, bringing together healthcare providers to better organize complexity, reduce friction losses and redundancies, and design coherent care arrangements both interprofessionally and interinstitutionally.

References

Hansen E, Heisig M, Leibfried S, Tennstedt F (1981) Seit über einem Jahrhundert, ... verschüttete Alternativen in der Sozialpolitik: Sozialer Fortschritt, organisierte Dienstleistermacht und nationalsozialistische Machtergreifung: der Fall der Ambulatorien in den Unterweserstädten und Berlin; 100 Jahre kaiserliche Botschaft zur Sozialversicherung; eine Festschrift. WSI-Studie zur Wirtschafts- und Sozialforschung. Bund-Verlag, Köln

Kalvelage B (1992) Korporatismus. In: Bauer R (ed) Lexikon des Sozial- und Gesundheitswesens, vol 2, Oldenbourg, München

Möhring-Hesse M (2015) Solidaristische Gefahren: Oswald von Nell-Breunings sozialpolitische Impulse für die Gegenwart. https://doi.org/10.15496/publikation-49106

Neubauer G (1984) Konkurrenz der Steuerungssystem in der Gesetzlichen Krankenversicherung. In: Herder-Dorneich P (ed) Soziale Ordnungspolitik, vol 1. Überwindung der Sozialstaatskrise: Ordnungspolitische Ansätze, 1st edn. Nomos, Baden-Baden pp 149–167

Sen A (2002) Ökonomie für den Menschen: Wege zu Gerechtigkeit und Solidarität in der Marktwirtschaft (C. Goldmann, Übers.) (Ungekürzte Ausg) dtv/Dt. Taschenbuch-Verl., München. http://www.socialnet.de/rezensionen/isbn.php?isbn=978-3-423-36264-1

Voges W (2005) Indikatoren im Lebenslagenansatz: das Konzept der Lebenslage in der Wirkungsforschung. ZES-Report, 11(1), 1–6. https://nbn-resolving.org/urn:nbn:de:0168-ssoar-357391 (ZES-Report)

Weisser G (1978) Gesellschaftspolitik. In: Katterle S, Mudra W, Neumann L, Neumann LF (eds) Beiträge zur Gesellschaftspolitik: Philosophische Vorfragen—beratende Sozialwissenschaft—soziale Sicherung—Mitbestimmung—Verteilungs- und Vermögenspolitik—Ordnungspolitik—besonders Einzelwirtschaftspolitik. Verlag Otto Schwartz & Co, Göttingen, pp 359–398

Introduction to Health Care Economics 45

Manfred Fiedler

Contents

45.1 What the Science of Economics Is About

Economics is a social science that focuses on meeting individual and collective (human) needs. A key issue is that the resources required to meet these needs, as well as the necessary labor, are not available in unlimited quantities and are therefore scarce (Weise et al. 1991). If the goods and resources needed to satisfy needs are not sufficiently available—whether permanently or temporarily, locally or generally—in relation to the qualified demand, competition arises over their use. Economics thus deals with the phenomenon of scarcity and with the instruments and methods for resolving the distribution dilemma resulting from scarcity.

M. Fiedler (✉)
Department of human medicine, Witten/Herdecke University, Witten, Deutschland
e-mail: manfred.fiedler@uni-wh.de

D. Schmitz et al. (eds.), *Chronic Care—Science and Practice*,
https://doi.org/10.1007/978-3-662-72298-5_45

45.2 Central Basic Concepts

45.2.1 Need—Requirement

A need is what a person fundamentally requires. Maslow's concept (1943), which distinguishes five types of needs, is widely recognized.

- Physiological needs (food, drink, housing, or clothing)
- Safety needs (physical integrity, health, personal and social security, such as income, employment)
- Social needs (friendship, family, connection with others)
- Personal needs (respect, self-esteem, social status, personal freedom)
- Self-actualization/meaning in life

Although this concept is often interpreted as hierarchical ("hierarchy of needs"), the types of needs do not represent a strict ranking. Nevertheless, we generally refer to physiological and safety needs as basic needs, whose fulfillment must be ensured for all people by society in order to enable an adequate life in terms of wellbeing.

In contrast to the concept of need is the concept of demand. Demand is the individual as well as societal conceptualization of how a need should be met. For example, the need for drinking can be satisfied by different beverages. In economic terms, requirement is thus the need made concrete in the form of demand.

45.2.2 Demand and Supply

Macroeconomic demand is the aggregated form of the requirements of individuals for a particular service or good. This is not a constant value, but is based on certain factors, primarily the price of a good and the individual preferences of each person within the scope of their available income and assets. The simple understanding that a higher price leads to lower demand must be qualified when it comes to goods that fulfill basic needs. For example, if rental prices rise, individuals cannot avoid this, but must instead reduce their demand for other goods, even if their prices have not increased.

In contrast, there is the supply of goods/services. Here, too, the statement that a higher achievable price leads to a higher supply only holds if the influence of individual suppliers is low. In the context of branding, for example, the deliberate restriction of supply can be used to achieve a higher market price. The product cycle theory of the Austrian economist Schumpeter shows that as a product matures, the number of potential suppliers decreases, and thus the influence of each supplier on quantity and price increases (Schumpeter 1950).

45.3 Market Economy versus Non-Market Economy in Healthcare

In the economics of healthcare, two perspectives can be distinguished, leading to significant differences in methods and instruments: market economy and non-market economy. From the market economy perspective, the optimal allocation of goods through market competition—that is, the formation of prices, supply, and demand through competition in a virtual place of economic activity (the market)—is also applied to healthcare. The non-market economy perspective refers to the analysis of economic sectors and areas in which market instruments lead to socially or economically inadequate or undesirable outcomes, and where other instruments for the allocation of scarcity are therefore considered. Given the particular importance of health services for ensuring participation and the integrity of individuals, these are declared political goods in many countries, with the aim of making at least some health services equally available to all citizens (non-excludability and non-rivalry). In this context, health services are distributed, for example, by convention, through prioritization of resource use, or according to the principle of social equity of need. Public property rights are also often defined so that scarcities can be actively reduced.

45.4 The Special Conditions of Demand for Health Services

The demand for health services has special characteristics that, in addition to the debate over whether they should be treated as political goods, are significant for the organization of health services. Fundamentally, health services are *uno-actu services*. Consumption and provision occur simultaneously; they cannot be stored. However, all personal services, such as haircuts, personal care, or wellness massages, share this characteristic. At the same time, they are only to a limited extent, or not at all, temporally flexible. Services for acute illnesses must be provided promptly, life-threatening conditions immediately, and chronic conditions continuously. This also limits the choice. Health services are not substitutable for one another, except in the selection of therapy. For example, in the case of a heart valve disease, a bowel operation cannot be chosen instead of heart surgery.

A health service, in the classical sense, is a productive transformation process. In the context of work system analysis—input, transformation, and output/result—patients are the object to be changed, who are altered through various medical, therapeutic, and nursing interventions. There is thus an identity between the person commissioning/receiving the service and the object to be transformed. For people, especially those with severe chronic illnesses, this means that they are continuously the subject of economic actions. Health services therefore affect everyday life and, in many cases, are of a fundamental, existential nature.

Every health service fundamentally has a non-professional component. For example, those affected must demonstrate therapy adherence (adherence, compliance); they perform part of the service themselves by, for instance, taking medication at the right time and in the right amount or following certain diets.

Finally, health services have a more or less significant non-professional component in the professional performance, such as parental caregiving for a sick child, emotional support and assistance during critical phases of illness, support with therapy, care, and everyday assistance for people with chronic illnesses.

45.5 Consumerism and Supply-Induced Demand

In connection with the involvement of those affected in service provision, reference is often made to the concept of *consumerism*. The term was originally understood as an empowerment concept. Patients are not the object of healthcare service provision, but rather the key decision-makers regarding their own health matters. This understanding, as important as it is in the relationship between service providers and those affected, also has a second aspect, which is based on the notion of the consumer (Khullar et al. 2020). Health services are interpreted as consumer goods, and self-determination in the treatment process becomes a process of personal responsibility with regard to the economic burden of decisions about the treatment process.

This understanding is contradicted by the concept of supply-induced demand. According to this, the knowledge and information gap between healthcare professionals and patients is central to their mutual relationship. The healthcare professional essentially holds the competence to define diagnoses. Therapeutic pathways are also within their competence, and to a large extent, this is also a legal matter, for example, when medically or nursing-necessary interventions are omitted or, conversely, when there is no indication. Studies show that when, for example, services are capped by a budget, many patients experience cuts to services *across the board*, including medically necessary services (Brot–Goldberg et al. 2017).

The concept of supply-induced demand is based on a particular feature of health services. Demand often remains diffuse because preferences for health services are not initially specified; rather, the as-yet-undefined health impairment serves as the reason for seeking treatment. This also applies to decisions about treatment and the course of treatment. Many aspects can only be assessed to a limited extent. From an economic perspective, we usually only know the price for the entire treatment at the end, unlike for individual interventions, because the course of treatment varies from patient to patient. This becomes particularly clear in the reimbursement of hospital treatment based on diagnosis-related case rates. The price to be billed is determined by the discharge diagnosis, the course of treatment—such as the number of hours of ventilation—and relevant comorbidities of the patient.

In the literature, the concept is also interpreted to mean that, as a result of rational decisions by providers, self-created demand leads to medically unnecessary overutilization (Hodek and Greiner 2010). This aspect, however, is not the subject here, especially in light of the contradictory scientific discourse, but rather the exclusive focus is on the hierarchy of competence in the relationship between healthcare professionals and patients.

45.6 Principles of Health Service Remuneration

How and which services are remunerated depends on the specific definition of the service (see Contribution 46), but also on the type of health system organization (see Contribution 43).

In principle, four forms of service remuneration can be distinguished: budget/salary, capitation, case-based payment, and fee-for-service (see Fig. 45.1).

1. With a *fixed budget*, the service provider receives a fixed sum, regardless of the actual number of services provided. For the provider, it is initially rational to have a minimum number of patients, cases, and thus services. The budget principle is quite common internationally for hospital remuneration. What is crucial is the link to a service mandate or contract, i.e., the obligation to treat patients within the scope of the mandate.
2. The *capitation* is paid regardless of the number of cases and services, based on the number of enrolled insured persons, or, in the case of a specific insurance arrangement, based on the number of insured persons to be cared for. Capitation payments can thus be used as a care agreement within the framework of a managed care contract. Depending on how the service providers are organized and how they settle ser-

Number of / type of payment	Patients	Cases - Contacts	Services
Fixed budget/salary	min	min	min
Per capita flat rate	max	min	min
Flat rate per case	max	max	min
Payment for individual services	max	max	max

Fig. 45.1 Forms of remuneration. (Adapted from Thiemeyer 1986a, b)

vices among themselves, this lump-sum financing method in such a context resembles the fixed budget.

3. With *case-based payment*, a defined treatment process is compensated with a lump sum, regardless of the actual partial services provided. The number of patient cases is thus relevant for revenue, and depending on the level of differentiation, so is the average remuneration. Case-based payment limits the incentive to expand services, but depending on its design, it can still lead to the construction of cases or revenue-oriented indication setting.
4. *Fee-for-service* involves financing each defined service provided with and to patients. To simplify billing, it is often implemented by financing service bundles, i.e., by grouping individual, factually related services that are regularly provided together. Fee-for-service is, on the one hand, technically complex to bill, and on the other hand, the incentive to expand services is very high. Fee-for-service is often used in so-called self-pay models (out-of-pocket), as well as being the predominant form of remuneration in outpatient medical care.

In reality, these forms of remuneration are often combined. For example, in outpatient medical remuneration, case-based, bundled, and fee-for-service payments are all used. In addition, global budgets or regional budgets are used as a method of financing, which are intended to limit total expenditures and can therefore affect the level of the aforementioned payments.

The above expectations regarding behavior are also purely economic perspectives, which assume economically rational behavior. In reality, other motives are formative in healthcare, such as professional ethics, as well as issues of liability law and patient safety. A remuneration system designed from this pluralistic economic perspective must take two aspects into account: First, it must support the health professional's decision-making, or at least not shape it economically. Second, it must be understood by health actors and perceived as fair and appropriate.

References

Brot-Goldberg ZC, Chandra A, Handel BR, Kolstad JT (2017) What does a deductible do? The impact of cost-sharing on health care prices, quantities, and spending dynamics. Q J Econ 132(3):1261–1318. https://doi.org/10.1093/qje/qjx013

Hodek J-M, Greiner W (2010) Kostensteigerung im Gesundheitswesen. Gesundh Sozialpolit 6:26–36

Khullar D, Darien G, Ness DL (2020) Patient consumerism, healing relationships, and rebuilding trust in health care. JAMA 324(23):2359–2360. https://doi.org/10.1001/jama.2020.12938

Maslow AH (1943) A theory of human motivation. Psychol Rev 50(4):370–396. https://doi.org/10.1037/h0054346

Schumpeter JA (1950) Kapitalismus, Sozialismus und Demokratie, 6th edn., 501 93/0324. Francke, Göttingen

Thiemeyer T (1986a) Gesundheitsleistungen—Steuerung durch Markt, Staat oder Verbände? Soz Fortschr 35(5/6):97–104

Thiemeyer T (1986b) Das ärztliche Honorar als Preis. In: Gäfgen G (Hrsg) Jahrestagung des Vereins für Socialpolitik, Gesellschaft für Wirtschafts- und Sozialwissenschaften: Bd 1985. Ökonomie des Gesundheitswesens: Jahrestagung des Vereins für Socialpolitik, Gesellschaft für Wirtschafts- und Sozialwissenschaften in Saarbrücken 1985. Duncker & Humblot, Berlin, pp 255–270

Weise P, Brandes W, Eger T, Kraft M (1991) Neue Mikroökonomie, 2., vollst. überarb. u. erw. edn. Physica-Lehrbuch. Physica-Verl, Heidelberg

Principles of Business Administration of Institutions for the Care of Chronically Ill People

46

Manfred Fiedler

Contents

46.1 Business Type Theory

In German health social law, we find the principle of so-called diversity of providers of facilities which expresses the accessibility of different types of enterprises to the *market for health services*. Here, we are dealing with three fundamental types of enterprises, which are also common internationally: public, (non-profit) charitable, and (profit-oriented) private enterprises. Even though this is only insufficiently explicated scientifically, the underlying understanding is that different types of businesses or enterprises have different economic modes, which in turn lead to different outcomes in healthcare provision. A more scientific-analytical understanding is provided by the concept of business type theory (also morphology of individual enterprises), developed by the so-called

M. Fiedler (✉)
Department of human medicine, Witten/Herdecke University, Witten, Deutschland
e-mail: manfred.fiedler@uni-wh.de

D. Schmitz et al. (eds.), *Chronic Care—Science and Practice*,
https://doi.org/10.1007/978-3-662-72298-5_46

Cologne School (in particular Weisser, Engelhardt, Thiemeyer, Schulz-Nieswandt). Starting from the external structure, such as market/economic order, basic and specific legal frameworks, entrepreneurial and operational actions can be explained by typifying internal structural characteristics. According to Engelhardt (1973), these include the purpose and objectives of the enterprise. Furthermore, characteristics of providors or owners as well as management, leadership structures and employees, and finally the size of the enterprise, legal form, internal organization, and business interconnections. Business type theory thus provides a more differentiated tool for analyzing the structures and economic actions of individual enterprises.

46.2 Enterprises in Healthcare Provision

1. From Individual Practice to Corporate Enterprise
   When German reunification was completed in 1990, two very different structures were found in outpatient care. In East Germany, a system structured by polyclinics, outpatient clinics, and individual practices stood in contrast to a system in West Germany that was primarily characterized by individual medical practices. Early on, the individual practice was established as the reference business form for outpatient medical care, even though this was relativized by the Health Structure Act of 1993. This business form requires outpatient physicians and psychotherapists to see their work not only as a professional task but always also as an entrepreneurial one. In conjunction with professional and performance law, the individual medical practice also controls the provision of services in outpatient care through prescriptions. This hierarchizes the relationships between professional groups and assigns the individual practice the responsibility for professional decisions for non-medical, such as therapeutic, interventions. Moreover, the division into medical specialties means that, especially for people with multiple chronic illnesses, different individual medical practices are responsible.
   In recent years, legal changes have created options for other business types (German Council of Experts for the Assessment of Developments in the Healthcare System 2018). These include, above all, group practices and medical care centers (Medizinische Versorgungszentren - MVZ). Although both business types may appear similar at first glance, there are fundamental differences related to their respective business purposes. While the group practice represents the association of contract physicians, where the medical license remains tied to the contracting parties—who often, though not necessarily, belong to the same specialty—the MVZ aims for interdisciplinary collaboration. Furthermore, when a partner leaves, the medical license remains with the MVZ if it is bought by the remaining partners. By acquiring additional licenses, the MVZ can also grow. Although the MVZ must be managed by a physician, the classic freelance status is no longer the focus when providing medical services. For example, hospitals, municipalities, and non-profit sponsors can establish an MVZ. Even though the MVZ is an enterprise of outpatient medical care, it enables entre-

preneurial networking of different service areas, for example, across sectors, but also with regard to social services or long-term care services.

Thus, the MVZ business type can provide the possibility of at least a legal integration of service areas in municipal healthcare provision that have previously been separated under social law, which can in principle be advantageous for people with chronic illnesses.

However, there are also two concerns:

There is a risk that the networked service providers may shift services within the network to the detriment of patients and social insurance funds in order to optimize service structures within the framework of remuneration regulations. This can also lead to an implicit undermining of the personal and institutional freedom of choice of those affected.

Although the last twenty years have seen a trend towards the formation of corporate groups by non-profit organizations or municipalities, in institutional long-term care and inpatient acute care, there has been an increase in profit-oriented providers, a withdrawal of municipalities from direct service provision, and a steady decline in non-profit providers. Thus, when public and non-profit corporate groups are formed, it can be assumed that their establishment primarily follows classic considerations, namely the achievement of economies of scale and scope (economies), in order to counter the economic advantages of regionally organized healthcare corporations. It is not scientifically established that networking in municipal healthcare provision, in view of supraregional profit-oriented strategies that pursue profit-oriented corporate objectives, leads to the desired results both economically and in terms of healthcare policy.

2. Public Economy versus Profit Economy

   In healthcare provision, public objectives predominate, as expressed in health social law. At the level of municipal economy health services are interpreted as services of general interest, which are necessary for citizens to lead a daily life of well-being and dignity (Luthe 2017). The EU Commission defines this understanding as services of public interest. These can be provided either by public institutions, enterprises, or companies, or by third parties. In this understanding, healthcare providers have a supply mandate, i.e., a public instrumental function to fulfill public objectives. We are dealing with an economic space of action, which is defined by societal economical goals. The increasing importance of profit-oriented business types in a societal economic sphere thus at least constitutes a field of tension. In this context, we speak of the pike in the carp pond. The profit-oriented enterprise (the pike) is supposed to put pressure on the non-profit, societal enterprises to provide services more efficiently. This is mainly achieved when the public enterprises also behave like pikes. In the end, only the pikes survive. In the political intention to create good conditions for profit-oriented enterprises, the non-profit, societal economy carps are either eaten, i.e., disappear from the market, or also become pikes.

   Both the national and international discussion about the remuneration of hospital services through case-based lump sums makes it clear that this includes the optimization of both cost and revenue structures. Those affected become economic risks if they entail above-average service expenditure, and economic opportunities if they promise at least an average contribution margin for the business result. In a profit-oriented business sphere, strategies such as risk selection, selective increase in case numbers, revenue optimization—such as upcoding, i.e., increasing revenues by upgrading the treatment case—are promising. A coexistence of over-, under-, and misprovision becomes more likely.

46.3 On Health Services

To better analyze the aforementioned questions, the nature of health services as such will be presented in conclusion, with a focus on the economic issue of the cost-revenue relationship.

1. On the Definition of Services in Healthcare
   From a work analysis perspective, a service always consists of partial services. What I define as a service is therefore not predetermined by nature. For example, the serving of meals in institutional care can fundamentally be performed either by a nursing professional as part of ongoing nursing care, or separated from the nursing process by a housekeeping staff member. For certain individuals who require assistance with eating, such as patients with swallowing disorders, this must be performed by a nursing professional for patient safety reasons. In the first case, the service is not listed separately, but only as part of nursing care; in the second case, we are dealing with an additional service that is provided separately through outsourcing and remains a distinct service even if, in individual cases, it is again performed by a nursing professional.
   Another perspective is to consider the treatment case. With regard to the overall treatment process, the service begins with the initial professional contact and ends with the completion of case-related treatment. The economic assessment should therefore refer to the overall service, which consists of the professional partial services of the individual organizations and professions. The respective remuneration must be structured in such a way that it supports the achievement of the desired treatment outcomes.
   A further perspective focuses on the systemic nature of health services. Since health services are predominantly time-critical and only limitedly schedulable, the readiness to provide services—which is a non-service—must be included. This applies not only to emergency care as such, but also to the provision of personnel and material resources for potential needs. A simple example may illustrate this: For the care of premature infants, it is necessary to have qualified staff and the physical infrastructure of a neonatology unit available, even if, fortunately, no premature infant is born.
2. On the Nature of Services in Chronic Illness
   The characteristics of services change for people with chronic illnesses, as they have an ongoing need for care. In the case of an acute illness, the intensity of treatment

generally decreases over the course of care. At the beginning of treatment, high costs are incurred, which decrease by the end of treatment; this results in a left-skewed, right-tailed cost curve (Fig. 46.1). In chronic illnesses, the need for services is continuous. Depending on the characteristics of the illness, services and thus costs are incurred steadily or recurrently (wave-shaped cost curve, Fig. 46.2), or, in the case of progressive diseases, with an increasing need for services and costs over time (Fig. 46.3).

Further, the characteristics of treatment for additional acute illnesses change. In this case, the chronic illness constitutes as a comorbidity, where the service for treating the acute illness must be adapted, for example, during a surgical procedure in people with thrombosis risks or those with dementia.

Finally, the treatment of the chronic illness must be continued in an adapted manner, taking into account the therapeutic measures for the acute illness, such as in diabetes mellitus or in people with kidney disease (requiring dialysis). In addition to a higher intensity of services, there is often a longer treatment duration, for example in wound healing disorders, or because rehabilitative interventions are less effective in people with limited mobility. Fundamentally, this means that the operational requirements for designing cross-specialty and interprofessional cooperation in the acute treatment of a chronically ill person are significantly increased.

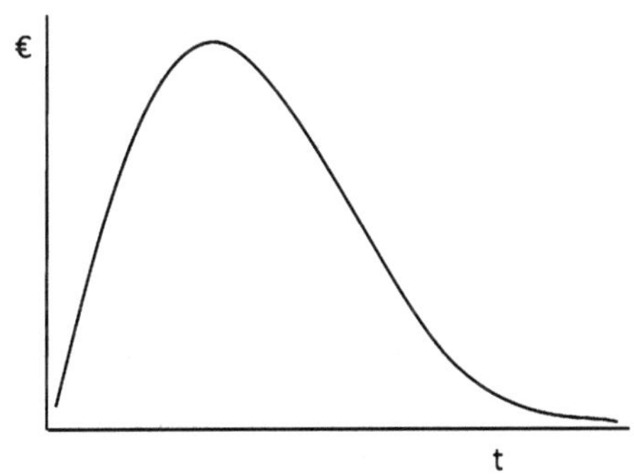

Fig. 46.1 Typical cost curve in acute illness (t = time course, own illustration)

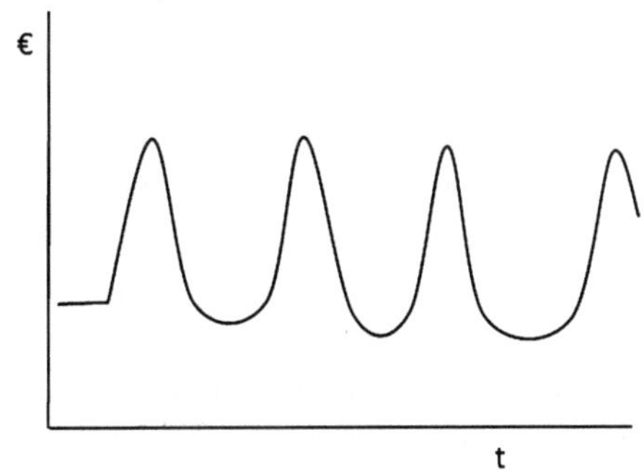

Fig. 46.2 Typical cost curve in chronic illness with recurring phases of higher care needs (t = time course, own illustration)

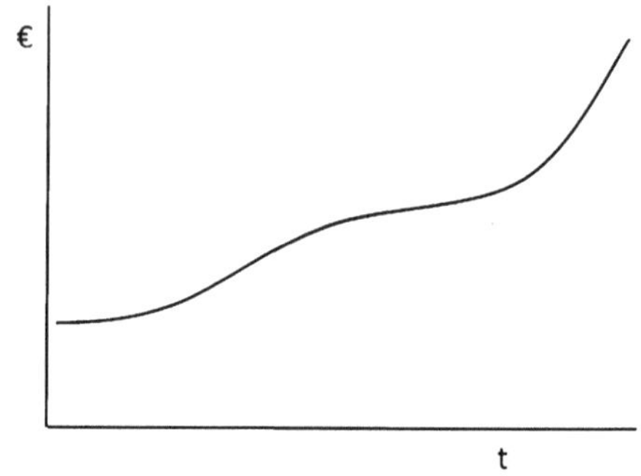

Fig. 46.3 Cost curve in progressive to terminal chronic illness (t = time course, own illustration)

3. Special Service Offerings
   The particular characteristics of chronic illnesses lead to specialized service offerings. These will be briefly illustrated with two examples.
   - Chronic illnesses have typical disease consequences. For example, people with chronic dizziness or mobility impairments are particularly at risk of falling in everyday life. Since these are mostly older individuals, geriatric trauma departments have been established in recent years to provide complex care for this group. Diabetes patients develop neuropathies and chronic wounds, the treatment of which must be integrated into clinical care (for example, to avoid amputations of limbs).
   - In some chronic illnesses, the disease progresses in episodes, which can be experienced as crises by those affected, such as in multiple sclerosis or certain mental illnesses. In this case, we are not dealing with a wave-shaped service pattern, but with isolated service peaks that, in terms of timing and intensity, resemble those of acute treatment.

46.4 Internalization and Externalization

Every organization has a formal business purpose, which is usually set out in statutes, articles of association, or similar documents. For profit-oriented companies, one purpose is profit generation; in addition, there is a business activity, such as the inpatient care of people in need of nursing. Non-profit organizations are, by definition, purpose-driven enterprises; they pursue a public purpose selflessly. Economically, the focus is not on profit, but rather on achieving at least a break-even result.

In addition to this immediate business purpose, every economic activity has direct or indirect effects on the business environment, so-called external effects (Mishan 1974), which are associated with economic activity without being recorded by the organization as costs or revenues, or as economic burdens or benefits. These effects can be monetary or non-monetary, intangible effects. External effects may also materialize with a time lag (intertemporal) or outside the regional context of the economic activity (extraterritorial).

An example will illustrate this. Residents living near a hospital with an emergency department experience increased noise pollution due to ambulance traffic (intangible costs). Conversely, the hospital provides the local population with greater security in medical emergencies (intangible benefit). Finally, the hospital's economic activity directly and indirectly increases regional economic output, secures jobs, and raises regional tax revenues (external monetary benefit).

The externalization of effects is inherent to economic activity, because a business, as an inseparable part of the biophysical and social environment, always influences it in various ways. For this reason, external effects can also become the subject of deliberate corporate strategy. Companies or organizations whose strategies are primarily determined by the interests of owners, i.e., shareholder value, are more likely to pursue the externalization of economic disadvantages onto third parties or into the future. In contrast, companies and organizations that consciously incorporate the impact of economic activity on third parties—on stakeholder groups involved in economic activity—into their strategies are more likely to seek to minimize the externalization of negative effects and to deliberately pursue positive effects for stakeholders. *Stakeholder thinking* (Philips 2011) refers to social groups that are directly affected by business activities. At first glance, it thus appears to be an ethical corrective to profit-driven behavior. However, in a sensitized economic environment, it can also be functionalized as a strategy for self-legitimation and thus as part of the company's marketing strategy.

Thus, we can initially understand shareholders and stakeholders as antagonistic pairs of concepts with resulting conflicting economic objectives, or alternatively, we can view *stakeholder thinking* as a complementary economic objective intended to secure the company's purpose.

46.5 Principles of Societal Accounting

To assess whether business objectives are being achieved, there are two main instruments:

- first, economic planning—at the company level, the business plan; at the departmental level, the partial business plan; and at the level of individual services, the calculation,
- second, the monitoring and evaluation of goal achievement in the form of controlling, cost-revenue accounting, and the balance sheet.

These instruments are focused on monetary indicators within the company. The classical profit and loss statement is intended to plan the company's economic success for a fiscal year as a profit plan and to present it retrospectively as a profit and loss account. The balance sheet, in turn, presents the assets and entrepreneurial capital as of a specific date, including the annual result from the profit and loss statement.

To determine whether a service can be provided economically, there are various forms of cost-effectiveness analysis. The classical form is full cost accounting, in which all direct costs for a partial service or a specific business unit are recorded and allocated. Indirect costs, such as for the finance department, human resources management, purchasing, etc., are allocated according to a defined key, such as direct personnel costs. These are set against the revenues generated or expected for the services provided. Other methods of cost accounting focus only on direct or variable costs (partial cost accounting). With full cost accounting, there is a risk that if a service is discontinued or a service area is closed, revenues for internal service areas will be lost, so their costs can no longer be fully covered. With partial cost accounting, where only a certain contribution margin needs to be achieved, the opposite risk arises: incorrect decisions may be made if certain indirect costs, such as energy costs, are insufficiently considered.

A broader, society-oriented cost-effectiveness analysis, by contrast, represents a supplement that, aside from legitimizing aspects, is also relevant for the development of the service portfolio and, furthermore, touches on regulatory and business law aspects.

It can refer to both internal factors, such as employee health as an outcome of improved working conditions, and external factors, such as the impact on income and employment in the region. By including monetary and non-monetary aspects beyond the essentially one-dimensional profit and loss statement, it can also be described as a multidimensional or extended cost-effectiveness analysis (ECA) (Neubauer and Wächter 2011; Priddat 2008). This multidimensionality refers not only to its content, but also to its target groups. While the annual financial statement, consisting of cost-performance accounting and the balance sheet, is initially aimed at shareholders and creditors, the ECA also addresses other internal and external stakeholders, such as employees, local residents—especially with regard to intangible effects—politicians, and local government.

The significance of an ECA that includes societal aspects can be illustrated by an example. The number of births required for an obstetrics department to operate profitably is more than 1,000 births per year. The economic requirement arises less from normal births and more from the care of high-risk pregnancies, or more precisely, from the ability to perform emergency C-sections at any time. In emergencies, the department must be reachable within 40 minutes. At the same time, specialized staff must be available immediately. In rural areas, the number of births is decreasing while travel distances are increasing. The contradiction between business management and societal requirements becomes clear. It can only be resolved through coordinated action across organizations.

A decisive factor in conducting the ECA is which factors are documented, whether they are meaningful and relevant, can be collected sustainably, and, finally, are accurate. When some companies prepared social balance sheets in the 1970s (Dierkes 1974), these were criticized for not providing sufficient evidence of changed societal behavior by companies, but merely listing corresponding activities. It also remains unclear how monetary goals are weighted against non-monetary goals within the company and what significance, for example, stakeholder-oriented goals have compared to the objectives of the company's core business. This question also arises when different target areas are operationally recorded and weighted against each other in terms of their respective goal achievement.

State and non-state certificates can be considered equivalent to an ECA, through which a company's (self-)commitment to certain economic behavior or specific service characteristics is confirmed and subject to verification. In healthcare, these include, for example, certificates such as "family-friendly intensive care unit," "baby-friendly hospital," or, in the USA, the so-called Magnet Hospital as a seal of outstanding nursing quality and working conditions with positive effects on patient care (Aiken et al. 2008). Certification is an instrument for distinguishing oneself qualitatively from other competitors, which, for example, legitimizes higher service prices for organic labels, or, as in healthcare—where advertising for the core service is not permitted—enables market advantages through secondary attributes.

46.6 The Value of the Business Type Discussion for Healthcare Provision

The fact that the discussion about business types in healthcare is not useless becomes evident in several respects.

1. Diversity of ownership is enshrined multiple times in German health law. However, the benefits of this diversity are rarely discussed in academic literature. Moreover, focusing solely on the ownership of healthcare organizations does not do justice to the variety of business types. An organization led by a healthcare professional differs in terms of professional leadership approach and corporate objectives from a corporate-run entity, even if both are formally profit-oriented.
2. In contrast, there is the public responsibility for healthcare provision that exists in almost all high-income countries. Except for the USA, all high-income countries achieve a public financing share from taxes or social insurance of 60% or more. Even in the USA, the public financing share accounts for about 8% of GDP.
3. Economic activity thus takes place in a public sphere of action that binds organizations and companies to public health objectives.
4. Studies show that there are differences in the qualitative delivery of services. Which business types are suitable for adequately achieving the objectives associated with public provision must be specified empirically, including with regard to the respective characteristics of the business types. In this context, we consider not only ownership morphologically, but also other characteristics such as management or staff.
5. A shortage of skilled workers, increasing demand for services, and limited financial and material resources present major challenges for the healthcare system. One of the currently preferred strategies to address these challenges is greater networking, integrated care, interprofessional collaboration, and interinstitutional cooperation. It is therefore also a matter of identifying which business types are both innovative and capable of cooperating in a spirit of trust, sharing their own resources and competencies.

References

Aiken LH, Buchan J, Ball J, Rafferty AM (2008) Transformative impact of magnet designation: England case study. J Clin Nurs 17(24):3330–3337. https://doi.org/10.1111/j.1365-2702.2008.02640.x

Dierkes M (1974) Die Sozialbilanz: Ein gesellschaftsbezogenes Informations- und Rechnungssystem. Edition Gesellschaft + Unternehmen. Herder & Herder, Frankfur am Main/New York

Engelhardt WW (1973) Die Unternehmens- und Betriebsmorphologie als Teildisziplin der Allgemeinen Betriebswirtschaftslehre. Jahrb Absatz Verbrauchsforsch 19:311–332

Luthe E-W (2017) Gesundheitliche Daseinsvorsorge heute—theoretische Perspektiven. In: Wendt WR (ed) Gesundheit. Politik—Gesellschaft—Wirtschaft Ser. Soziale Bewirtschaftung von Gesundheit: Gesundheitswirtschaft im Rahmen sozialer Versorgungsgestaltung. Springer Fachmedien, Wiesbaden, pp 21–68

Mishan EJ (1974) The economics of disamenity. Nat Resour J 14(1):55–86. https://core.ac.uk/download/pdf/151601321.pdf. Accessed 22 Sept 2023

Neubauer G, Wächter H (2011) Die "Erweiterte Wirtschaftlichkeitsrechnung" (EWR)—ein Ansatz zu einer interdisziplinären Innovationsplanung. Z Arbeitswiss 65(1):67–76

Philips RA (Hrsg) (2011) Stakeholder theory: impact and prospects. Cheltenham England, Edward Elgar http://site.ebrary.com/lib/alltitles/docDetail.action?docID=10482018

Priddat BC (2008) Die "Erweiterte Wirtschaftlichkeitsrechnung" (EWR)—ein Ansatz zu einer interdisziplinären Innovationsplanung. Z Öffentl Gemeinnützig Unternehm 31(2):152–173

Sachverständigenrat zur Begutachtung der Entwicklung im Gesundheitswesen (2018) Bedarfsgerechte Steuerung der Gesundheitsversorgung. Bonn. https://www.svr-gesundheit.de/fileadmin/Gutachten/Gutachten_2018/Gutachten_2018.pdf. Accessed 04 July 2018

Methods of Health System Evaluation and Health Indicators

47

Dennis Häckl and Tobias Schäffer

Contents

47.1 Background and Classification

The evaluation of health systems is a crucial process that assesses the performance and effectiveness of health systems to ensure high-quality care, patient safety, and efficient use of resources. The effectiveness of a health system is assessed using various

D. Häckl (✉)
Health Economics and Management, Leipzig University, Leipzig, Deutschland
e-mail: dennis.haeckl@uni-leipzig.de

T. Schäffer
Health Economics and Management, Leipzig University, Leipzig, Deutschland
e-mail: tobias.schaeffer@uni-leipzig.de

D. Schmitz et al. (eds.), *Chronic Care—Science and Practice*,
https://doi.org/10.1007/978-3-662-72298-5_47

evaluation methods and health indicators. These provide important insights into the health status of a population, the quality of healthcare delivery, and progress toward achieving health-related goals. In addition to the entire health system, various evaluation methods and indicators are also suitable for assessing individual segments of the overall system. This allows for the evaluation of almost arbitrarily detailed segments, such as sectors of care, individual care programs, or treatment methods for specific indications. Accordingly, it must be clarified in advance what is to be the subject of the evaluation. The evaluation of the health system or a segment thereof generally considers four components in the form of:

- Structure: The structure component assesses the organizational aspects of health systems, including the distribution and availability of healthcare facilities, personnel, and infrastructure.
- Process: The process component evaluates the interactions between healthcare providers and patients, adherence to clinical guidelines, and the quality of services delivered.
- Outcome: The outcome component measures the impact of health services on the health of the population, including morbidity, mortality, and overall well-being.
- Cost: The cost component encompasses the costs associated with treatment.

The relevance of evaluation methods and indicators arises from the primary goal of a health system, which is to promote and improve the health and well-being of individuals and society as a whole.

47.2 Objectives and Areas of Application

In addition to the subject of the evaluation, it must be defined in which dimension an evaluation is to be conducted. The most common evaluations are carried out in the following dimensions:

47.2.1 Evaluation of Individual Dimensions of Health Services

- Effectiveness in healthcare refers to the extent to which interventions or technologies achieve desired (therapeutic) outcomes. In addition to the clinical or care-related relevance of the observed effect, statistical tests are used to assess significance. Statistical significance indicates whether an observed effect is actually present or occurs merely by chance.
- Efficiency in healthcare refers to the ratio of achieved (therapeutic) outcomes to the resources used to achieve them. Efficiency deals with optimizing resource allocation to ensure high-quality care. The resources required for this should be appropriate, so that unnecessary duplicate examinations and the associated costs are avoided.

- Quality of healthcare is the extent to which health services and interventions provided to patients meet established standards, guidelines, and best practices. The aim of the evaluation is to identify strengths and weaknesses of care in the quality dimensions (structure, process, outcome). The indicators form the basis for quality assurance or quality management in the service-providing units.
- Access to healthcare refers to the availability of needed health services, including preventive, diagnostic, curative, and rehabilitative care. This includes various factors that can facilitate or hinder a person's use of health services, such as availability, affordability, geographic proximity, waiting times, cultural acceptance, and the absence of discrimination or barriers. Inadequate access to healthcare can lead to delays in diagnosis and treatment (and thus increased subsequent costs), uncontrolled chronic diseases, and poorer health outcomes.
- Patient safety encompasses the prevention of harm to patients during the provision of health services. This includes measures and initiatives by providers and healthcare organizations to minimize the risk of adverse events, medical errors, and injuries associated with the medical care of patients. Patient safety also includes the protection of sensitive and confidential health data in modern healthcare.
- Patient-centeredness is an approach to healthcare that emphasizes the active involvement of patients in their own decisions and treatment plans. It is about understanding and respecting patients' preferences, values, needs, and goals while providing high-quality and individualized care.
- The identification of improvements is also a possible dimension of a health system evaluation. By identifying areas in need of improvement, the evaluation of health systems fosters a culture of continuous quality improvement that enhances the overall delivery of health services.

47.2.2 Support for Health Policy and Reforms

The results of health system evaluations serve as the basis for evidence-based health policy. This includes ensuring that policy decisions are made on the basis of the best available evidence from research studies, clinical trials, systematic reviews, and other reliable sources of information. A challenge for evidence-based health policy is a clear understanding of policy objectives, the availability of relevant measurement instruments, and the increasing abundance of studies/publications (including so-called *research waste*) (Puljak 2019). In particular, it is important to understand how these objectives are to be defined, operationalized, and measured. The aim is to avoid implementing measures based on opinions, ideology, or anecdotal evidence.

47.3 Methods of Health Economic Evaluation and Health Indicators

The methodology of health system evaluation and health indicators enables the answering of numerous questions. The following section presents and explains the most important methods and indicators.

47.3.1 'Classical' Health Economic Evaluations

Health economic evaluations are systematic and analytical processes used to assess the economic impact of measures, treatments, programs, or strategies in healthcare (Schöffski and Graf von der Schulenburg 2012). Their primary goal is to relate the costs and outcomes of different interventions in order to support decision-making and resource allocation in healthcare. Health economic evaluations typically compare at least two interventions. There are four types of health economic evaluation. Table 47.1 summarizes these and their respective calculations.

- Cost-Benefit Analysis
  - In cost-benefit analysis, the costs and benefits of health interventions are assessed in monetary terms. From an economic perspective, an intervention is advantageous if the benefits outweigh the costs. Since the result is measured in monetary units, interventions or investments in healthcare can be compared with those in other sectors. However, a key challenge is translating medical outcomes into monetary values.
- Cost-Effectiveness Analysis
  - Cost-effectiveness analysis focuses on comparing costs and health-related outcomes, which are often expressed in natural units such as life years gained,

Tab. 47.1 Characteristics of health economic evaluation methods. (Egger et al. 2021, p. 88; Icks et al. 2010, p. 919)

	(a) Cost-Benefit Analysis (C1-C2/B1-B2)	(b) Cost-Effectiveness Analysis (C1-C2/E1-E2)	(c) Cost-Utility Analysis (C1-C2/U1-U2)	(d) Cost-Minimization Analysis
Costs	Monetary units (€, $ etc.)	Monetary units (€, $ etc.)	Monetary units (€, $ etc.)	Monetary units (€, $ etc.)
Benefit	Monetary units (€, $ etc.)	Natural units (mmHg)	Utility value between 0 and 1 (QALYs, etc.)	Held constant
Calculation	$\frac{(N_1-K_1)}{(K_2-N_2)}$	$\frac{(K_1-K_2)}{(E_1-E_2)}$	$\frac{(K_1-K_2)}{(U_1-U_2)}$	$C_1 - C_2$
Variables	C = costs; B = benefit valued in monetary terms; E = effect (benefit in natural units); U = unit of utility value; 1 = intervention under evaluation; 2 = alternative intervention			

symptom-free days, or clinical endpoints. For example, the effectiveness of an intervention aimed at lowering blood pressure can be quantified using the measurement millimeters of mercury (mmHg). The required data must either be collected within a study or sourced from existing literature. Cost-effectiveness analysis primarily considers the specific benefit of an intervention rather than the overall health status.

- Cost-Utility Analysis
  - Similar to cost-effectiveness analysis, cost-utility analysis compares costs and health-related outcomes, but the results are expressed in terms of (artificially generated) utility values. Quality-adjusted life years (QALYs) are a widely used measure that enables comprehensive quantification of the impact of health interventions on both the quantity and quality of life. QALYs are an index formed from life years gained and changes in quality of life. Accordingly, the concept of health-related quality of life is central to the calculation. In some countries, costs per QALY are mandated as a decision-making aid for health economic evaluations and thus have a direct impact on the design of healthcare provision (National Institute for Health and Care Excellence [NICE] 2022; Versteegh et al. 2016).
- Cost-Minimization Analysis
  - Cost-minimization analysis compares the direct costs of alternative interventions that lead to equivalent health outcomes. Thus, the benefit for both alternatives is considered equivalent and held constant. This type of analysis focuses on identifying the least expensive option among equally effective treatments.

47.3.2 Health Technology Assessment (HTA)

A Health Technology Assessment (HTA) is a systematic and multidisciplinary evaluation process that assesses the clinical effectiveness, safety, cost-efficiency, and societal impact of health technologies. These technologies include medical devices, pharmaceuticals, diagnostic tests, medical procedures, and other healthcare interventions. An HTA is generally based on a systematic literature review that considers both controlled study conditions and real-world care settings. In addition, the cost-effectiveness and social, ethical, and legal frameworks of the new technology are taken into account in the evaluation. The main objective of HTA is to provide evidence-based information to support decision-making in healthcare at various levels, including policy decisions, healthcare reimbursement, and clinical practice guidelines.

47.3.3 Health Indicators

Health indicators are quantitative measures that allow for the assessment of the health status of a group of people, the prevalence of risk factors, or the performance of health systems. When health indicators are considered at the national level, comparisons between nations can be made (European Observatory on Health Systems and Policies 2023). For more specific questions, health indicators can be developed for a small segment of the population, most commonly using a particular indication as the criterion. Health indicators serve several important functions:

- Monitoring and surveillance: Health indicators enable continuous monitoring of health trends, disease patterns, and the utilization of health services, thereby contributing to the early detection of public health issues.
- Benchmarking: Health indicators allow for comparisons between regions, countries, or health systems, helping to identify best practices and areas in need of improvement.
- Evaluation of interventions: Health indicators assist in assessing the impact of measures, programs, and strategies in healthcare to ensure they achieve the intended outcomes or to identify evidence of unintended effects.
- Further development of the health system: Policymakers use health indicators to identify potential for improvement and inequalities, to develop evidence-based strategies, and to drive the advancement of the healthcare system.

Various standardized indicators are available for monitoring the health of a population. At the initiative of the European Union (EU), the European Health Indicators were defined. This list includes indicators on demographic and socioeconomic factors, health status, health factors, as well as health resources and health promotion. The indicators on health status provide information on the national prevalence of individual chronic diseases such as diabetes or COPD, as well as the self-perceived assessment of the health status of those affected.

In addition, since 1991, there has been a set of indicators at the federal and state level for the health framework report of the states.[1] The total of 297 indicators covers population-specific framework conditions, the health status of the population, health-related behaviors, health risks from the environment, healthcare facilities, utilization of services, healthcare personnel including training, expenditures and financing, as well as costs.

Morbidity

Morbidity is a health indicator that refers to the presence of diseases or health conditions and provides insight into the burden of disease and the general health status of a population. Monitoring morbidity helps in assessing the prevalence or incidence, distribution, and impact of various health conditions and serves as a guide for prevention, management, and treatment of diseases. Indicators related to morbidity include:

[1] The data are available free of charge (https://www.gbe-bund.de/).

- The prevalence rate is the proportion of a population suffering from a specific disease (or condition) at a given point in time. This indicator helps to quantify the overall burden of a disease in a population.
- Point prevalence is the proportion of individuals in a population suffering from a disease (or condition) at a specific point in time. It provides a snapshot of the disease burden at a particular moment.
- Period prevalence is the proportion of individuals who suffer from a disease or condition at any time during a specific period. It offers a broader overview of the disease burden over a longer timeframe.
- The incidence rate is the proportion of newly diseased individuals occurring in a specific population during a defined period.
- Cumulative incidence is the total proportion of newly diseased individuals occurring in a specific population during a defined period. The proportion is calculated using the number of healthy individuals at the start of the study.

Mortality

Mortality is a measure that reflects the number of deaths in a specific population during a defined period, usually expressed as a rate per 1,000 or 100,000 people. Mortality rates provide a snapshot and offer valuable information about the impact of diseases, the effectiveness of health interventions, and the social determinants of health (see Contribution 16). There are several key mortality indicators that play an important role in assessing health and developing strategies:

- Cause-specific mortality rates focus on deaths attributable to specific causes, such as infectious diseases (e.g., HIV/AIDS, malaria), non-communicable diseases (e.g., cardiovascular diseases, cancer), accidents, and injuries. Analysis of cause-specific mortality provides insight into the disease burden and the effectiveness of the healthcare system.
- A standardized mortality ratio compares the observed number of deaths in a specific population with the expected number of deaths based on age-specific mortality rates of a reference population. If the observed mortality rate is above or below the expected rate, this is referred to as excess mortality or reduced mortality, respectively. This assessment allows for the evaluation of the quality of healthcare and health outcomes in specific groups.
- The indicator of years of potential life lost estimates the total years of life lost due to premature death in a population.
- Age-specific mortality rates measure the risk of death in different age groups and provide valuable information about health inequalities across different life stages.
- Sex-specific mortality rates measure the risk of death among the male and female population, respectively. This allows for the evaluation of gender-specific health disparities.

Supply-Side Indicators of Healthcare Provision

The indicators on the supply side of healthcare provision focus on assessing the availability, capacity, and resources of healthcare services and facilities. These indicators provide information about the infrastructure, personnel, and necessary resources for effective and efficient healthcare delivery. Monitoring supply-side indicators is crucial for planning and managing healthcare services, ensuring adequate access to care, and optimizing resource allocation.

The following key indicators are important for assessing the supply side of the healthcare system:

- Healthcare facilities as the number of hospitals, outpatient clinics, and health centers, as well as specialized centers.
- Healthcare personnel as the number of physicians, nurses, and other healthcare professionals (pharmacists, laboratory technicians, and other medical specialists).
- Medical equipment and technology for diagnostic purposes, such as X-ray machines, ultrasound devices, and laboratory equipment, as well as the availability of advanced imaging techniques like magnetic resonance imaging and computed tomography.
- The availability of a list of essential medicines as defined by the World Health Organization (WHO) (WHO 2023), incidents of medicine shortages or supply bottlenecks.
- Bed capacity as the number of hospital beds available for inpatient care, as well as the availability of specialized beds in intensive care units.
- Health infrastructure as the physical infrastructure supporting healthcare delivery, including buildings, facilities, and medical equipment.
- Distribution of healthcare facilities and personnel across different regions to assess accessibility.
- Distribution of the healthcare budget as the share of the government budget allocated to healthcare provision and infrastructure development, as well as private and public investments in health infrastructure and technology.
- Telemedicine services as the availability of telemedicine and virtual health services for remote consultations and healthcare delivery, as well as the implementation of digital tools for patient management, appointment scheduling, and health education.

Risk Factors

Risk factors are important health indicators that provide information about the occurrence of certain diseases or health conditions. Evaluating risk factors helps identify population groups at increased risk for specific diseases. Risk factors may include behavioral or environmental risks for adverse health outcomes. In addition, they can reflect the risk of developing a secondary or comorbid condition in the presence of a chronic disease.

Health-Related Quality of Life

Health-related quality of life (HRQoL) is a multidimensional health indicator. It measures how people perceive their physical, mental, emotional, and social well-being in relation to their health status and healthcare. HRQoL is often assessed using standardized questionnaires or surveys that capture various aspects of an individual's well-being. These surveys typically cover several domains, including physical functioning, mental health and emotional well-being, social functioning, role limitations, pain and discomfort, and general health perception. Examples of validated questionnaires include the Short Form Health Survey (SF-36), the EQ-5D, the Health Assessment Questionnaire Disability Index (HAQ-DI), or the Medical Outcomes Study HIV Health Survey.

47.3.4 Quality Indicators

Quality indicators are important reference points for service providers and policy makers in their pursuit of safe, effective, patient-centered, timely, efficient, and equitable healthcare. They cover a range of dimensions, from clinical outcomes and patient safety to patient satisfaction and cost efficiency. Clinical quality indicators provide information about the effectiveness of medical interventions and the prevention of adverse events. Patient-centered indicators highlight the human aspect of care and the overall patient experience. In healthcare, quality is primarily defined in relation to a standard, which means the number of indicators may potentially correspond to the number of standards (Prütz 2012). For example, the standard of avoiding overprovision can be evaluated by the number of ambulatory care-sensitive cases in hospitals. Since quality is a central element in the ongoing development of the healthcare system, the guidelines of the Federal Joint Committee, as stipulated in §§ 136 ff. SGB V, require the Institute for Quality Assurance and Transparency in Healthcare to provide an annually updated quality indicator database for the German healthcare system.

47.4 Challenges and Limitations

Health indicators play a crucial role in assessing the performance of health systems, guiding policy decisions, and improving health outcomes. However, they present challenges, as health is a complex concept that cannot always be fully captured by a single indicator.

Many indicators focus on specific health areas without covering the entire spectrum. The availability of accurate, reliable, and up-to-date data is essential for meaningful health indicators. In some regions or sectors, data collection may be limited, or certain population groups may be underrepresented. The interpretation of health indicators requires context, as changes in indicators may be due to various factors, such as improved quality of healthcare or changes in diagnostic criteria. Health indicators can obscure health inequalities and inequities between different population groups. Aggregated data, depending on socioeconomic status, race, ethnicity, or geographic location, may not provide insight into differences in health outcomes.

Health indicators may neglect qualitative aspects and long-term effects of interventions. External factors such as economic conditions, environmental changes, or technological advances can also influence outcomes.

References

Egger M, Razum O, Rieder A (2021) Public Health Kompakt. De Gruyter. https://doi.org/10.1515/9783110667378

European Observatory on Health Systems and Policies (2023) Health system reviews. https://eurohealthobservatory.who.int/publications/health-systems-reviews. Accessed 31 Aug 2023

Icks A, Chernyak N, Bestehorn K, Brüggenjürgen B, Bruns J, Damm O, Dintsios C-M, Dreinhöfer K, Gandjour A, Gerber A, Greiner W, Hermanek P, Hessel F, Heymann R, Huppertz E, Jacke C, Kächele H, Kilian R, Klingenberger D et al (2010) Methoden der gesundheitsökonomischen Evaluation in der Versorgungsforschung [Methods of health economic evaluation for health services research]. Gesundheitswesen (Bundesverband der Ärzte des Offentlichen Gesundheitsdienstes) (Germany) 72(12):917–933. https://doi.org/10.1055/s-0030-1262859

National Institute for Health and Care Excellence (2022) NICE health technology evaluations: the manual. https://www.nice.org.uk/process/pmg36/resources/nice-health-technology-evaluations-the-manual-pdf-72286779244741. Accessed 31 Aug 2023

Prütz F (2012) Was ist Qualität im Gesundheitswesen? Ethik in der Medizin 24(2):105–115. https://doi.org/10.1007/s00481-012-0189-5

Puljak L (2019) Methodological research: open questions, the need for ‚research on research' and its implications for evidence-based health care and reducing research waste. Int J Evid Based Healthcare 17(3):145–146. https://doi.org/10.1097/XEB.0000000000000201

Schöffski O, Graf von der Schulenburg J-M (2012) Gesundheitsökonomische Evaluationen. Springer. https://doi.org/10.1007/978-3-642-21700-5

Versteegh M, Knies S, Brouwer W (2016) From good to better: new Dutch guidelines for economic evaluations in healthcare. PharmacoEcon 34(11):1071–1074. https://doi.org/10.1007/s40273-016-0431-y

WHO (2023) The selection and use of essential medicines 2023: executive summary of the report of the 24th WHO Expert Committee on the selection and use of essential medicines (24.–28. April). Genf. https://www.who.int/publications/i/item/WHO-MHP-HPS-EML-2023.01

Public Health—Needs and Forward-Looking Services with Regard to Community Health Nursing and Digitalization

48

Lisa Schmidt and Frank Weidner

Contents

48.1 Milestones from 'Social Hygiene' to 'New Public Health'

While health-related problems in the population before the end of the 19th century, if considered at all, were viewed primarily from a perspective that could be described as natural scientific, industrialization, the expansion of cities, the associated rise in uncontrollable spread of diseases, and growing social inequality gradually led to an increasing focus on socially determined causes of illness. As a result, public health as such

L. Schmidt (✉)
Frankfurt University of Applied Sciences, Fachbereich 4: Soziale Arbeit und Gesundheit—Health and Social Work, Frankfurt am Main, Deutschland
e-mail: l.luft@fb4.fra-uas.de

F. Weidner
Professur für Pflegewissenschaft mit dem Schwerpunkt Gesundheitsförderung und Prävention, Koblenz, Deutschland
e-mail: fweidner@uni-koblenz.de

D. Schmitz et al. (eds.), *Chronic Care—Science and Practice*,
https://doi.org/10.1007/978-3-662-72298-5_48

moved more into the spotlight. This shift in perspective gave rise to a new, interdisciplinary, and practice-oriented discipline—the so-called social hygiene. Its goal was to maintain the health of entire population groups, taking into account their respective social circumstances, and to encourage citizens to adopt behaviors that would sustainably improve their health (Schmidt-Semisch and Schorb 2021). This change in perspective was also evident in the course of social legislation (Müller et al. 2018). It became increasingly clear that health-promoting behavior cannot be sustainably encouraged by mere information or sanctions. Driven by new health challenges such as the rise in chronic diseases and inspired by the internationally developed and 1986 adopted Ottawa Charter for Health Promotion by the World Health Organization, another key milestone or developmental step took place—from the previous approach of so-called *Old Public Health* to the forward-looking approach of *New Public Health*. While the former focused exclusively on health risks, causes of disease, and subject-oriented behavioral changes (Rosenbrock 2021), *New Public Health* now encompasses a much broader perspective, focusing especially on the reasons for causes and developments of diseases as well as the social determinants of health (Klemperer 2020; Rosenbrock 2021). Thus, the reduction of health-damaging factors and the identification and promotion of health resources became central to these efforts. Another new focal point was the needs-based, target group-oriented, and contextually relevant design of interventions, so that cooperative learning and participatory approaches are increasingly applied (Klemperer 2020). Social inequalities also came more into focus, as socially disadvantaged population groups, for example, tend to exhibit more health-damaging behaviors or encounter such conditions, often lacking the means to autonomously change their living circumstances in a health-promoting way. This is, for example, due to low educational attainment or insufficient financial resources (Rosenbrock 2021).

Hurrelmann and Razum (2012) identify population-based prevention and health promotion as a primary goal of public health and, in this context, emphasize the importance of adopting the broadest possible perspective on health-relevant issues, which should include all involved health disciplines. In recent years, participatory approaches to the development of interventions have also gained significant importance in order to better address the needs and wishes of the target groups (Baratt 2008) and to increase the acceptance of measures as well as social equity of opportunity. Ethical, economic, and organizational issues are also increasingly coming into focus, as are the collection of health data and the evaluation of interventions, which are also identified as central tasks of public health (Rehfuess et al. 2021). Thus, public health is understood, in line with the internationally recognized definition, as "the science and practice of preventing disease, prolonging life, and promoting health through organized efforts of society" (RKI 2016).

There is also a connection to political actors, as the discipline provides data and recommendations, sometimes in the form of decision-ready templates, for policymakers. These are an important basis for developing solutions to population-based health problems, taking into account economic and organizational aspects (e.g., Schmidt-Semisch and Schorb 2021). However, with reference to Rosenbrock (2021), it should be noted as a limitation that economic aspects, despite available evidence, often receive greater emphasis, and the stronger focus on curative care and medicine repeatedly leads to primary preventive measures tending to be subordinated to medical treatment.

48.2 Public Health in the Scientific Landscape

An international comparison shows that Public Health in Germany was addressed with a time lag and with a natural orientation towards existing approaches, which initially originated predominantly in the Anglo-American sphere. The independent development of the discipline, further professionalization, and scientific grounding remain central focal points among Public Health stakeholders. The first establishment of academically oriented continuing education in Germany took place at the university level in the 1990s (Fischer et al. 2023; Schmidt-Semisch and Schorb 2021).

According to Schmidt and Schorb (2021), it has been disadvantageous that this young discipline has so far been supported neither by a political movement nor by strong professionalization, and that constructive collaboration among the scientific fields involved in Public Health has been hampered by the lack of an overarching paradigm. Although the initial placement at universities was considered a positive starting point, the attachment to medical faculties has had a negative impact on Public Health to this day. Schaeffer et al. (2010) describe that this placement resulted in the neglect of the formation of independent, subject-specific schools, and, similar to the also emerging discipline of nursing science, there was insufficient emancipation from medicine. Furthermore, a generally dominant physician-centrism is noted in the German healthcare system, and the monopoly position of medicine is seen, among other things, as partly responsible for the fact that the development of the Public Health discipline stalled early on due to tendencies of erosion. However, Schaeffer et al. (2010) also see an opportunity here to conceptualize Public Health and nursing science together as new *health sciences* or *health professions* and to build structures in close cooperation in order to be able to hold their own against the almost overpowering field of medicine. As early as 1994, Schaeffer pointed out the differences in the professionalization potential of both disciplines, but also discussed their ability to connect with each other. These synergies now appear to have been recognized, as topics relevant to nursing science are increasingly being considered from a Public Health perspective (Fischer et al. 2023).

Parallel to the academization of Public Health in Germany, the international establishment of Evidence-Based Public Health (EBPH) began in the 1990s, which developed out of Evidence-Based Medicine (EBM) (Sacket et al. 1996). The aim here is to translate current research findings into practice in such a way that interventions can be better assessed in terms of their effects (Rehfuess et al. 2021). The central methods and instruments of evidence-based practice in Public Health are studies, reviews, and guidelines. EBPH focuses on entire population groups and investigates the effectiveness of preventive measures in their geographic and sociocultural context. These are generally highly complex relationships that can only be studied with great effort and many accessible data in controlled designs. In this context, a multidisciplinary approach is also essential, as it makes sense to apply expertise, experience, and methods from as many relevant fields as possible and to establish links to other disciplines such as economics and social sciences. Therefore, structured approaches, interdisciplinary cooperation, and consultations for formulating evidence-based action criteria for decision-making are of central importance (Rehfuess et al. 2021).

Evidence-based practice has now become highly significant, as the design of measures for prevention, health promotion, and health protection has become more important not only for recipients of services but also in terms of practical and effective implementation. The focus here is not only on the potential benefits but especially on the assessment or exclusion of possible risks (Rehfuess et al. 2021).

According to Rehfuess et al. (2021), successes regarding the importance of evidence-based practice in Public Health include the fact that measures and interventions can be implemented increasingly in a more targeted and effective (and also time-saving) manner. It is also positive that Public Health has, to some extent, found its way into the funding programs of the German Research Foundation (Schaeffer et al. 2010).

Despite these initial successes, there is still an urgent need for clarification, especially regarding the definition of Evidence-Based Public Health. Based on a systematic literature review, Rehfuess et al. (2021) found that there is a diversity of terms ranging from "evidence based" to "evidence informed," and that this diversity of terms consequently leads to a correspondingly heterogeneous interpretation of the concept of evidence-based practice (ibid., pp. 518 f.). It is also criticized that the memorandum of the Federal Centre for Health Education (De Bock et al. 2020) narrows the subject of EBPH to the perspectives of prevention and health promotion. Instead, orientation towards international examples is recommended. The memorandum was published in 2020 with the recommendation to develop a standard as well as a cross-disciplinary understanding regarding the implementation of evidence-based practice in Germany. Against the background of this increasingly legally anchored demand for evidence-based practice and the associated preference for corresponding methods, it should be considered that this trend may lead to the already insufficient development of independent Public Health theories being further neglected (Schaeffer et al. 2010).

In addition to the outstanding need to harmonize heterogeneous terms, Schmidt-Semisch and Schorb (2021) outline another challenge: the ongoing phase of clarifying substantive priorities and the lack of prioritization of methods for developing a Public Health strategy. For example, it would be desirable to develop a comprehensive set of methods for health sciences in order to progress from a multi- to a pluridisciplinary approach. This shared understanding could also lead to the respective knowledge base and discipline-specific methods of the fields being more mutually recognized, without neglecting the further development of discipline-related paradigms.

48.3 Public Health and Community Health Nursing

In addition to Public Health, Community Health is intended to address questions regarding the impact of social inequality and differing living conditions on the development, maintenance, and improvement of health, as well as the increased effectiveness of health-promoting and preventive interventions for specific population groups. The aim, for example, is to identify problems, risks, and disadvantages faced by population groups and to tailor interventions more closely to their needs and requirements (Faller et al. 2022). Community Health Nursing (CHN) is cited as a new professional role linked to this, and is mentioned in the coalition agreement of the German federal government for the 2021–2025 legislative period. Initial approaches to qualification, job profiles, and areas of deployment in Germany were initiated several years ago by the Robert Bosch Foundation (RBS 2023) together with the DBfK and the Agnes-Karll-Gesellschaft für Gesundheitsbildung und Pflegeforschung. An expert report on the legal prerequisites and possibilities for establishing Community Health Nursing (CHN) in Germany was presented by Igl and Burgi 2021. The authors examine the developments, tasks, and competencies of CHN, but still see a number of professional and social law hurdles that must be overcome in order to fully realize the potential of CHN in Germany—as is common in some other countries.

Three central areas of deployment for CHN are being discussed in Germany. First, there is the independent provision of services in primary care; second, contributions to the public health service; and third, closely linked to the first two areas, planning and management tasks in municipal public services (Agnes-Karll-Gesellschaft für Gesundheitsbildung und Pflegeforschung 2022). The intention is to employ academically trained nursing professionals with a master's degree. The tasks of CHN are oriented towards health-promoting and preventive, advisory, planning, and management functions. In the context of primary care, medical tasks under § 64 d SGB V are also being discussed. In the public health service and municipal public services, epidemiological, data-driven, and regional planning, monitoring, and management tasks are added (Völkel and Weidner 2020).

The Robert Bosch Foundation, together with numerous healthcare providers, has supported and piloted several PORT center projects. These are health centers integrated into both the municipality and primary care, where CHN are intended to serve as first points of contact and networkers, enabling specific population groups to access healthcare in a low-threshold and needs-oriented manner (RBS 2021). Here, certain diagnostic, therapeutic, advisory, and coordinating activities are also intended to play a central role. The aim is, among other things, to ensure early treatment and counseling, to provide or facilitate needs-based interventions and services in interdisciplinary cooperation, and, where such services do not exist, to help create them.

CHN often operates at the interface between individual case management and group-based or regionalized care management. This is intended, not least, to compensate for structural problems and to establish new care structures. The role of CHN in municipal public services adds a regional planning and management perspective to this (Völkel and Weidner 2020).

The first definition of Community Health Nursing comes from the American Nurses Association (ANA) in 1980: "the synthesis of nursing practice and public health practice applied to promoting and preserving the health of populations." (Nies and McEwen 2019). In Germany, functions such as the community nurse are also included. It is suggested that a definitional and functional distinction be made between these roles and professional profiles in order to clarify the respective areas of responsibility, thereby promoting optimal collaboration and ensuring good communication among stakeholders (Agnes-Karll-Gesellschaft für Gesundheitsbildung und Pflegeforschung mbH 2022).

48.4 Digital Public Health

The rapidly advancing development in the field of digitalization, as in other areas of healthcare, is having a significant impact on how Public Health as a science is changing and, ultimately, how research and practical concerns are being addressed using digital and virtual possibilities (Zeeb et al. 2020). In reform approaches to the healthcare system, such as in the context of the Robert Bosch Foundation's 'Neustart' initiative, digitalization is consistently conceived as a renewal of information, communication, and administrative processes in primary care (RBS 2021). Against this background, developments in Digital Public Health can be seen as another forward-looking component that will become increasingly important for the practical implementation of Public Health measures. Currently, however, Digital Public Health is still in a phase of exploration and development (Zens et al. 2020; Zeeb et al. 2020). The current focus is on relevant development, application, and knowledge processes related to digitalization in terms of population health and public healthcare. Data processing and the use of information and communication technologies are being discussed, but less so their concrete application, such as telemedicine (Zeeb et al. 2020). The review article highlights that not only is a definition still lacking, but a fundamentally controversial discourse is also underway. The question is raised as to whether Public Health needs to be fundamentally readjusted in light of digitalization, or whether digitalization can be integrated and contribute to achieving Public Health goals. Thus, in addition to *Digital Public Health*, terminologies such as *mobile (M-)Health, E-Public Health*, or *Health 2.0* are also used. These terms each emphasize different technologies and thus have varying degrees of proximity to the traditional discipline of P*ublic Health* (Zeeb et al. 2020). It is also noted that there is a need for research on the opportunities and limitations of establishing Digital Public Health, as there are currently hardly any evaluation studies available. The development of evaluation criteria is also considered inadequate. For example, it would be essential to take a closer look at aspects such as user perspectives, the acceptance and feasibility of digital offerings, and the aspect of equal opportunities (Zeeb et al. 2020).

Among the advantages of increased digitalization in Public Health, it is discussed that data, for example in the planning or evaluation of Public Health measures, can be generated and processed more effectively in digital form. In addition, the practical use of programs and apps that encourage regional information sharing, networking, and mutual support can contribute to a health-promoting environment. Zens et al. (2020) see great potential in digital solutions, particularly for capacity building and municipal health promotion. Possible applications include monitoring disease and health processes, health risk assessment, preparedness for potential emergencies and public health challenges, as well as in prevention and health promotion. For example, apps for tracking health-related behaviors are being considered. The emerging topic of digital health literacy is also playing an increasingly important role. Especially during the COVID-19 pandemic, it became clear how important it is for broad segments of the population to be reached with reliable and trustworthy health information, including via social media.

Last but not least, possible disadvantages and potential risks of digitalizing Public Health are also being recognized, particularly with regard to the protection of collected health data, especially when it is of a personal nature. Possible social inequalities should also be considered, as studies show that digital health offerings mainly reach groups that are already privileged in terms of health (Schaeffer et al. 2018).

48.5 Outlook

Without a doubt, there is today, after the end of the COVID-19 pandemic, an increased general interest in public health. This is accompanied by expansion programs for the public health service, reform initiatives for primary care, and a certain renaissance of municipal public services with regard to aging, the rise in chronic and multiple illnesses, as well as ensuring the provision of nursing care. All of this is also intended to better prepare for and respond to global and demographic challenges that pose risks to people's health. Public health could play a greater role here, both as a science and as a field of practice, than has previously been attributed to it. Together with forward-looking developments in this country such as the CHN in the context of nursing science, as well as the carefully considered opportunities of digitalization, a range of additional potentials could be unlocked for the healthcare system in Germany.

References

Agnes-Karll-Gesellschaft für Gesundheitsbildung und Pflegeforschung mbH (Hrsg) (2022) Community Health Nursing Aufgaben und Praxisprofile. https://www.dbfk.de/de/themen/Community-Health-Nursing.php. Accessed 20 May 2023

De Bock F, Dietrich M, Rehfuess E (2020) Evidenzbasierte Prävention und Gesundheitsförderung. Memorandum der Bundeszentrale für gesundheitliche Aufklärung (BZgA). Bundeszentrale für gesundheitliche Aufklärung, Köln. https://doi.org/10.17623/BZGA:2020-EPGF-DE-1.0

Faller G, Walter-Klose C, Betscher S, Becker J (2022) Community Health als neuronales Netz. In: Department of Community Health (DoCH) (ed) Community Health Grundlagen, Methoden, Praxis. Juventa, Weinheim/Basel pp 22–35

Fischer F, Kuhn J, Kuhlmey A (2023) Public Health und Pflegewissenschaft: Zwei Disziplinen mit gemeinsamen Zielen. Bundesgesundheitsblatt 66(5):477–478
Hurrelmann K, Razum O (2012) Handbuch Gesundheitswissenschaften. Beltz Juventa, Weinheim/Basel
Igl G, Burgi M (2021) Rechtliche Voraussetzungen und Möglichkeiten der Etablierung von Community Health Nursing (CHN) in Deutschland, Schriften zum Sozialrecht 61. Nomos. https://doi.org/10.5771/9783748924319
Klemperer D (2020) Sozialmedizin—Public Health—Gesundheitswissenschaften: Lehrbuch für Gesundheits- und Sozialberufe, 4., überarb. u. erw. edn. Hogrefe, Bern
Müller R, Wehkamp K-H, Larisch J (2018) Public Health—Global Health: neu denken, neu konzipieren. In: Schmiedebach H-H (ed) Medizin und öffentliche Gesundheit: Konzepte, Akteure, Perspektiven. De Gruyter, Oldenbourg, pp 47–64
Nies MA, McEwen M (eds) (2019) Community/public health nursing. Promoting the health of populations, 7th edn. Elsevier, St. Louis/Missouri
Rehfuess EA, Zhelyazkova A, von Philipsborn P, Griebler U, De Bock F (2021) Evidenzbasierte Public Health: Perspektiven und spezifische Umsetzungsfaktoren. Bundesgesundheitsblatt 64(5):514–523
Robert Bosch Stiftung (ed) (2021) Gesundheitszentren für Deutschland. Wie ein Neustart in der Primärversorgung gelingen kann. https://www.neustart-fuer-gesundheit.de/publikationen. Accessed 10 June 2023
Robert Bosch Stiftung (2023) Gesundheit: Community Health Nursing. https://www.bosch-stiftung.de/de/projekt/community-health-nursing. Accessed 20 May 2023
Robert Koch Institut RKI (2016) Definition „Public Health". https://www.rki.de/DE/Content/Institut/Public_Health/Beitrag_Jubilaeumsbuch.html#doc8449980bodyText1. Accessed 20.05.2023
Rosenbrock R (2021) Was ist New Public Health? Bundesgesundheitsblatt 44:753–762
Schaeffer D (1994) Zur Professionalisierbarkeit von Public Health und Pflege. In: Schaeffer D, Moers M, Rosenbrock R (eds) Public Health und Pflege. Zwei neue gesundheitswissenschaftliche Disziplinen. WZB, pp 103–128
Schaeffer D, Moers M, Hurrelmann K (2010) Public Health und Pflegewissenschaft—zwei neue gesundheitswissenschaftliche Disziplinen. Eine Zwischenbilanz nach 15 Jahren. WZB Discussion Paper SP I 2010-301
Schaeffer D, Hurrelmann K, Bauer U, Kolpatzik K (Hrsg) (2018) Nationaler Aktionsplan Gesundheitskompetenz. Die Gesundheitskompetenz in Deutschland stärken. Berlin: KomPart 2018. https://www.nap-gesundheitskompetenz.de/. Accessed 10 May 2023
Schmidt-Semisch H, Schorb F (2021) Einleitung: Public Health zwischen Multi-, Inter- und Transdisziplin. In: Schmidt-Semisch H, Schorb F (eds) Public Health. Sozialwissenschaftliche Gesundheitsforschung. Springer VS. https://doi.org/10.1007/978-3-658-30377-8_1
Völkel M, Weidner F (2020) Community Health Nursing. Meilenstein in der Primärversorgung und der kommunalen Daseinsvorsorge. In: Bundeszentrale für politische Bildung (ed) Pflege Praxis-Geschichte-Politik. APUZ—Aus Politik und Zeitgeschichte, pp 318–329
Zeeb H, Pigeot I, Schüz B (2020) Digital Public Health—ein Überblick. Bundesgesundheitsblatt 63(2):137–144
Zens M, Shajanian Zarneh Y, Dolle J, De Bock F (2020) Digital Public Health—Hebel für Capacity Building in der kommunalen Gesundheitsförderung; Ausgangslage, Entwicklungsfragen, TEAviisari als modellhafte Implementierung. Bundesgesundheitsblatt 63(6):729–740

Community Health Care: Stakeholders, Concepts, and Needs-Based Service Development

49

Manfred Fiedler

Contents

49.1 The Municipality as a Site of Care

The majority of care for people affected by chronic illness takes place in their living environment. This necessitates an understanding of care that includes the home, the immediate residential environment (neighborhood), as well as the municipality as a territorial administrative organization.

Another aspect is the frequency and urgency that require health and health-related services to be accessible within the everyday environment. Finally, aspects of care design must take into account social and socio-economic resources, as well as the competencies of those affected that are limited by chronic illness.

Typical municipal care cases include services for so-called minor illnesses. Although the term "minor illness" is scientifically imprecisely defined, we understand it to mean

M. Fiedler (✉)
Department of human medicine, Witten/Herdecke University, Witten, Deutschland
e-mail: manfred.fiedler@uni-wh.de

D. Schmitz et al. (eds.), *Chronic Care—Science and Practice*,
https://doi.org/10.1007/978-3-662-72298-5_49

illnesses that are easily diagnosable based on clinical presentation, do not require specialized expertise for diagnosis or treatment, and generally have a mild, well-manageable course (see Contributions 6 and 7). Depending on the chronic illness, however, such a minor illness can take a more severe course, which requires familiarity with the specific clinical picture of the affected individual.

Critical disease courses point to care in acute medical emergencies, as a service that must be provided without delay or with minimal delay to prevent avoidable health complications. For this reason, it must be organized locally, particularly through emergency care facilities (emergency medical services, emergency physicians, and emergency departments).

Especially in the case of chronic limitations, continuous access to recurring medical-therapeutic and nursing services must be organized as everyday-near services. In addition, services for chronic illnesses that require specialized medical care, such as diabetes mellitus, Parkinson's disease, or dementia, are locally organized secondary care services. Supplementary services to cope with the physical, social, and mental consequences of illness, especially when everyday functioning is impaired, should be designed to be close to everyday life and tailored as such.

49.2 The Concept of Community-Based Care

The above illustrates the importance of the municipal sphere for the emergence, management, and coping with illness. We therefore speak of community-based care, referred to as Community Health Care (CHC).

The term is common in practical and scientific discourse, but is nevertheless not universally agreed upon. Following Goodman et al., we understand Community Health as a multi-sector and multi-disciplinary collaborative enterprise that uses public health science, evidence-based strategies, and other approaches to engage and work with communities, in a culturally appropriate manner, to optimize the health and quality of life of all persons who live, work, or are otherwise active in a defined community or communities (Goodman et al. 2014, p. 5). Here, communities are understood not only as public institutions, but in the broadest sense as all those involved in health care, health security, and health promotion within the municipality or a region.

The WHO assigns municipalities a key role in health promotion in the Ottawa Charter (World Health Organization [WHO] 1986). Nuntaboot (WHO 2010) describes four crucial areas of Community Health Care:

- Health problems and risks,
- lifestyle-related issues regarding health behavior and care,
- environmental risks to health,
- finally, availability and accessibility of health services.

These are reflected in clinical care, patient-centered care, but also in health promotion and the empowerment especially of those affected by chronic illness and their social networks, the development and promotion of organizations and municipal networks working on initiatives to promote healthy working and environmental conditions, and finally, supplementary social services to ensure daily activities and support for caring relatives (see Contribution 19).

With this understanding, CHC is not an independent scientific field, but a political field of action shaped by a large number of different stakeholders. The design of this field of action is subject to the (established) structural conditions of the health system. For example, in Germany, the organizational responsibility for primary and secondary medical care lies with the Associations of Statutory Health Insurance Physicians, whereas in Finland, for instance, it is the direct responsibility of municipal authorities.

In Germany, we are also confronted with different responsibilities for prevention and health promotion, which, depending on the area, are divided among social insurance providers, employers, or the public health service (Öffentlicher Gesundheitsdienst - ÖGD).

49.3 The Municipality as an Actor in Care

The areas in which CHC is perceived as a relevant municipal field of action depend on the relevant interests and, above all, on the integration of health-related issues within the framework of the municipal political structure (arena). For example, in Northern Europe, municipalities are, according to the self-conception of Nordic health policy, to a high degree self-organizers of community-based health policy, whereas in Germany the municipal role is significantly more limited, as other stakeholders possess health law-related competencies independent of the municipality.

In Germany, the role of municipalities within CHC is increasingly less about operating hospitals and care facilities. Furthermore, health care for people in special health situations is relevant. As a traditional, independent field of health policy, practical public health care should be mentioned, which in the second half of the 19th century primarily included public health policing tasks to prevent and contain infectious diseases and to enforce public hygiene measures (Fiedler and Schmitz 2021). The Public Health Service as a municipal mandatory task predominantly fulfills these functions, as was the case during the coronavirus pandemic 2020–2022, even though the exercise of state health supervision has been supplemented by other tasks, such as school health examinations. Thus, in the context of scientific and practical discourse, the understanding of health hazard prevention has been broadened, for example, by focusing on the protection of vulnerable groups from non-communicable diseases within the framework of the risk group concept. Health care is also increasingly recognized as part of municipal public services. How this is perceived, however, remains unclear. Given the prevailing understanding of the municipal responsibility for public services and the structural diversity of the health policy arena, it can currently be assumed that the municipality plays a rather passive role in the form of ultimate responsibility for health security and provision. This can be observed, for example, in municipal care counseling, which gains relevance as a stopgap due to insufficient services from other stakeholders. The social psychiatric service, as a legally defined municipal task, represents within the (social) psychiatric care system a supplementary instrument for—including preventive—counseling, crisis intervention, and pre- and post-care in institutional psychiatric interventions. Thus, it can be stated for Germany that CHC as a policy field takes place primarily in and through municipalities only as a selectively implemented policy concept.

49.4 Primary Care and Community Health Care

An integral component of CHC, in the broadest sense, is primary care. The Federal Centre for Health Education defines this as the first low-threshold points of contact for people with health problems (Zimmermann 2021). In Germany, these are predominantly general practitioners, office-based pediatricians, gynecologists, and ophthalmologists, i.e., primary medical care. Internationally, primary care is understood more broadly. For example, as early as 1978, the WHO defined Primary Health Care in the Declaration of Alma Ata as "essential health care based on practical, scientifically sound, and socially acceptable methods and technology made universally accessible to individuals and families in the community. […] It is the first level of contact of individuals, the family, and the community with the national health system bringing health care as close as possible to where people live and work, and constitutes the first element of a continuing health care process" (WHO 1978, Z.VI). This expresses access to the health system with fundamental reference to the everyday lives of those affected and their relatives, which also includes all everyday health-related activities beyond curative treatment. Thus, primary care can also be provided by nursing facilities, social services, and others, provided they are sufficiently qualified.

For people with chronic illnesses, the concept of primary care must be understood broadly. They are continuously dependent on specialist medical care, sometimes, as in the case of people with HIV or people with mental illnesses in special life situations, through specialized outpatient clinics in and attached to hospitals. For those in institutional long-term care, nursing staff often constitute or provide the first point of contact for care.

49.5 Concepts of Municipal Health Policy

Even though there is a lack of a clear understanding of CHC as a policy field both in Germany and internationally, it is nevertheless possible to identify areas for municipal health policy initiatives in local practice, which will be discussed here as examples.

In some German federal states, municipalities have been enabled to establish health conferences involving stakeholders from regional care provision. In North Rhine-Westphalia, these are regulated by the Public Health Service Act (ÖGDG-NRW) and are therefore predominantly moderated by the public health departments. Fundamentally, they serve the function of municipal health management, focusing on prevention and health promotion as well as the coordination of health care. Depending on the health policy arena of the respective municipality, they thus enable health policy initiatives for special needs beyond standard care.

In recent years, responsibility for long-term care planning has been transferred to municipalities to varying degrees depending on the federal state. In some federal states, care conferences have been established as an instrument, usually only on a voluntary basis.

The participatory structure of such conferences is sensible. However, due to the limited legally established decision-making authority, their impact on the municipal health system remains very diffuse. Moreover, the separation into different regulatory spheres does not appear to be effective. This is because both in care planning and in health coordination, subject areas overlap or are interconnected, such as with regard to the social determinants of health, especially for people with chronic illnesses, and issues of health social work.

This becomes evident in the area of inclusive urban development. The majority of people are, due to illness or serious injury, impaired in participation in the broadest sense. While in 2021 only 1.4% of those under 18 in Germany had a severe disability, among adults aged 55 and over, it is one in five (19.7%) (Statistisches Bundesamt 2023). Inclusive urban development is therefore a field that must primarily address the social and health care of people with chronic illnesses and enable them to lead as independent a life as possible.

A tool of increasing importance in this context can be so-called neighborhood health work, which, beyond traditional neighborhood work, focuses particularly on people who are especially at risk or particularly affected by chronic illnesses. An example of this is dementia networks, which are both neighborhood-based and regional alliances of those affected and the health and social care professionals involved in their care, addressing the specific care requirements of people with dementia. In Finland, in the 2010s, integrated health and social centers were established alongside primary care health centers, dedicated to health protection, promotion, and care for particularly vulnerable population groups, in which social work and health care are integrated.

49.6 Summary

CHC as a policy field is central to addressing and managing chronic illness. National and international concepts show that there are instruments and approaches for this, but fundamentally, it requires strengthening the municipality as a moderator or coordinator.

References

Fiedler M, Schmitz D (2021) Perspektiven der öffentlichen Gesundheitspflege: Berufspraktische Erwägungen für die Versorgung vulnerabler Menschen während COVID-19. In: Mai M (ed) Die Pflege und die Coronapandemie in Deutschland: Folgen für Profession und Versorgung, 1st edn. Verlag W. Kohlhammer, Stuttgart, pp 92–123

Goodman RA, Bunnell R, Posner SF (2014) What is "community health"? Examining the meaning of an evolving field in public health. Prev Med 67(Suppl 1):pp 58–S61. https://doi.org/10.1016/j.ypmed.2014.07.028

Statistisches Bundesamt (2023) 22711-0002:—Schwerbehinderte: Deutschland, Stichtag, Altersgruppen. https://www-genesis.destatis.de/genesis/online#astructure. Accessed 20 Aug 2023

World Health Organization (1978) Declaration of Alma-Ata. International Conference on Primary Health Care, Alma-Ata, USSR. http://www.who.int/publications/almaata_declaration_en.pdf?ua=1. Accessed 20 Aug 2023

World Health Organization (1986) Health Promotion: Ottawa Charter Charter adopted at an International Conference on Health Promotion, International Conference on Health, November 17-21, Ottawa, Canada

World Health Organization (2010) A framework for community health nursing education: Nuntaboot, Khanitta, Neu-Delhi

Zimmermann T (2021) Primäre Gesundheitsversorgung/Primary Health Care. https://doi.org/10.17623/BZGA:Q4-i096-2.0

Healthy (Health-Equitable) Cities: Approaches to Participation and Inclusion in the Neighborhood

50

Christian Bleck

Contents

50.1 Background

The living conditions in cities give rise to specific influences on health, which particularly affect people with chronic illnesses. Although considerations of the relationships between the circumstances of a city and the health of its population date back at least to the 16th century and gained renewed importance during the industrialization of the 19th century (Baumgart et al. 2018), it is only since the mid-1980s that the active health-promoting role of cities has been systematically addressed. One of the driving forces for

C. Bleck (✉)
Professur Wissenschaft Soziale Arbeit, Fachbereich Sozial- und Kulturwissenschaften, Hochschule Düsseldorf, Düsseldorf, Deutschland
e-mail: christian.bleck@hs-duesseldorf.de

D. Schmitz et al. (eds.), *Chronic Care—Science and Practice*,
https://doi.org/10.1007/978-3-662-72298-5_50

health promotion in cities can be seen in the *Healthy Cities* initiative launched by the World Health Organization (WHO) in 1986 (Böhme and Stender 2020).

For research and practice contexts relating to healthy cities, the term combination Urban Health or CityHealth has become established, which can be understood as the "application of public health theory and practice to the health of urban populations" (Fehr 2020, n.p.). On the one hand, health is increasingly being related to the influences of living conditions and the residential environment. On the other hand, health has gained importance in all policy areas through the WHO's *Health in All Policies* adopted at the 8th Global Conference on Health Promotion in 2013, thus becoming a cross-cutting issue in municipal policy. This is also linked to a focus on health equity (Köckler and Geene 2022), which is fundamental to the everyday lives of people with chronic illnesses. Justice represents a significant normative orientation for public health and, specifically, for urban health. This is even more pronounced, from a critical societal perspective on health inequality, in the still emerging concept of health-equitable cities. Based on these perspectives of healthy and health-equitable cities, this chapter will outline possible approaches to participation and involvement at the neighborhood level, as well as the significance of the municipality and social work.

50.2 Healthy and Health-Equitable Cities

If the WHO defines health as a "state of complete physical, mental and social well-being and not merely the absence of disease or infirmity" (own translation, WHO 2020, p. 1), it is obvious that the environmental and living conditions of a city are also essential influencing factors. The characteristics of cities have specific effects on the well-being of their inhabitants, with a frequent distinction made between influences of the social and physical environment. For example, the high population density in cities is a social environmental factor that can have a positive effect on networking potential, but a negative effect on the potential for conflict. Positive or negative influences of the physical environment refer in particular to the natural environment (e.g., green spaces) and the built environment (e.g., urban density), or to physical-chemical environmental factors (e.g., noise levels, air and water quality). In view of these—here named as examples—influences of urban environments on health, questions about the prerequisites for healthy cities are obvious. According to the WHO, a *Healthy City* is one in which the health and well-being of citizens are appropriately considered in decision-making processes. Healthy cities are thus committed to the health of their citizens and, with the involvement of many municipal stakeholders, develop structures and processes for its sustainable improvement (Böhme and Stender 2020). With regard to people with ongoing, sometimes progressive illnesses, it should also be noted that the aforementioned environmental influences can be particularly burdensome or beneficial, and their well-being must also be considered in light of potential vulnerability.

As an interdisciplinary field, the branch of Urban Health derived from Public Health focuses on health in urban spaces with a cross-sectoral, integrative perspective on the diverse structures and processes relevant to this (Trojan and Fehr 2020). In terms of content, Urban Health refers, for example, to the health status of population groups, environmental influences in the city, health promotion, or disease prevention in cities, including their municipal governance processes (Fehr 2020). These topics also play a role in rural areas under different conditions, for which the field of Rural Health has developed. Looking at the functions of Urban Health, three core tasks can be identified, following Rainer Fehr and Alf Trojan (2018):

(1) The recognition of urban population groups in their specific life situations, which are shaped by the urban environment;
(2) the analysis of urban living environments that are significant for health; and
(3) the municipal governance of health-relevant structures, measures, and services.

In recent years, the concept of health equity has also been applied to cities, as it has been argued that the strategies and programs of public and urban health research do not go far enough (Bůžek et al. 2022). Although questions of health (in)equality of opportunity certainly play a role here, and the model of the social determinants of health (Dahlgren and Whitehead 1991) is a well-known foundation of public and urban health programs, it is criticized that the power and dominance structures underlying social inequality and the determinants of health are not sufficiently addressed (Bůžek et al. 2022). This not only emphasizes that health-promoting and health-burdening living conditions in cities and their neighborhoods are unequally distributed and that there are links between living conditions and health, but also explicitly asks which social conditions lead to this.

Although the connection between health equity and the city has only recently been discussed more intensively within a critical societal framework of urban health conditions, the concept of health equity is by no means new. Its roots can be found in the social medicine of the 19th century, and the WHO has repeatedly addressed it since its founding in 1946; in its first constitution as well as in its later declarations and charters, such as the Ottawa Charter (1986), in which *Health for All* was programmatically formulated as a task for the international community of states (Dzudzek and Strüver 2020). Thus, concepts for healthy cities also refer to health equity, although with more or less concrete theoretical justification based on theories of justice.

The idea of health-equitable cities is intended to serve as an additional orientation, drawing attention to the fact that access to and protection of the health of all citizens is of particular importance for social justice (Rauprich 2009). Thus, from an explicitly justice-theoretical perspective, health can be regarded as an essential prerequisite "for having a normal range of life opportunities in a society. A fair share of this range is a cornerstone of social justice" (Rauprich 2009, p. 519). Accordingly, greater attention should be paid to the fact that "illness and health cannot be considered independently of the power relations that intersect a society in an intersectional way" (Dzudzek and Strüver

2020, p. 266), which in turn particularly affect those with chronic illnesses. At the same time, approaches to healthy and health-equitable cities should not and cannot be strictly separated; rather, the perspective of health equity should serve to sensitize approaches to healthy cities. Therefore, the following will not distinguish between healthy and health-equitable cities, but will introduce the term *healthy (health-equitable) cities* using parentheses. This is intended to express that, to date, healthy and health-equitable cities cannot be clearly distinguished from each other in either theory or practice, and that approaches to healthy cities can also intend health equity. On the other hand, the use of parentheses maintains a differentiating marker, indicating that not all concepts of healthy cities are simultaneously founded on health equity.

50.3 Participation and Involvement in Healthy (Health-Equitable) Cities at the Neighborhood Level as well as the Roles of the Municipality and Social Work

50.3.1 Neighborhood as Local Environment

The term "neighborhood" is predominantly used to refer to the local environment in the sense of people's residential surroundings, although the theoretical references differ between disciplines. It refers to a manageable residential area, depending on the size of a municipality, such as a city or residential district, a smaller community, or a village (Bleck et al. 2018).

Focusing on the neighborhood brings into view the immediate, locally distinct living conditions of people, including not only the physical-material environment but also the social environment of citizens. The neighborhood can therefore also be considered a special social space. Such an understanding assumes interrelationships between physical spaces and social actions, addressing both individually perceived life-world perspectives and collectively experienced as well as socially and politically framed environmental structures and conditions (Bleck et al. 2018).

Considering the neighborhood as a local and social space is significant in the context of healthy (health-equitable) cities because the influences of the social and physical environment on citizens' health are primarily felt locally and can also be influenced at this level. For questions of health equity, this level is also relevant because differentiation processes occur within cities, leading to different conditions for the health of their citizens in the local environment. Thus, environmental conditions "are unequally distributed in the various sub-areas of the city, which can lead to situations of environmental distributional injustice" (Köckler and Sieber 2020, p. 928).

50.3.2 Involvement and Participation

The neighborhood thus has a special significance for the implementation of ideas of healthy (health-equitable) cities, which is also associated with specific approaches to involvement and participation. Involvement and participation are ambiguous terms that are understood differently not only in various disciplinary contexts but also in German-speaking compared to English-speaking contexts. In the German-language discussion, there are conceptual understandings in which either participation integrates both aspects, or this is the case starting from the concept of involvement. In this contribution, participation is understood as a specific component of involvement, with the concept of involvement referring to fundamental rights of social belonging and participation referring to processes of engagement (Bartelheimer et al. 2020). At the same time, it is evident that there are reciprocal connections and consequences between involvement and engagement. Depending on the context and situation, involvement can lead to engagement or engagement can lead to involvement (Krön et al. 2019).

Involvement and participation should be regarded as mutually relevant in healthy (health-equitable) cities. On the one hand, healthy (health-equitable) cities, in line with their perspective on justice, are oriented toward involvement and engagement, because involvement addresses the rights of social belonging that apply to all people, and participation, as a fundamental democratic principle, addresses their engagement in municipal contexts. On the other hand, involvement and participation, in the sense of a biopsychosocial understanding of health, and also in the sense of a state of physical, mental, and social well-being (WHO 2020), have a direct impact on the health of (chronically ill) people. Therefore, considerations regarding the promotion of healthy (health-equitable) cities with the aim of involvement and participation of their citizens are justified, and at the same time, the role of the municipality must be examined in this context.

50.3.3 On the Role of the Municipality

If health is influenced by a multitude of factors that are not solely within the sphere of influence of the health sector (AGGSE 2020), then municipalities have a special role to play on the one hand, because only at the municipal level is there sufficient insight into the local structures, conditions, needs, and requirements. On the other hand, municipalities bear a particular responsibility, as—derived from the principle of the welfare state (Art. 20, Sec. 1 Basic Law) and guided by municipal self-government (Art. 28, Sec. 2 Basic Law)—they are responsible for public services, even though each municipality can decide for itself what it considers relevant in this regard at the local level.

Furthermore, if justice as a central principle also means that access, distribution, and procedural justice are ensured in health-relevant areas (Bunge and Böhme 2019), then municipalities have special functions:

1.) Enabling access to relevant societal sectors (e.g., services, safety, and transportation),
2.) fair distribution of environmental burdens and resources,
3.) enabling participation in relevant information, planning, consultation, and decision-making processes (ibid.).

With these three orientations, the participation and involvement of citizens can evidently be taken into account and pursued as target horizons.

Specifically, municipal administration plays a pivotal role in shaping health-promoting environments and living conditions, as it can, in the context of public services, analyze, plan, steer, and moderate to stimulate and jointly develop and implement health-promoting structures and processes together with citizens (AGGSE 2020). This concerns health-promoting urban planning and development as a cross-cutting municipal task, which involves various topics and affects almost all departments of municipal administration, such as urban development, health, environment, mobility, sports, education, social affairs, and finance (ibid.). At the same time, this requires, especially at the neighborhood level, collaboration with numerous institutions and stakeholder groups outside the municipal administration from the fields of education, health, and social services, business, property owners, civil society initiatives, and citizens, as well as organizations or individuals relevant to the respective neighborhood. This presupposes the integration of various sectoral planning processes and instruments in order to incorporate health concerns and relevant local environmental and living conditions. However, the integrated, explicitly cross-departmental action required for this within municipal administration is still not sufficiently practiced (Böhme et al. 2023).

While it must be explicitly emphasized that the promotion of health in cities does not lie solely within the municipal sphere of responsibility, but is often dependent on frameworks set by the federal and state governments, municipalities do possess essential levers for shaping these processes. Christa Böhme and Klaus-Peter Stender (2020) have identified the following quality elements of *health-promoting neighborhood development*, which are summarized here with additional points of my own:

1. *Neighborhood-based reporting*, as an indicator-based analysis of the health situation in the neighborhood to develop measures for neighborhood-specific health promotion.
2. *Integrated development and action plans* for systematic, participatory, health-promoting neighborhood development based on neighborhood-specific analyses, objectives, and measures.
3. *Cross-departmental collaboration* for establishing, continuing, and implementing health-promoting neighborhood development within municipal administration with regard to health as a cross-cutting issue.
4. *Health-related networks* as a starting point and platform for planning and coordinating activities for neighborhood-based health promotion with broad participation of health-relevant stakeholder groups, such as providers of health and community work,

schools, childcare facilities, sports clubs, self-help groups, physicians, health insurance funds, and relevant municipal administration professionals.

5. *Local coordination office for health promotion* as a driving force for a variety of steering and coordination tasks in a health-promoting neighborhood development process at the neighborhood level and in the intermediary sector, with necessary tasks such as coordination, moderation, networking, project development, activation, participation, and public relations.
6. *Neighborhood-specific project development and implementation* with different objectives and content depending on the respective framework conditions, needs, and requirements, such as nutrition, physical activity and sports, stress management, addiction prevention, and even structural areas such as housing, environment, and transportation.

With regard to these quality elements, it can be stated on the one hand that several elements potentially support the participation and involvement of citizens, provided that, firstly, they are not only informed but also able to participate in decision-making and are granted more or less decision-making authority depending on the context, and secondly, that not only the project processes but also their outcomes or resulting measures focus on the social affiliations of citizens in their living environments.

On the other hand, municipal administration plays a decisive role in implementing these elements, directly in reporting, integrated concepts, and cross-departmental collaboration, but also in further initiating or supporting roles. The social work profession can also—among various other specifically relevant professions—be involved in the context of several of the quality elements mentioned. However, it brings a particular competence profile for healthy (health-equitable) cities, especially with regard to neighborhood-specific project development and implementation at the neighborhood level.

50.3.4 On the Role of Social Work

Within the context of healthy (health-equitable) cities, social work is well-suited—based on a broad concept of health such as that of the WHO—to support the health of citizens in their neighborhoods through participatory means. This is because social work is characterized by a multi-perspective and transdisciplinary approach and, in its fields of practice—including with people with chronic illnesses—always operates at the interface between the individual and society. In doing so, it particularly addresses the everyday coping and life management tasks of people living in challenging environments and circumstances.

Secondly, social work as a profession is predestined to promote the justice claims of healthy (health-equitable) cities, as it is professionally and ethically guided by the principles of human rights and social justice, and critically addresses social and political structures that can contribute to specific processes of exclusion, especially for people with chronic illnesses.

Thirdly, social work can contribute to the promotion of healthy (health-equitable) cities in neighborhoods in a particularly participation- and involvement-oriented way, as it can draw on its original professional foundations and experiences, which are anchored in concepts of community work, neighborhood work, and social space orientation and practice. This also provides it with specific action concepts and competencies to implement the life-world approach adopted in the Ottawa Charter, which focuses on the health-promoting framework conditions of people in their everyday environments.

At the neighborhood level, social work can contribute to the development of healthy (health-equitable) cities through various approaches. This can occur, for example, through fields of action that directly and explicitly relate to health, which are differentiated in health-related social work in the social sector, social work in the health sector, and clinical social work, and may address areas such as health promotion and prevention, health self-help, and clinical-therapeutic interventions (Rademaker 2023). However, in the understanding of health as a cross-cutting issue, contributions at the neighborhood level can also originate, on the one hand, from classic community or neighborhood work and, on the other hand, from neighborhood-based openings and offerings of institutions in other fields of social work (e.g., youth work, integration assistance, elderly care).

It should be noted that there cannot be *one* strategy for neighborhood-based projects on possible paths to healthy (health-equitable) cities, as these depend on the local conditions, needs, and requirements. Typically, however, the first step involves an analysis of the circumstances in the neighborhood, for which the space and the questions to be addressed by the analysis must first be defined. From the outset, it should be clarified which affected citizens and groups can be appropriately involved, in what ways, and with regard to their specific characteristics. Neighborhood or social space analyses often take into account social and infrastructure-related data, which are collected for the area under study via official municipal statistics, possibly as part of municipal health reporting, in order to gain insights into possible needs in the neighborhood. From the perspective of social work, with its focus on participation and involvement, needs-based analyses that capture the subjective views of citizens on the structures, services, and quality of their neighborhood are particularly important. Methods can be used for this purpose that qualitatively explore the perspectives of citizens on site through direct engagement, for example, in the context of workshop series—such as the pin method, neighborhood walks, future workshops, or planning cells (e.g., Trojan et al. 2013; Bleck et al. 2013).

Although neighborhood-based analyses and subsequent activities in the context of healthy (health-equitable) cities must be individually tailored to local circumstances, resources, needs, etc., it is essential in principle to clarify which understanding of health and which perspectives are to be used to examine environmental and living conditions in the immediate vicinity. In terms of health equity, the influences of various dimensions of social inequality in connection with health at the local level should be considered. Theoretical models that describe the relationships between social status, environment, and health can be helpful—building on this, the so-called "Spatial Urban Health Equity Indicators Model (SUHEI)," which relates three types of indicators (environmental stressors, environmental resources, and vulnerable populations) to each other (Köckler et al. 2020). In addition, the specific conditions for participation and involvement, as well as power relations, should be critically reflected upon in a life-situation-oriented manner, not only with regard to the neighborhood but also to the neighborhood project itself. The role that chronic illnesses play in this context depends on the project framework. There are neighborhood activities in which a selected chronic illness is at the center, such as dementia-friendly neighborhoods. More often, however, neighborhood projects will address selected health topics based on needs and requirements, from which people with chronic illnesses will also benefit.

50.4 Conclusion

The perspective of healthy (health-equitable) cities is directed at both health-promoting and health-inhibiting environmental conditions, as well as at the living situations, the dimensions of social inequality at play within them, and the underlying power relations that lead to different prerequisites for individual health. Approaches to healthy (health-equitable) cities are primarily effective at the neighborhood level, because it is there that citizens experience the influences of social and physical environments, and essential opportunities exist to concretely promote their participation and involvement in their living environment. Therefore, it is the task of municipal administration to analyze the framework conditions for health at a small scale and, in cooperation with local stakeholder groups, to structurally promote them. Social work, with its professional roots and experience in community and neighborhood work, as well as its holistic view of people's everyday and living conditions, can play a special role here when it qualitatively explores health-related needs in a participatory manner with citizens in the neighborhood and, on this basis, develops and offers individual and group-oriented services in a networked and cooperative manner with other professions (e.g., medicine, physiotherapy, nursing) that are oriented toward people's life-worlds. There is potential for further development in the integration of activities at the level of municipal administration and neighborhood projects. Not only should the results of analyses from urban development and planning be transferred to the neighborhoods, but conversely, the diverse experiences and knowledge from neighborhood-based projects should also be incorporated into urban development and planning processes. Ultimately, healthy (health-equitable) cities can only live up to their aspirations if they take the health of their citizens seriously as a cross-cutting issue, oriented toward participation and involvement, and in cooperation across different urban levels and sectors.

References

Arbeitsgruppe Gesundheitsfördernde Gemeinde- und Stadtentwicklung—AGGSE (ed) (2020) Empfehlungen für eine gesundheitsfördernde und nachhaltige Stadtentwicklung: Fünf Thesen der Arbeitsgruppe Gesundheitsfördernde Gemeinde- und Stadtentwicklung (AGGSE).

https://backend.repository.difu.de/server/api/core/bitstreams/5af026fa-a671-4fc5-a42d-a022ab969b45/content. Accessed 10 July 2023
Bartelheimer P, Behrisch B, Daßler H, Dobslaw G, Henke J, Schäfers M (2020) Teilhabe—eine Begriffsbestimmung. Springer VS, Wiesbaden
Baumgart S, Hornberg C, Fehr R (2018) Räumliche Planung und StadtGesundheit—eine wechselvolle Geschichte. In: Fehr R, Hornberg C (eds) Stadt der Zukunft—Gesund und nachhaltig: Bestandsaufnahme und Perspektive. oekom, München, pp 33–54
Bleck C, van Rießen A, Knopp R (2013) Der Blick Älterer auf 'ihr Quartier'—Methoden und Instrumente für die sozialräumliche Arbeit mit älteren Menschen. Sozialmagazin 38(5–6):6–17
Bleck C, van Rießen A, Knopp R, Schlee T (2018) Sozialräumliche Perspektiven in der stationären Altenhilfe. Eine empirische Studie im städtischen Raum. Springer VS, Wiesbaden
Böhme C, Stender K-P (2020) Gesundheitsförderung und Gesunde—Soziale Stadt—Kommunalpolitische Perspektive. In: Bundeszentrale für gesundheitliche Aufklärung (BZgA) (ed.) Leitbegriffe der Gesundheitsförderung und Prävention: Glossar zu Konzepten, Strategien und Methoden. https://doi.org/10.17623/BZGA:Q4-i043-2.0. Accessed 10.07.2023
Böhme C, Franke T, Preuß T, Heinrichs E, Schreiber M, Kumsteller F, Köckler H, Hornberg C (2023) Kooperative Planungsprozesse zur Stärkung gesundheitlicher Belange—modellhafte Erprobung und Entwicklung von Ansätzen zur nachhaltigen Umsetzung: Abschlussbericht. Umweltbundesamt. https://digital.bibliothek.uni-halle.de/pe/download/pdf/3263857?originalFilename=true. Accessed 07 July 2023
Bunge C, Böhme C (2019) Umweltgerechtigkeit. In: Bundeszentrale für gesundheitliche Aufklärung (BZgA) (ed.) Leitbegriffe der Gesundheitsförderung und Prävention: Glossar zu Konzepten, Strategien und Methoden. https://doi.org/10.17623/BZGA:Q4-i136-2.0. Accessed 07 July 2023
Bůžek R, Hübl S, Kamphaus L, Dzudzek I (2022) Wenn die Verhältnisse unter die Haut gehen: Urbane Gesundheit relational gedacht. sub\urban 10(1):41–71
Dahlgren G, Whitehead M (1991) Policies and strategies to promote social equity in health. Institute for Future Studies, Stockholm
Dzudzek I, Strüver A (2020) Urbane Gesundheitsgerechtigkeit. Geogr Z 108(4):249–271
Fehr R (2020) Urban health/StadtGesundheit. In: Bundeszentrale für gesundheitliche Aufklärung (BZgA) (ed) Leitbegriffe der Gesundheitsförderung und Prävention. Glossar zu Konzepten, Strategien und Methoden. https://doi.org/10.17623/BZGA:Q4-i124-2.0. Accessed 01 July 2023
Fehr R, Trojan A (2018) Nachhaltige StadtGesundheit—Warum wir das Konzept brauchen und wie wir es für Hamburg thematisch gefasst haben: Eine Einführung. In: Fehr R, Trojan A (eds) Nachhaltige StadtGesundheit Hamburg. oekom, München, pp 11–24
Köckler H, Geene R (2022) Gesundheit in allen Politikfeldern / Health in All Policies (HiAP). In: Bundeszentrale für gesundheitliche Aufklärung (BZgA) (ed.) Leitbegriffe der Gesundheitsförderung und Prävention: Glossar zu Konzepten, Strategien und Methoden. https://doi.org/10.17623/BZGA:Q4-i157-1.0. Accessed 07 July 2023
Köckler H, Sieber R (2020) Die Stadt als gesunder Lebensort? Stadtentwicklung als ein Politikfeld für Gesundheit. Bundesgesundheitsbl Gesundheitsforsch Gesundheitsschutz 63:928–935
Köckler H, Simon D, Agatz K, Flacke J (2020) Gesundheitsfördernde Stadtentwicklung. Inf Raumentwickl 1:98–109
Krön A, Rüßler H, Just M (2019) Teilhaben und Beteiligen auf Quartiersebene: Aufbau von Partizipationsstrukturen mit älteren Menschen. Barbara Budrich, Opladen/Berlin/Toronto
Rademaker AL (2023) Gesundheitsbezogene Soziale Arbeit im Sozialwesen. In: van Rießen A, Bleck C (eds) Handlungsfelder und Adressierungen der Sozialen Arbeit. Kohlhammer, Stuttgart, pp 342–350

Rauprich O (2009) Gesundheitsgerechtigkeit. Zur Theorie von Norman Daniels. Bundesgesundheitsbl Gesundheitsforsch Gesundheitsschutz 52(5):519–526

Trojan A, Fehr R (2020) Nachhaltige StadtGesundheit: konzeptionelle Grundlagen und aktuelle Initiativen. Bundesgesundheitsbl Gesundheitsforsch Gesundheitsschutz 63(8):953–961

Trojan A, Nickel S, Wolf K, Süß W (2013) Partizipation als strategisches Element in der quartiersbezogenen Gesundheitsförderung. In: Trojan A, Süß W, Lorentz C, Wolf K, Nickel S (eds) Quartiersbezogene Gesundheitsförderung: Umsetzung und Evaluation eines integrierten lebensweltbezogenen Handlungsansatzes. Beltz, Weinheim, pp 270–279

World Health Organization (2020) Basic documents. Forty-ninth edition. World Health Organization, Geneva

Public Health Crises and Public Health Emergency Preparedness

51

Manfred Fiedler and Hans Lemke

Contents

51.1 On the Health Crisis

The coronavirus pandemic has made public health crises a subject of scientific debate. Until the pandemic, legal regulations in this area were primarily anchored in infection control laws and in regulations for major loss events as the health-related component of disaster management.

M. Fiedler (✉)
Department of human medicine, Witten/Herdecke University, Witten, Deutschland
e-mail: manfred.fiedler@uni-wh.de

H. Lemke
Ärztlicher Leiter Rettungsdienst Stadt Dortmund und
Leiter Notaufnahme Klinikum Dortmund A.D., Dortmund, Deutschland

D. Schmitz et al. (eds.), *Chronic Care—Science and Practice*,
https://doi.org/10.1007/978-3-662-72298-5_51

A health crisis represents a health-related demand on individuals, care facilities, and systems that has the potential to cause qualitative and quantitative, temporary or permanent, overload. On a personal level, a health crisis can mean the collapse of individual coping and management strategies, and furthermore, a massive impairment of access to health services and, for those with chronic illnesses, a significant restriction or collapse of existing care arrangements.

Beyond this, we speak of a public health crisis when a health-related demand affects at least one social group in such a way that health care for this group is particularly at risk because the care systems are quantitatively or qualitatively overwhelmed by the demands. In this understanding, a public health crisis has both a spatial reference and a temporal dimension (Fiedler and Schmitz 2021):

With regard to the temporal dimension, they can be distinguished as event-related crises—whose time of occurrence and impact (duration and severity) are indeterminate—from those that develop over a longer period, and whose occurrence and effects are fundamentally predictable in the future. We refer to the former as incidental and the latter as developing (emerging), or, since they are already recognizable today, as immanent health crises.

Incidental public health crises include, for example, waves of infection, which, depending on their spatial extent, may also have a pandemic character (see Fig. 51.1). They also include major loss events such as plane crashes, train accidents, terrorist attacks, as well as extreme weather events with high casualty numbers and, where applicable, impacts on health infrastructure.

Immanent health crises are often structurally embedded crises, such as the effects of demographic change, but also crises caused by other social-medical developments, such as the emerging issue of antibiotic resistance.

The spatial reference refers to the dimensional extent of personal and regional impact of a health crisis. For example, the World Health Organization defines an epidemic as a

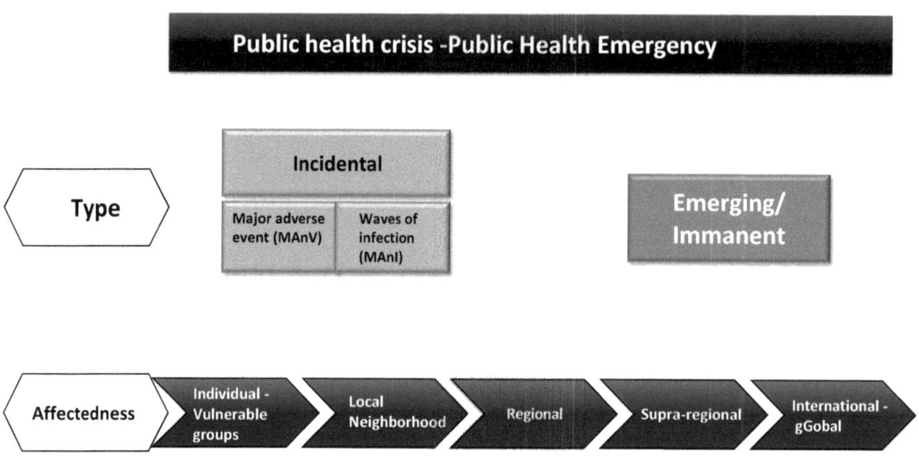

Fig. 51.1 Public health crises. (Own illustration)

pandemic when at least two world regions are affected. While Hurricane Katrina in the USA in 2004 devastated several states on a large scale, the flood disaster in Germany in 2021 was limited to a specific region.

51.2 Incidental Health Crises

51.2.1 Major Loss Events

Major loss events represent the intermediate stage between routine emergency services and a disaster situation. In addition to causing significant property damage, they can also result in a large number of casualties within a short period. This situation is defined as a mass casualty incident (MCI).

Major loss events such as the Ramstein air show disaster in 1988 have demonstrated the importance of establishing targeted structures on site to coordinate the deployment of emergency services and involved institutions. The primary focus is not on the rapid transport of many affected individuals, but rather on their stabilization at the scene. After this initial care, targeted transport to suitable hospitals follows. The goal is to return to individualized care at the incident site as quickly as possible.

The Ramstein disaster, with over 1,000 victims, had far-reaching effects on emergency services, particularly regarding the reorganization of procedures for mass casualty incidents. The first emergency physicians to arrive temporarily structure and coordinate the scene until the arrival of the lead emergency physician. Their responsibilities include assessing the situation and required resources and reporting to the control center, establishing local command structures, initiating hospital alerts, and organizing the rescue, triage, and controlled transfer of the injured (see Fig. 51.2).

While the focus in a major loss event is on caring for the victims, a terrorist situation is defined as a *life-threatening operational situation* because the responders themselves are in an unclear risk environment. Upon recognizing a terrorist situation, the prehospital care strategy must be changed from *Stay and Play* to *Load and Go* in order to minimize the risk to emergency and rescue personnel as well as to the still-functioning infrastructure from a potential *Second Hit*. Hospital entrances must be secured, and patient allocation should be managed exclusively through the emergency department (ZNA). Initial triage must take place in a tent or outdoors in front of the hospital to avoid endangering hospital infrastructure.

51.2.2 Waves of Infection—Mass Casualty Incident of Infected Persons

In high-income countries, waves of infection—defined as a higher-than-expected number of cases within a certain period—initially represent a limited system risk. Only when an outbreak can no longer be controlled and institutional or locally limited measures are

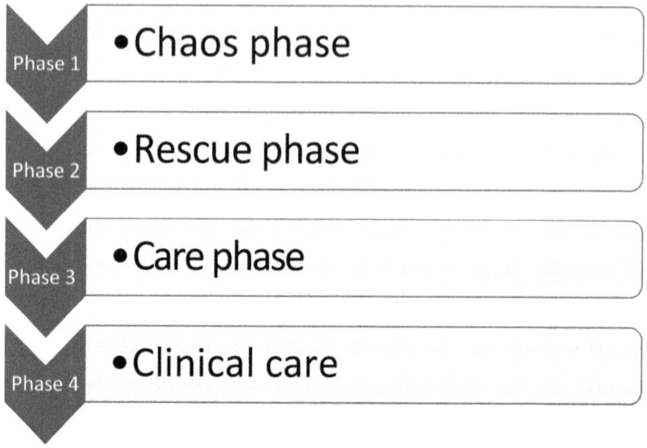

Fig. 51.2 Phases of major loss event management. (Based on Lechleuthner et al. 1990)

insufficient to prevent further spread do we speak of an epidemic. Infectious diseases possess characteristics that can turn them into a public health crisis. These include: contagiousness, i.e., transmissibility within contact groups; transmission routes, such as via physical contact, air, or contaminated food; a lack of baseline immunity to the infectious disease; and, finally, the consequences of the disease, need for treatment, available treatment options, and mortality. Particularly dangerous are infectious diseases with high contagiousness, a high proportion of severe cases, and a high mortality rate when therapeutic options are limited. The WHO defines a pandemic as an outbreak that spreads to at least two of the five WHO world regions.

Whereas the focus in major loss events is on managing the initial incident, in the case of pronounced waves of infection, access routes to hospitals for both walk-in and ambulance-assigned patients must be clearly marked and monitored. These access routes to the emergency department must remain strictly separated from other patient flows.

51.3 Immanent Health Crises

Immanent health crises are already embedded within the health system, but develop over time and therefore have a prognostic probability of occurring in the future. Unlike incidental health crises, they can thus be assessed in terms of their timing and their impact on the health system. As a result, they can be influenced in terms of their extent and severity through measures taken in the present. In U.S. practice, since the 2010s, the increase in drug and medication addiction (the opioid crisis) has been declared a public health crisis in individual states and nationwide. The causes lie in social and economic developments, in conjunction with a significant increase in the prescription of opioid-containing pain medications whose effects were underestimated.

51.4 Concept of Preparedness

51.4.1 Theoretical Background

The terrorist attacks on the USA in 2001, pandemics such as SARS-CoV-1, MERS-CoV, or H1N1, and finally devastating natural disasters like Hurricane Katrina, prompted an increasing scientific discourse on the question of how health systems can be prepared to prevent and manage public health crises.

By 2017, the WHO developed a guideline intended to assist nation-states in developing preparedness at the national and even municipal level, also taking into account health crises caused by technological or social factors (WHO 2017), and established the Global Preparedness Monitoring Board, which was to assess worldwide activities for preparing for health crises and published its findings (Global Preparedness Monitoring Board 2019). At the same time, the European Center for Disease Control (ECDC) also published the PHEP concept (European Center for Disease Prevention and Control [ECDC] 2017).

According to McCabe et al., the principles for PHEP can be identified as Willingness, Readiness, and Ability (McCabe et al. 2010). Willingness refers to the necessary commitment and political will at various levels of action to prepare for identified future health challenges, to provide the necessary resources, and for those involved in crisis management to enter into a trusting and mutually supportive cooperation. Ability refers to the individual, institutional, and systemic prerequisites for being able to respond to health crises in a timely manner—simply put: staff, structure, and stuff. Readiness, finally, is the individual, organizational, and municipal/regional capability, in terms of quality standards, qualifications, or knowledge, to have answers to health crises.

The basis for practical implementation is an understanding of public health care and the associated competencies for action (ECDC 2017). In Germany, the tasks of preparing for and responding to (Respond) health crises are not uniformly distributed, either in terms of state regulations or with regard to municipal structures, and are usually not conceptually or substantively concentrated in a single leading authority within the municipalities.

The PHEP concept (see Fig. 51.3) focuses on the spatially related political levels of action, where public authorities are at least responsible for organizing the involvement of stakeholders at each level. A fundamental aspect of health crises is that they always affect both individuals and localities, meaning that the public health service must be a central actor within a transparent community health care concept.

51.4.2 Practical Implementation

Neither the WHO concepts nor those of the ECDC have been implemented into national structures in Germany. This applies both to the understanding and prevention of incidental health crises and to the systematic influence on the effects as well as the avoidance or mitigation of inherent health crises. This deficiency became apparent during the coronavirus pandemic in the form of inconsistent, rolling legislation, predominantly top-down, ad hoc measures with a health-police character, and a lack of personnel, organizational, and structural competencies in the public health service (Fiedler and Schmitz 2021).

Beyond this, there are also shortcomings in terms of preparedness for major loss events. The main deficits are due to:

- inconsistent legal frameworks
- non-continuous communication structures
- insufficient regulations or legal requirements regarding major incidents
- inadequate definition of interfaces in the areas of leadership and organization

Hesse has developed the web-based **Interdisciplinary Care Registry** IVENA e-Health and made it mandatory for all control centers and hospitals, providing management-relevant information on the occupancy of central emergency departments, hospital capacities, or available large diagnostic devices. Only six other federal states have adopted the system so far. The Federal Association of Medical Directors of Emergency Services has established a nationwide hospital registry, in conjunction with IVENA, which can be used in major incidents to refer patients to the nearest suitable specialist clinics. For

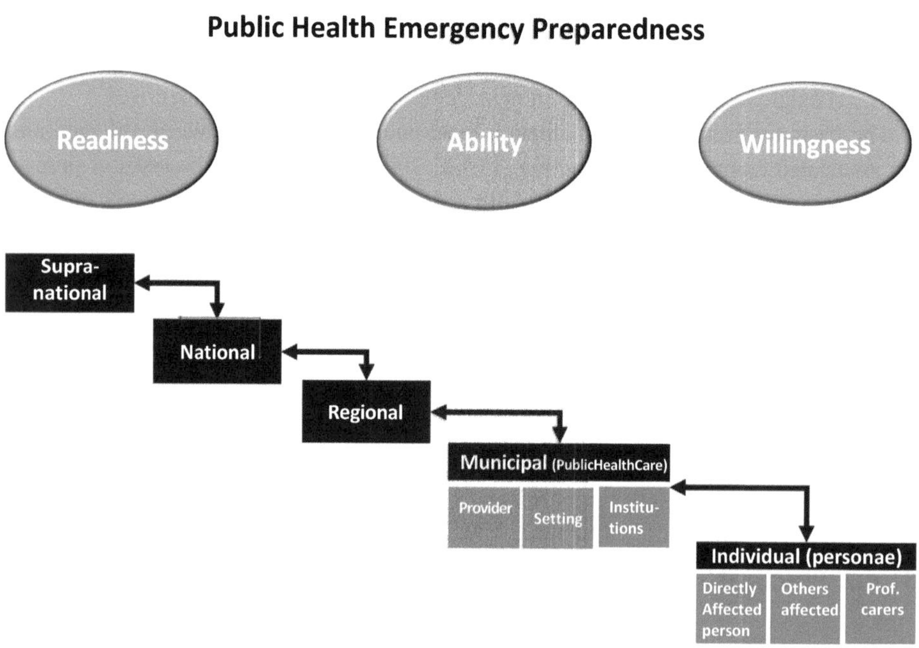

Fig. 51.3 PHEP. (Own illustration)

example, North Rhine-Westphalia uses a stand-alone solution (IG-NRW [Information System for Hazard Prevention NRW]), resulting in a lack of interfaces with *IVENA*. Communication across state borders is hampered, which can have dramatic consequences in the event of an incident.

51.5 People with Chronic Diseases in Health Crises?

People with chronic illnesses are fundamentally vulnerable and are particularly affected by health crises. The example of the COVID-19 pandemic makes this abundantly clear, as people with chronic pre-existing conditions experienced disproportionately severe courses and a higher mortality rate when infected. At the same time, they generally depend on continuous access to health care facilities. Crisis-related disruption of care can lead to the progression of existing or the development of (additional) chronic diseases.

To protect people with chronic illnesses before and during health crises, a persona-based approach is needed—that is, the typifying identification of vulnerable population groups within the framework of community-based PHEP, in order to enable essential care pathways in the respective crisis scenarios.

References

European Center for Disease Prevention and Control (2017) Public health emergency preparedness: core competencies for EU_Member States (ECDC Technical Report). Stockholm

Fiedler M, Schmitz D (2021) Perspektiven der öffentlichen Gesundheitspflege: Berufspraktische Erwägungen für die Versorgung vulnerabler Menschen während COVID-19. In: Mai M (ed) Die Pflege und die Coronapandemie in Deutschland: Folgen für Profession und Versorgung, 1st edn. Verlag W. Kohlhammer, Suttgart, pp 92–123

Global Preparedness Monitoring Board (2019) A world at risk: annual report on global preparedness for health emergencies. Genf

Lechleuthner A, Bouillon B, Schweins M, Dauber A (1990) Die vier Phasen eines Massenanfalls von Verletzten (MANV) – Ein Konzept für Management, Fehleranalyse und Qualitätssicherung. Notarzt 6:160–165

McCabe OL, Barnett DJ, Taylor HG, Links JM (2010) Ready, willing, and able: a framework for improving the public health emergency preparedness system. Disaster Med Public Health Prep 4(2):161–168. https://doi.org/10.1001/dmp-v4n2-hcn10003

WHO (2017) A strategic framework for emergency preparedness, Geneva

One Health—Environment and Health in the Context of Chronic Diseases

52

Daniela Schmitz and Simone Hatebur

Contents

52.1 Definition & Background

One Health (OH) is an approach of the World Health Organization that defines the sustainable design of health as a multisectoral and collaborative task at the interface of human, animal, and environmental health. Human health can only be integratively shaped in harmony with a healthy environment and animal world (see Fig. 52.1). There is no uniform definition; the central focus is on the close connection of these three areas.

D. Schmitz (✉)
Department of human medicine, Witten/Herdecke University, Witten, Germany
e-mail: Daniela.Schmitz@uni-wh.de

S. Hatebur
Faculty of Health, Witten/Herdecke University, Witten, Germany
e-mail: simone.hatebur@uni-wh.de

D. Schmitz et al. (eds.), *Chronic Care—Science and Practice*,
https://doi.org/10.1007/978-3-662-72298-5_52

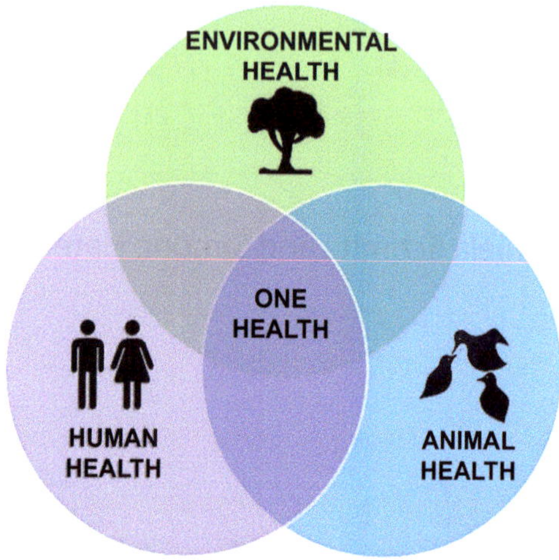

Fig. 52.1 One Health concept. *Source* Creative Commons by Thddbfk, CC-BY-SA 4.0

The implementation of this shared task requires multiple sectors, disciplines, and communities with stakeholders from business, science, politics, and education. These stakeholders are expected to gather, disseminate, and communicate the necessary knowledge for this complex task so that common threats to health and ecosystems can be addressed and contribute to sustainable development (OHHLEP et al. 2022).

The OH approach was developed in the early 2000s. The starting point was the increasing spread of zoonoses, i.e., diseases transmitted from animals to humans by viruses (e.g., dengue virus), bacteria (e.g., Lyme disease), or parasites (e.g., toxoplasmosis). Zoonoses can also be transmitted from humans to animals, such as tuberculosis or influenza, which are mutually transmissible in both directions.

The precursor to OH was the curative approach One Medicine (OM), an interdisciplinary cooperation between human and veterinary medicine. The original idea is attributed to Rudolf Virchow, who saw no *dividing lines* between human and veterinary medicine, as there is no natural barrier between humans and animals. For example, measles and rinderpest (BSE) share a common ancestral pathogen, which, through mutations, specialized in the two hosts: humans in the case of measles infection and rinderpest in animals. OH expands OM by including environmental factors (natural and built environment) and aims for transdisciplinary collaboration (see contribution 03) (Sinclair, 2019).

52.2 Elements & Principles

OH aims to protect health and unites the perspectives of individual, public, and global health from a resilience-oriented approach. In addition to health science aspects, perspectives from social sciences and agricultural sciences are also integrated, as health is also influenced by climate, ecosystems, food safety, the handling of antibiotic-resistant

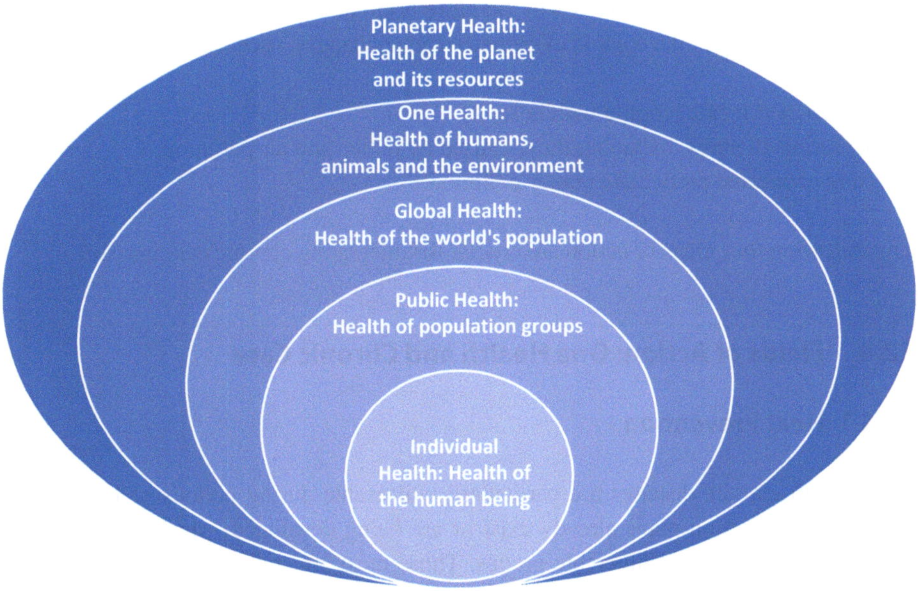

Fig. 52.2 Layer model of health concepts. (Adapted from Marty 2021)

pathogens, and biodiversity. Another term in the scientific discourse surrounding OH is Planetary Health, which is more politically accentuated and, based on the three pillars of sustainability—ecology, economy, and social—seeks to achieve health equity for current and future generations (Zinsstag et al. 2021). The perspective adopted by OH can be visualized using the layer model (see Fig. 52.2):

To implement the essential principles of OH, cross-sectoral and interdisciplinary communication is required, based on a shared understanding and participation of all involved. Consequently, the education system must aim for the development of relevant competencies that enable joint action and the development and implementation of structural prevention measures.

52.3 People with Chronic Diseases in the One Health Concept

Previous publications on OH have focused on maintaining health and preventing disease. Living with chronic illnesses has received less attention. According to the model in Fig. 52.2, individual health—and thus living with chronic illnesses—forms the core for all surrounding approaches, including how life with chronic illnesses can be shaped at the interface of environment and health. In particular, older, multimorbid individuals are vulnerable to environmentally induced changes. These may be due to the consequences of climate change as well as environmental emissions (Bauer and Becker 2021). In the future, living with chronic illness will therefore bring new coping requirements for those affected, especially in the context of climate-related changes, such as:

- physical and mental coping with heat
- increasing allergies, including those caused by pollen and air pollution
- rising ozone and particulate matter pollution.

The following four areas of action are crucial for integrating chronic care into OH.

52.4 Fields of Action: One Health and Chronic Care

52.4.1 Heat Prevention

People with chronic diseases are particularly vulnerable during periods of heat. Initial municipal heat action plans already exist or are being developed, which also take into account the situation of vulnerable groups. Those most affected are elderly people over 75 years of age who are immobile, have a lower socioeconomic status, and live alone on higher floors. The heat problem is exacerbated by chronic diseases of the heart, kidneys, or lungs, as well as by dementia or depression (Günster et al. 2021).

Despite an adequate warning system from the German Weather Service, the implementation of measures by regional health actors is often incomplete, a situation worsened by the occurrence of heat waves during holiday periods when staffing levels are lower (Bauer and Becker 2021). In addition, there is a lack of screening instruments in both outpatient and inpatient settings to identify at-risk individuals early. Due to staff shortages, proactive outreach by general practitioners cannot be implemented nationwide. Communication between nursing services and general practitioners also needs to be intensified. Bauer and Becker therefore propose that, in the event of regional extreme heat, health authorities declare a heat emergency to handle it as a disaster situation. This would also enable aid organizations to support the care of people with chronic diseases. A shift in perspective is needed here regarding the term "disaster": away from a focus solely on material damage toward an expansion to include humanitarian harm. To prevent heat-related risks, preventive measures for dealing with heat and its risks must be communicated to those affected, and, if necessary, medications and practice procedures at general practitioners' offices must be adjusted.

52.4.2 Zoonoses and Pandemics

Zoonoses occur regularly, although only a few escalate into endemics or even pandemics. Nevertheless, reliable research findings are needed when new diseases emerge and regarding their consequences for people with chronic diseases, in order to develop appropriate treatment and protective measures as well as preparedness (see contribution 51). Zoonotic viral diseases also occur more frequently during heat periods, such as dengue fever (Romanello et al. 2022).

As a measure to contain the coronavirus pandemic, social distancing was chosen due to the increased morbidity and mortality among older and chronically ill people, which led to increased loneliness and associated psychological stress. In the future, more proportionate measures will be needed than those enacted at the beginning of the coronavirus pandemic, for example in the form of preventive and therapeutic concepts, to minimize further psychological, physical, or social problems for chronically ill people caused by society-wide restrictions. In principle, the increased vulnerability of people with chronic diseases should be given greater consideration when implementing measures.

52.4.3 Nutrition

Nutrition plays a central role in the context of chronic diseases, as dietary habits can influence the course of disease both positively and negatively. Malnutrition, undernutrition, overnutrition, or deficiencies may result. In the case of poor nutrition, overweight, high blood pressure, and diabetes can develop—these are all non-communicable diseases that are the most common causes of death. From an overarching One Health perspective, food supply and security as well as the composition of the diet play a role. Globally, an unhealthy diet is one of the leading causes of death (Schulz and Simon 2021).

The close interconnection between environment and health is clearly evident in the use of pesticides in agriculture, which can lead to species extinction, in CO_2 emissions, and in the land required for livestock and animal feed. Species extinction can lead to undernutrition. For example, bee die-offs can result in crop failures and thus contribute to undernutrition among people dependent on those crops. Extreme weather in general, such as heat or hail, also negatively affects crop yields. Malnutrition or overnutrition due to excessive consumption of meat, sugar, and salt, and insufficient intake of fruits and vegetables, can negatively influence the course of chronic diseases. Overall, Swinburn et al. (2019) refer to this as a syndemic, which considers obesity, undernutrition, and climate change together. These three phenomena interact biologically, psychologically, and societally.

A resource- and environmentally-friendly solution is the low-meat and predominantly plant-based Planetary Health Diet. It reduces land use and environmental impact while also contributing to a healthy diet. A future shift toward a more plant-based diet could reduce the 55% of agricultural sector emissions that come from the production of red meat and dairy, while also preventing diet-related deaths per year. This could also reduce the risk of zoonoses (Romanello et al. 2022). Strategies to be developed in this field of action can only be effective if nutrition is considered in a broader context and people with chronic diseases are included in dietary planning.

52.4.4 Energy & Supply System

Dependence on fossil fuels intensifies the health impacts of climate change. These lead to air pollution, which can also negatively affect chronic diseases. In addition, CO_2 emissions cause a rise in temperature, which leads to species extinction and extreme weather events. Instead of relying on air conditioning, which exacerbates the problem through resource consumption, urban planning should increasingly focus on greening city centers, which has a cooling effect.

The healthcare sector is responsible for five percent of all CO_2 emissions worldwide (Romanello et al. 2022). These result from transport and logistics to healthcare facilities, the mobility of staff within the facilities, and the energy consumption within organizations. To ensure that the supply system also consumes less energy and emits less CO_2, there are initial initiatives such as the climate-friendly hospital. The energy consumption of a hospital bed is roughly equivalent to that of four single-family homes. Savings are conceivable in the areas of procurement, IT, food, waste, energy (ventilation, cooling, heating, lighting, see German KLIK guide), and logistics.

Ultimately, this contribution should be understood as an outline of the complex interconnection between human, animal, and environmental health, intended to raise awareness of the needs and increased vulnerability of people with chronic diseases when developing measures. The required competencies for implementation can be described as integrated problem-solving competence, which consists of a critical assessment of future scenarios, consideration of one's own and contextual values in action, recognizing and overcoming obstacles to change processes, and empathetic interpersonal competence (see contribution 19).

References

Bauer J, Becker C (2021) Geriatrie – Neue Herausforderungen für die medizinische Versorgung älterer Menschen. In: Traidl-Hoffman C, Schulz C, Herrmann M, Simon B (eds) Planetary Health: Klima, Umwelt und Gesundheit im Anthropozän. Medizinisch Wissenschaftliche Verlagsgesellschaft, pp 122–130

Günster C, Klauber J, Robra B-P, Schmuker C, Schneider A (2021) Versorgungs-Report: Klima und Gesundheit. Medizinisch Wissenschaftliche Verlagsgesellschaft, Berlin

Marty E (2021) What is planetary health? https://www.forbes.com/sites/johndrake/2021/04/22/what-is-planetary-health. Accessed 23 Aug 2023

One Health High-Level Expert Panel (OHHLEP), Adisasmito WB, Almuhairi S, Behravesh CB, Bilivogui P, Bukachi SA et al (2022) One health: a new definition for a sustainable and healthy future. PLoS Pathog 18(6):e1010537

Romanello M, Di Napoli C, Drummond P, Green C, Kennard H, Lampard P, Scamman D, Arnell N, Ayeb-Karlsson S et al (2022) The 2022 report of the Lancet Countdown on health and climate change: health at the mercy of fossil fuels. Lancet 400(10363):1619–1654

Schulz CM, Simon B (2021) Anthropozän – Die Überschreitung planetarer Grenzen. In: Planetary Health (ed) Klima, Umwelt und Gesundheit im Anthropozän, Medizinisch Wissenschaftliche Verlagsgesellschaft, Berlin, pp 7–27

Sinclair JR (2019) Importance of a one health approach in advancing global health security and the sustainable development goals. Rev Sci Technol 38(1):145–154

Swinburn BA, Kraak VI, Allender S (2019) The global syndemic of obesity, undernutrition, and climate change: the Lancet commission report. Lancet 393(10173):741

Zinsstag J, Waltner-Toews D, Tanner M (2021) Why one health? In: Zinsstag J, Schelling E, Crump L (eds) One health: the theory and practice of integrated health approaches, 2nd edn. Wallingford, CABI, pp 15–25

Status Quo and Development Trends in Digital Health

53

Sven Meister and Felix Hoffmann

Contents

S. Meister (✉)
Lehrstuhl für Gesundheitsinformatik, Fakultät für Gesundheit/Department Humanmedizin, Universität Witten/Herdecke, Witten, Germany
e-mail: sven.meister@uni-wh.de

S. Meister
Abteilung Gesundheitswesen, Fraunhofer-Institut für Software- und Systemtechnik ISST, Dortmund, Germany

S. Meister
Purpose:Health e.V., Dortmund, Germany

F. Hoffmann
APOLLON Hochschule der Gesundheitswirtschaft, Bremen, Germany
e-mail: Felix.Hoffmann@apollon-hochschule.de

F. Hoffmann
Purpose:Health e.V., Dortmund, Germany

D. Schmitz et al. (eds.), *Chronic Care—Science and Practice*,
https://doi.org/10.1007/978-3-662-72298-5_53

53.1 Status Quo of Digitalization and the Impact of Societal Change

Digitalization is a frequently used and now overused term. It is widely stated and written that digitalization is not an end in itself. But what, then, is digitalization, what is its current status, and where might its possible lines of development lead?

We begin this chapter by classifying the digital-***-word family and examining the current state of digital health. Here, we use the conventional narrative style in order to set a counterpoint in the following chapter and to engage in critical discourse, driven by the question of whether and how chronic care can find support in this context.

53.1.1 From Digital to Digitalization to Digital Transformation

In the following, we want to devote ourselves to classifying the term digitalization. Fig. 53.1 provides an overview of the historical development. It becomes clear that the concept of digital representation—i.e., zeros and ones—was already used by Leibniz. The term digitalization puts us in a dilemma, as it can mean both the conversion of analog data and information into a digital representation and the initiation of a transformation or change process. Conversion of analog data versus process change—the English language offers us greater differentiation with the terms *digitization* and *digitalization*. We less frequently speak of digital transformation, which Ebert and Duarte describe as the introduction of "disruptive technologies to increase productivity, value creation, and social prosperity" (Ebert and Duarte 2018, p. 16). Furthermore, it is characterized by inevitability, speed, irreversibility, and uncertainty (Oswald et al. 2022). Finally, digital transformation addresses the growing societal implications.

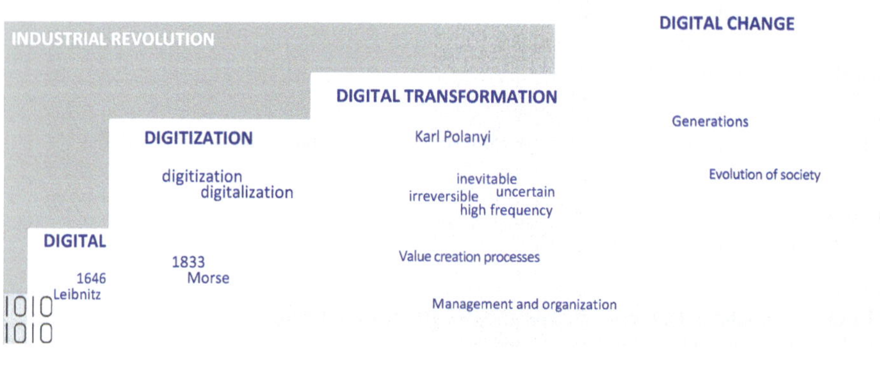

Fig. 53.1 From the industrial revolution to digital transformation. (Own illustration)

Thus, the original conversion from analog to digital may mean that societal influence changes our understanding of purpose and value orientation. Likewise, the self-concept of purpose and value orientation can influence the degree of digitalization.

53.1.2 Status Quo in Healthcare

There can be a world of difference between legal norms and the actual operationalization of digitalization, as is also the case in healthcare. It is evident that since 2018, when Germany was ranked second to last in a study on digitalization, a multitude of laws have been advanced by the Federal Ministry of Health (BMG). These include the Hospital Future Act, the Digital Healthcare Act, the Patient Data Protection Act, and others with explicit reference to digitalization. At the same time, it should not be overlooked that the history of digitalization in healthcare—in Germany as well, with reference to the GKV Modernization Act of 2004—goes back further, as shown in the following Fig. 53.2.

Technical solutions were created and care—initially with little interprofessional collaboration—was arranged around the technology. Patients were placed at the center, but usually without regard for the human factor, which is an inherently important component for care and nursing. This complex was ultimately condensed in the digitalization strategy available since 2023, which also aims to give research a voice through increased use of health data (Federal Ministry of Health 2023).

53.1.3 VUCA and BANI as Counterpoints to a Non-Reactive Strategy

Chronic care requires a long-term view of care perspectives that takes into account the individual life and care context of patients (see contribution 17). In this situation, strategies offer the potential to provide guidance, but at the same time must also be able to respond to changes. The fact that the nature and extent of changes in society are constantly increasing is made clear by terms such as VUCA (volatile, uncertain, complex, ambiguous) or BANI (brittle, anxious, non-linear, incomprehensible). Continuity seems to be a virtually non-existent asset, and our lives are increasingly characterized by chaos.

With a non-adaptive strategy and a sluggish healthcare system, it appears virtually impossible to adequately respond to the long-term needs in care—here, in particular, chronic care. Furthermore, it must be critically questioned to what extent the predominant (mis)use of the term digitalization is appropriate to the challenges outlined above and the strategic target area.

Perhaps the thinking behind a strategy that addresses the aforementioned points does not require a solitary shift onto digitalization. In the following chapter, the authors will open a purpose-oriented line of development, which can be supported by digitalization but focuses on the common good of society.

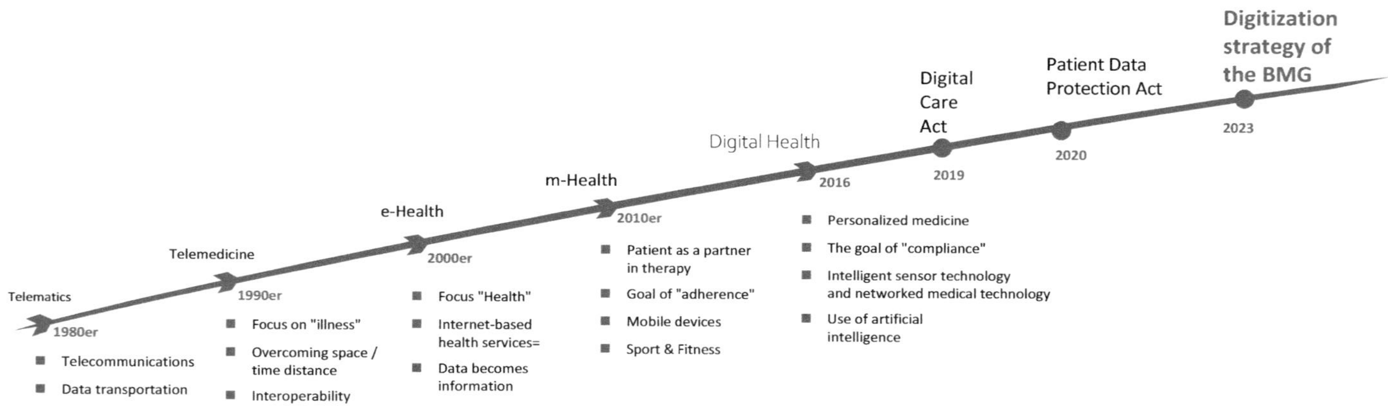

Fig. 53.2 Timeline of the development of digitalization in healthcare provision and research. (Own illustration)

53.2 Purpose Orientation for a Future-Oriented Digital Healthcare System

The development of a line of progress for digitally supported healthcare must allow for the question of what meaning and purpose underlie it. VUCA and BANI name essential aspects of our time that must be taken into account. We have already addressed the term digitalization as a supporting building block and will now turn to the concept of purpose.

53.2.1 Purpose Economy

Organizations generally have a purpose and reason for which they exist. These can be quite diverse, for example, the production of consumer goods or the provision of services. Typically, an exchange of services takes place, such as services for money. In this constellation, different people interact with each other, each with their own needs, which are mutually satisfied.

Let us approach the topic using the example of a hospital. It is obvious that a hospital provides healthcare services and thus fulfills an important function for sick or injured people. In addition, a hospital is also an employer for many people who earn their livelihood by providing healthcare services.

This is where purpose comes into play. The term *purpose* refers to the *why*—the reason a person or organization exists. In the case of a hospital, it can be assumed that the hospital's purpose is to:

1. ensure the best possible healthcare for the people in the respective region, and
2. provide meaningful and adequately compensated jobs for people in healthcare professions.

However, in most cases, it is not only employees and patients who interact in a hospital; there are also other stakeholders who influence the hospital's activities (see Fig. 53.3). On the one hand, this includes the state as the legislative authority, which sets the legal

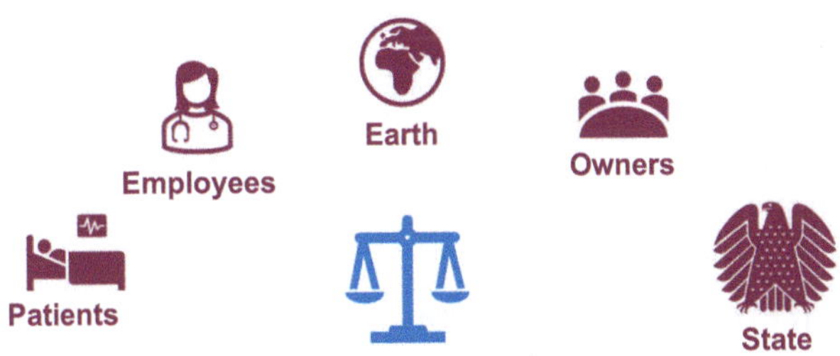

Fig. 53.3 Stakeholders in healthcare organizations. (Own illustration)

framework for healthcare, and indirectly also the planet Earth, which, although not a direct stakeholder, provides the essential basis of life for all people and thus indirectly sets important parameters for responsible action within the hospital.

On the other hand, there are also the owners, who have the final say in business decisions. The role of the owners will be examined in more detail below.

In many companies, the role of the owners is associated with the right to withdraw as much money as they wish from the company. Due to complex ownership structures such as exchange-traded funds (ETFs), it is not uncommon for owners not even to know which companies they hold shares in. The only information that is transparently available to many investors is the performance of their portfolio. And this is not surprising, since people generally invest in ETFs to make a profitable return on their assets.

Let us consider who makes the business decisions and how company profits are used. In the case of a hospital that is run as a public limited company and held by small investors through ETFs, it is not the small investor who makes the business decisions, but the ETF manager. As described above, the success of the ETF manager is measured by the performance of the ETF. It is therefore not surprising that, when making business decisions, they focus exclusively on whether the decision will increase the value of the investment or not.

In this way, the company transforms from a purpose-driven organization, which primarily aims to create social value, into a financial enterprise, which is primarily intended to satisfy the interests of the owners. Healthcare provision is no longer an end in itself, but becomes a means to an end.

53.2.2 Designing Purpose-Driven Organizations in Healthcare

Corporate law offers numerous possibilities to anchor the purpose of a company so deeply in its constitution that it results in a completely new understanding of ownership. All of these legal structuring options for purpose-driven organizations have in common that they provide for asset dedication and tie ownership to a community of values. Asset dedication means that the company's assets can no longer be distributed to the owners without compensation simply because of ownership, but are instead tied to the company for the realization of its purpose. Apart from this, purpose-driven organizations can operate in the market like any other company (Hoffmann and Schumacher 2022).

However, a suitable legal form alone is not enough to achieve entrepreneurial success. The legal constitution of the company is merely the foundation on which the company's social value can be built. Five areas of action are likely to play a decisive role in this regard.

Field of Action 1: Process Development

Care processes in healthcare must be designed to achieve the best possible outcome with the least possible use of resources. The particular importance of using resources sparingly arises not only for financial reasons, but especially for reasons of ecological sustainability. Humanity must sooner or later succeed in transforming from waste management to a circular economy, and this will be all the easier the lower the overall resource consumption is (Hoffmann and Khaladj 2022).

Field of Action 2: Standardization and Automation of Processes

Efficient and effective care processes are an important step toward good healthcare provision. However, optimized processes alone will not solve the problem of staff shortages, which will become even more acute in the coming years due to demographic reasons. In recent years and decades, numerous technologies have emerged that can independently carry out individual process steps or entire processes, thereby relieving human labor. The standardization and automation of processes—commonly referred to as *digitalization*—is an integral part of designing care processes.

Field of Action 3: Transformational Leadership

On the one hand, healthcare is characterized by the processing of a wide variety of information, and on the other hand, by rapid change. Decision-makers must respond quickly to changing environmental conditions. This requirement calls for appropriate communication and leadership structures to ensure decisions are made both quickly and correctly. Hierarchical leadership structures, as established in many industrial companies, cannot meet this need. Instead, more and more organizations are developing decentralized leadership structures, up to and including self-leadership, which enable rapid decisions while making the best possible use of the knowledge available within the workforce.

Field of Action 4: Qualification

The requirements for employees in healthcare will change, in some cases rapidly, in the coming years. This calls for qualification measures not only for young people in vocational training/academization, but also for those already employed, who must learn to cope with new demands.

Field of Action 5: Purpose Economy

A corporate constitution in which healthcare provision and the creation of meaningful and adequately compensated jobs take center stage, and the financial interests of the owners play only a subordinate role, is an important success factor.

53.2.3 Purpose:Health e. V.

The *Purpose:Health e. V. network* is an initiative that aims to shape the transformation of the healthcare sector. Most of its members are roughly in the middle of their professional careers and therefore not only bring the skills required for smart change concepts, but also, due to their remaining professional years, the motivation to actually make a difference.

The main activities of the network include connecting people who, as innovators, are taking completely new paths and can benefit from others who have already had similar experiences. In addition, the network conducts research projects to better understand the challenges and solution strategies surrounding the transformation of the healthcare sector.

53.2.4 Purpose-Oriented Healthcare and Chronic Care

Chronic care plays a central role in addressing the long-term medical needs of people with chronic illnesses. The care of these individuals can benefit from organizational structures that primarily serve the purpose and, through modern process, leadership, and communication structures, enable high-performing health research. Digitalization, in turn, offers further opportunities to bridge space-time distances in the context of chronic care and serves as a supporter of the core idea of purpose-oriented healthcare.

Purpose orientation has the potential to improve the care pathway for chronic care patients by focusing on purpose and meaning and aiming to promote a self-determined life. The care pathway connects various healthcare providers who follow purpose principles to enhance agency and overall well-being. The focus is therefore not only on the situational consideration of a single point in time, but on empowering individuals to longitudinally address all challenges in leading a self-determined life.

Patient empowerment is an essential element in dealing with chronic diseases and promoting quality of life (see Contributions 18 & 19). In order to develop the individual path of patients in a purpose-oriented way, appropriate education of medical professionals is required. Together, they must identify values, purpose, meaning, and goals for ongoing care with their patients and operationalize the results. This process encourages patients to focus on what truly matters to them—beyond their illness—toward a self-determined life. Digitalization and data can support this process by better incorporating the individual history of patients in the sense of a biography. An example at this point is the electronic patient record (ePA) according to § 291a SGB V.

Goals are the essential anchor point, both for purpose-oriented organizations and for providers and patients. These must be realistic and meaningful and should always foresee an active role for patients. Digitalization in the sense of personalized care leverages the ever-growing volume of health data. Their analysis, for example through artificial intelligence, can support the identification of relevant goals as well as their monitoring, such as the derivation of personalized treatment plans or the early detection of complications. In addition, digital tools facilitate remote monitoring and real-time feedback.

Within the framework of chronic care, purpose thus prioritizes the well-being, safety, satisfaction, and self-determination of patients and makes use of data through digitalization. This promotion of improved patient outcomes is accompanied by enhanced collaboration: interprofessional cooperation with the aim and purpose of comprehensive care at a fair price. Thus, purpose does not negate the concept of efficiency, but rather seeks to maximize effects through a minimum of resource-related waste, for example, by optimizing human resources, reducing waiting times, and optimizing intra- and inter-organizational processes.

53.3 Outlook

It seems understandable that we need change for a future-proof healthcare system. The shortage of skilled workers will persist, as will demographic change. As so often, digitalization alone is seen as the lever for change, as it spares us from having to question the entire system as a whole. Thus, the BMG's digitalization strategy for the healthcare sector offers only a few building blocks and refrains from a significant revolution. This seems obvious, as digitalization is never an end in itself and would simply require a care strategy first. The strategic approach is a central anchor point, because without strategy there is no purpose. The strategy *configures* the purpose goals, which must subsequently be communicated and operationalized.

Every strategy brings change. People usually tolerate this only in small doses and mostly only when the purpose and benefit for their own well-being can be clearly identified. This is not always possible, so on the one hand, more community-oriented education is needed, and on the other hand, a structured approach—called *change management*. Purpose orientation means putting even greater focus on the human factor. Changes must be identified early and communicated appropriately.

The development path for a future, digitally supported healthcare system must not shy away from building competencies. In the sense of self-determination theory, well-being or motivation is promoted by ensuring that autonomy is not restricted, social connectedness is fostered, and there is neither competence overload nor underload. *Learning on the job* is a typical pattern. However, in this process, people only acquire what they subjectively perceive as relevant. This perception does not necessarily have to align with organizational goals and could even counteract the intended purpose. Purpose-oriented healthcare organizations identify and manage competencies along roles in the form of a competency matrix. Only in this way can training and development needs for employees be sufficiently derived.

The ever-increasing push for digitalization must make us aware that interactions are changing. This is currently perceived as a reduction in *human-to-human interaction* in favor of *human-technology interaction*. This new form of interaction between humans and technology must be actively shaped. We must avoid people experiencing confrontation through technology. Likewise, mere coexistence of both is not value-creating for a purpose-oriented target vision. Cooperation and collaboration between humans and technology make it possible to generate efficiency, which in turn can be invested in strengthening human-to-human interaction.

Finally, a purpose-oriented development path that incorporates digital innovations must always be considered from an ethical perspective and in terms of technology assessment. The effects of such innovations on purpose—here, meaning and purpose in the context of chronic care—must be evaluated at an early stage. More and more, *Patient-Reported Experience Measures* and *Patient-Reported Outcome Measures* must be included, and new procedures must also be developed to take the perspectives of employees into account.

References

Bundesministerium für Gesundheit (ed) (2023) Gemeinsam Digital: Digitalisierungsstrategie für das Gesundheitswesen und die Pflege. https://www.bundesgesundheitsministerium.de/fileadmin/Dateien/3_Downloads/D/Digitalisierungsstrategie/BMG_Broschuere_Digitalisierungsstrategie_bf.pdf. Accessed 4 Aug 2023

Ebert C, Duarte CHC (2018) Digital transformation. IEEE Softw 35(4):16–21. https://doi.org/10.1109/MS.2018.2801537

Hoffmann F, Khaladj N (2022) Digital Health als Funktionsbereich in Krankenhäusern: Erfahrungen nach zweijährigem Betrieb der Stabsstelle für medizinische Prozessentwicklung am Klinikum Darmstadt. Gesundheitsökonomie & Qualitätsmanagament. https://doi.org/10.1055/a19085409

Hoffmann F, Schumacher H (2022) Rechtliche Gestaltungsmöglichkeiten der Purpose Economy im Gesundheitswesen. Public Health Forum 30(3):180–184. https://doi.org/10.1515/pubhef-2022-0034

Oswald G, Saueressig T, Krcmar H (eds) (2022) Digitale Transformation: Fallbeispiele und Branchenanalysen, 2., überarb. Aufl. Springer Gabler, Wiesbaden

Ethical Aspects of the Use of Technical Systems for Vulnerable Persons

54

Arne Manzeschke and Galia Assadi

Contents

54.1 Digitalized Life Worlds—Digitalized Care

From its beginnings with the simplest tools taken from nature to recent robots, 'gene scissors,' or artificial intelligences, the history of human development has always also been a technical one. The development and use of technical instruments has a lasting

A. Manzeschke (✉)
Evangelische Hochschule Nürnberg, Ethik und Anthropologie, Nürnberg, Germany
e-mail: arne.manzeschke@evhn.de

G. Assadi
Wissenschaftliche Mitarbeiterin am Institut für Pflegeforschung, Gerontologie und Ethik, Nürnberg, Germany
e-mail: galia.assadi@evhn.de

D. Schmitz et al. (eds.), *Chronic Care—Science and Practice*,
https://doi.org/10.1007/978-3-662-72298-5_54

impact on the relationship that people have with their inner (e.g., self-concept) and outer nature (e.g., body), and continuously changes it. Technology expands the realm of human possibilities and structures it at the same time, by prescribing possibilities for its handling and use while excluding others. In this way, technology helps determine how people act, which decisions they make, and in which orders they can live together—in the end, therefore, who they are. Consequently, we humans in our technologically shaped life worlds can increasingly only understand ourselves on the basis of technologically generated perceptions, judgments, and actions (Adam et al. 2016). This circumstance, which is often overlooked when technology is established, is increasingly coming into the public consciousness through digitalization as a novel technology.[1,2] People are creating digitalized life worlds (Gransche and Manzeschke 2020), whose gains in safety, comfort, or health they do not want to miss, but whose risks and limitations they wish to avoid as much as possible. The development and establishment of digital devices and structures therefore requires responsible design and corresponding procedures for reflection, deliberation, and evaluation at the micro, meso, and macro levels of society. To fulfill this responsibility, we as humans, in our respective roles and statuses, must on the one hand reflect anticipatorily and act despite all uncertainties. On the other hand, we must try to retrospectively understand how we have reached the technological point we are at now, what it means for us, and which alternatives we have rejected and why. In addition, especially in the context of healthcare, even higher demands are placed, because the decisions we make there affect ill people, who are particularly dependent and vulnerable.

What can support us in ethical orientation? What kinds of knowledge do we need, what forms of reflection can show us paths we should take, but also wrong turns whose pursuit would be associated with significant losses? These questions are to be addressed in a mode of reflection that does not aim for ready-made answers, but instead enables those affected by the questions to find their own *coherent answers* for themselves and their context. This form of ethical reflection does not require prefabricated expert judgments that merely need to be implemented, but rather orientation instruments with which the necessary knowledge can be gained and individual ethical decision-making and responsibility can be supported.

[1] On the concept of technology (Grunwald 2013, pp. 13–17). For the distinction between *Technik* and *Technologie*, see Wiegerling (2000).

[2] The attention that generative AI, such as ChatGBT, Lamda, and others, has received illustrates this fact quite well: research on AI has been ongoing for seventy years now. The transformative or even disruptive potentials have been discussed since the 1990s. But only now, as the technology becomes known to and usable by the general public, is it widely recognized in society that fundamental changes may be imminent.

54.2 On the Conceptual Place of Ethics—What Must One Know to Judge Ethically?

To enable this form of ethical reflection, the perspective is shifted. This is intended to make clear what is often (too) briefly addressed in (premature) ethical analyses of technologization in healthcare: the reflection on the conditions of possibility for well-founded ethical judgments. In order to have an orienting effect in the lived reality of the people involved, these judgments cannot simply be exhausted in the *application* of traditional theoretical forms of reflection to current situations. In the context of technical assistance for chronically ill people, this means a thorough engagement with the existing technical possibilities. In this way, the danger can be averted that hypothetical reflections, which present theoretical options but not technical realities (as in the case of so-called *care robots,* Manzeschke and Assadi 2023), stir up fears and increase the prevailing lack of orientation. It is necessary to clarify the anthropological and ethical implications of the technology in question, in order to enable digital maturity at different levels of actors. This requires knowledge about digital systems and structures that goes beyond their use, and instead illuminates fundamental interactions, options, and limitations from different perspectives. Furthermore, it is necessary to analyze the context in which technology is to be used and to identify its specific characteristics (Böhme 1997). Important insights into what happens between humans and technology can also be gained by addressing anthropological questions, as these help to understand which conceptions of the human and of (good) human life are inscribed in socio-technical structures and practices. In this way, it can be examined whether and in what form a technologization project touches on these conceptions. In order to judge soundly, the most comprehensive possible knowledge of the object of judgment is essential, which is why it is of central importance to examine in detail what happens between humans and digital technology. Interactions between humans and technology must be described systematically and concretely in order to understand which actions, reactions, and interactions occur. This requires a methodological approach with which the often abstractly outlined human-technology relationships (e.g., the robot assists, the system supports users) can be described concretely and examined for their implications.

Here, the analytical focus on technical systems and their ethical implications is expanded from the outset to include their environments and associated dynamics, such as economization, which has brought about significant changes especially in healthcare (Maio 2014). To understand each of these dynamics in their respective effects, they must first be analyzed separately. However, to arrive at ethically robust judgments, responsible actions, and attitudes in digitalized worlds, the complexity of the structures and dynamics must be taken into account as fully as possible in a second step. To this end, we present elements of an instrument with which the interactions between humans and technical systems can be described concretely and examined for their anthropological implications.

54.3 On the Relationship Between Humans and Machines—Roles and Relations

The development, design, and application of human-technology relationships are influenced by assumptions about humans and technology acquired through socialization in a broad sense (this encompasses long-term elements such as mentality, culture, tradition, but also more short-term ones such as e.g. conventions, customs, contemporary trends), which are not, and often cannot be, fully conscious to either developers or users. Both conscious and unconscious notions guide construction and usage processes by orienting human actions, thoughts, and feelings, and by influencing the interpretation of situations and the selection of appropriate behavioral options. Implicit conceptions of humans (images of humans) and machines (images of machines) thus exert an indirect influence on human-technology interaction and thereby determine its success or failure. However, it must also be considered in a broader sense that the influence is not limited to a single concrete interaction, but that technology, through its mediality (Hubig et al. 2013), gradually changes the entire self-concept and worldview of humans.

Images of humans and machines achieve their orienting effect by reducing the complexity of the social and the technical, which is made possible by three construction principles:

1. Images of humans and machines link certain assumptions considered characteristic of humans or machines, bundle these into types (through *abstraction*), and implicitly exclude other possible and plausible options *(selection)*.
2. This focuses attention on specific aspects or behaviors of humans or technical systems *(reduction)*, systematically disregarding other information that could be relevant to the success of the interaction. For example, ill individuals are primarily reduced to their illness.
3. The selected aspects are often interpreted as static or ahistorical qualities of humans or technology *(fixation)*. This increases the risk of inadequately interpreting the real dynamics, flexibility, and variability of human life and human forms of interaction and relationships, both with other humans and with technical systems.

If there is a lack of alignment between the images of humans and machines held by designers of technical systems and those held by users, these images can hinder successful development and implementation and create orientation problems, which is why they should be critically reflected upon and, if necessary, corrected. This critical reflection is a form of active orientation within and about increasingly complex human-machine relationships, taking into account the fact that human orientation always presupposes a form of being oriented (Stegmaier 2008). The acquired orientation influences perception, emotional and rational interpretation, ethical evaluation of the situation, as well as practical handling of it, and can only be identified through targeted analysis.

To enable this form of analysis, we propose an orientation framework that allows for the concrete description and analysis of the use case scenario, the human-technology relationship, and the roles assigned to humans and technical systems. This provides an anthropologically and technically informed understanding of concrete human-technology relations, serving as a basis for ethical evaluation. In order to assess what actually occurs between humans and technology, and whether these events are desirable or should be prevented, a description of the specific use case must be created that makes clear what (social) objective is being pursued through the use of a technical system. The more detailed the description, the better the human-technology relationship and its implications can be understood. This verbal form of representation is formalized in a use case diagram *(use case diagram)*. In this form of modeling, which originates from computer science (Kecher 2005), every single action performed by the system is depicted. Thus, on the one hand, the abstract objectives named in the use case scenario (e.g., technology is to contribute to promoting autonomy/technology is to enable participation) are described in the form of discrete (technical) actions and interactions, and on the other hand, the relationships between individual actions on the human and technical sides are clarified. This approach enables a precise understanding of the functioning of technical systems as well as the expectations placed on users and technical systems. Furthermore, it allows for questions regarding the technical and social preconditions that must be met in order to realize interactions in the planned form—questions that are often unconsciously assumed or not explicitly addressed in ethical analysis. To gain a sound understanding of the images of humans and machines articulated in the *use case scenario* and the *use case diagram*, these are analyzed using the *concept of roles*. The concept of roles is used in both technical and non-technical disciplines to explain (social and/or technical) orders of interaction. The multidisciplinary use and structural analogy of role concepts opens up interdisciplinary communication, although the differences between disciplinary conceptions must be taken into account. The concept of roles serves in four ways as a hinge that makes explicit and thus open to reflection the connection between areas that are often conceived in isolation and dualistically:

1. Connection between humans and technology (the concept of roles is present in both domains).
2. Connection between humans and society (acquisition and internalization of expectations linked to roles through socialization processes).
3. Connection between concrete interaction situations and social order (the adequate performance of a role stabilizes social order, whereas deviant behavior calls this order into question).
4. Connection between past and present—since present-day representations of roles express expectations developed and stabilized in the past, the often excluded historical and social preconditions for human-technology interactions become more apparent.

By referring to roles and the expectations articulated through them, the attributed potentials, needs, and deficits of role holders can be identified. The potentials and deficits associated with the roles of humans and machines, in turn, allow conclusions to be drawn about the norms linked to them and articulated through them. Behavioral norms formulate the rules associated with a role and, in turn, refer to abstract values (such as freedom, justice, equality). Approaching the issue through norms and values also enables reflection on the context of the respective interaction, since both norms and values always refer to a specific historical and social scope of validity.

This structured analysis of human-technology relationships allows for a better understanding of the events between humans and technology that are to be ethically evaluated. The basis for reflection is significantly expanded to include both individual and structural aspects of the respective context of use that are relevant for ethical assessment. In the present case, in abstract terms, this concerns the healthcare sector, as the question here is to clarify the legitimacy of using technical systems with vulnerable groups. To this end, the concept of vulnerability will first be outlined.

54.4 The Human Being as a Vulnerable Creature

The conceptual origins of vulnerability lie in the field of disaster research and thus in technical contexts, where the term was first developed conceptually at the end of the 1970s (O'Keefe et al. 1976). It was primarily applied in the analysis of complex systems (such as climate), with particular focus on identifying potential systematic weaknesses. Building on these beginnings in climate and environmental research, the term has, in recent decades, diffused into the human and social sciences. From an anthropological perspective, a number of key questions arise in reflecting on human vulnerability: Is vulnerability understood as an exceptional situation or as a regular condition? Should vulnerability be understood as binary or as a matter of degree? What is the basis of vulnerability and how is it addressed? Based on these questions, two positions can be distinguished in simplified terms.

54.4.1 Vulnerability as a Disruptive Factor

In theories that primarily characterize humans by their capacity for autonomy and thus sketch them mainly as animal rationale (e.g., Kant, Hegel, Rawls, Beauchamps and Childress), vulnerability is conceived as an exceptional state that confronts humans with aspects of their biological, psychological, and social constitution that cannot be overcome through rational reflection. Since the physical and psychological integrity of the autonomous human is usually taken for granted in these theories, vulnerability, illness, and dependency appear as disruptions to be remedied or, if that is not possible, alleviated.

Thus, on the one hand, vulnerable groups can be distinguished from non-vulnerable groups (binary classification). Technology is conceived here as an assisting instrument in the service of overcoming or mitigating vulnerable states, as a tool for restoring a *normal state* of physical integrity and autonomy. If this is not possible, technology is often seen as an aid to reduce human dependency or as a substitute for human support when such support is unavailable. This perspective is reminiscent of the view common in technology-oriented disciplines, which uses vulnerability as an analytical category to identify the threat potential to the functionality of systems (Wachsmuth et al. 2012). From the perspective of technology assessment, a vulnerability analysis contributes to answering the question of how threats to system functionality can be excluded and resilience potentials strengthened or built up.

With regard to human vulnerability, technology is tasked with compensating for the loss of capability and enabling people to once again participate autonomously in everyday life. Vulnerability is primarily understood as a danger, and accordingly, technology is constructed as an instrument of risk mitigation, in order to at least partially control the undesirable and yet unavoidable fact of vulnerability.

54.4.2 Vulnerability as an Anthropological Constant

While autonomy-centered theories conceive of vulnerability as a disruptive fact that should ideally be overcome with the help of technology, relational theories conceptualize it as an inescapable characteristic of human existence (Levinas 2008; Waldenfels 2000). Relational theories emphasize that corporeality and vulnerability can only be conceived together, and that vulnerability must be understood as a precondition for corporeality. Based on the thesis that subjective life can only be understood as conditional life and is thus dependent on supportive norms and relationships, every life is characterized in principle as vulnerable and at risk (Butler 2009). Vulnerability is understood as an ambivalent characteristic of the conditio humana, which emphasizes the inescapable dependence on others, but at the same time frames this as openness and thus as an opportunity for growth, learning, and development (Matthews and Tobin 2016). Against this background, technology appears not only as an instrument for fulfilling human objectives, but as a precondition for human existence. Technology shapes the relationships that people have with themselves and with others. Technical structures, which can be understood as social conditions of human life, thus help determine who the vulnerable human being can be and how people can live together. Here, technology determines, among other things, which aspects of the human are considered relevant, which are disregarded (because they cannot be technically captured), and which are deemed negligible.

To understand how we can act ethically responsibly and what kind of relationship we should have with people and technology, we must first find answers to the question of how we understand ourselves.

54.5 Ethics and Vulnerability—How Can and Should Technology Enable a Responsible Approach to Vulnerability?

The status attributed to vulnerability at the anthropological level helps determine which ethical questions are raised, which ethical obligations we seek to fulfill, and which boundaries we consider non-negotiable. Structurally analogous to the differences in anthropology, two traditions of thought can also be distinguished in the field of ethics. These, too, can be characterized by the pair of concepts autonomy and relationality. They either emphasize human autonomy as a precondition for ethical judgment and action, or human relationality, sociality, and vulnerability, which are both the basis for action and decision-making and the source of obligation. To illustrate the aforementioned differences, these are briefly listed below.

Ethics of Autonomy

- Focus on individual autonomy
- Physical integrity
- Justice (conceived as distributive or performance-based justice between actors conceptualized as isolated)
- Focus on concrete actions while simultaneously facing the challenge of including enabling structures in ethical deliberation
- Avoidance of manipulation and deception
- Data protection and data security as obligations resulting from respect for privacy
- Responsibility is linked to sovereignty. The person who performs the concrete action is considered responsible.

Relational Ethics

- Focus on enabling relationships. Capturing the vulnerable person within their network of relationships
- Embodiment (relationality, openness, capacity for sensation)
- Justice with regard to structures that enable the greatest possible diversity of life and experience forms
- The relationship between caregiver and caretaker is not only discussed from the one-sided perspective of change on the part of the caretaker, but its influence on the caregiver also becomes apparent.
- Prohibition of discrimination
- Sensitivity to complexity
- Emphasis on and appreciation of emotions as a resource for thinking and acting, not as a disruptive factor

54.6 Technology as a Response to the Recognition of Vulnerability

Support for chronically ill individuals can generally expect to receive swift consent. This does not fundamentally change with the use of technical systems. However, a closer look at our concepts of vulnerability quickly reveals that a more nuanced, ultimately dialectical approach is required. The use of technical systems actually intensifies the problem and the necessity for a comprehensive analysis of the socio-technical arrangements and the underlying self-conceptions and motivations driving them. Without a concrete, well-founded, anthropologically and technically informed understanding of human-technology relations, ethical judgments usually remain abstract and prove to be of little practical relevance or sustainability. We advocate for an anthropological reflection that should necessarily precede ethical reflection, especially since digital technologies also challenge us on an anthropological level by questioning previously valid distinctions between human and machine. The result of this form of reflection is a concrete scenario that unites different perspectives, which not only abstractly states what technical systems are supposed to accomplish in practice (the system assists, etc.), but, through micro-level analysis of individual actions between human and technical system, first makes the interaction between human and technology comprehensible for designers and users. This scenario serves as the basis for ethical evaluation, which can be carried out using an established model such as MEESTAR (Manzeschke et al. 2013). This form of ethical evaluation requires a concrete scenario that is assessed according to different moral dimensions. Additionally, MEESTAR offers an integration of various social-structural perspectives (individual, organizational, societal), allowing technology to be evaluated both in terms of its concrete implications for the respective users and with regard to its societal effects.

References

Adam MH, Gellai S, Knifka J (2016) Technisierte Lebenswelt: Über den Prozess der Figuration von Mensch und Technik. Transcript, Bielefeld

Böhme G (1997) Ethik im Kontext. Über den Umgang mit ernsten Fragen. Suhrkamp, Frankfurt am Main

Butler J (2009) Gefährdetes Leben. Suhrkamp, Frankfurt am Main

Gransche B, Manzeschke A (eds) (2020) Das geteilte Ganze. Horizonte Integrierter Forschung für künftige Mensch-Technik-Verhältnisse. Springer VS, Wiesbaden

Grunwald A (2013) „Technik“. In: Armin Grunwald (ed) Handbuch Technikethik. J. B. Metzler, Stuttgart-Weimar, pp 13–17

Hubig C, Huning A, Ropohl G (eds) (2013) Nachdenken über Technik: Die Klassiker der Technikphilosophie und neuere Entwicklungen. Edition sigma, Baden-Baden

Lévinas E (2008) Totalität und Unendlichkeit. Versuch über die Exteriorität. Karl Alber, Freiburg/München

Kecher C (2005) UML 2.0. Das umfassende Handbuch. Rheinwerk-Verlag, Bonn
Maio G (2014) Geschäftsmodell Gesundheit. Wie der Markt die Heilkunst abschafft. Suhrkamp, Frankfurt am Main
Manzeschke A, Assadi G (2023) Künstliche Emotion – Zum ethischen Umgang mit Gefühlen zwischen Mensch und Technik. Ethik in der Medizin. Springer
Manzeschke A, Weber K, Rother E, Fangerau H (2013) Ethische Fragen im Bereich altersgerechter Assistenzsysteme: Ergebnisse der Studie. VDI/VDE Innovation, Berlin
Matthews S, Tobin B (2016) Human vulnerability in medical contexts. Theor Med Bioeth 37(1):1–7
O'Keefe P, Westgate K, Wisner B (1976) Taking the naturalness out of natural disasters. Nature 260
Stegmaier W (2008) Philosophie der Orientierung. Walter de Gruyter, Berlin/New York
Wachsmuth J et al (2012) Sektorale Vulnerabilität: Energiewirtschaft. In: Schuchardt B, Wittig S (eds) Vulnerabilität der Metropolregion Bremen-Oldenburg gegenüber dem Klimawandel (Synthesebericht). nordwest2050- Berichte Heft 2, Projektkonsortium, pp 95–112
Waldenfels B (2000) Das leibliche Selbst. Vorlesungen zur Phänomenologie des Leibes. Suhrkamp, Frankfurt am Main
Wiegerling (2000) Der Titel lautet: Klaus Wiegerling: „Technik". In: Ralf Schnell (ed) Metzler Lexikon Kultur der Gegenwart. J. B. Metzler, Stuttgart-Weimar, pp 501–502

Instruments for Evaluating the Usefulness and Effectiveness of Digital Technologies

55

Patrizia Held and Ulrike Lindwedel

Contents

55.1 Background—Problem Statement

Digital technologies have become an essential element in healthcare, aiming to bridge the gap between medical care and the self-management of people with chronic illnesses (see contribution 36). To assess the effectiveness and usefulness of such technologies, appropriate evaluation instruments are required to ensure that digital solutions truly provide added value and benefits for care and are accepted by all stakeholders. However, due to the diversity of people with chronic illnesses, which is accompanied by various impairments and competencies, evaluations of effectiveness and usefulness face challenges for which no standardized approach can be proposed. It is important to consider

P. Held · U. Lindwedel (✉)
Hochschule Furtwangen, Institut Mensch Institut Mensch, Technik und Teilhabe, Furtwangen, Deutschland
e-mail: ulrike.lindwedel@hfu.eu

P. Held
e-mail: patrizia.held@hfu.eu

D. Schmitz et al. (eds.), *Chronic Care—Science and Practice*,
https://doi.org/10.1007/978-3-662-72298-5_55

the use of technology from multiple perspectives and in a transdisciplinary manner in order to evaluate the impact and actual added value for the individual care of people with chronic illnesses.

This chapter presents and discusses various instruments for assessing the usefulness and effectiveness of digital technologies in the context of chronic care, taking into account the great heterogeneity of people with chronic illnesses.

55.2 Instruments for Assessing Usefulness

The prerequisite for achieving high usefulness and acceptance of digital health technologies lies in understanding the users and the context of use. Especially in the context of chronic care, a lack of knowledge about users leads to offerings and their underlying technology being developed past the needs of people with chronic illnesses. The involvement of experts alone is not sufficient to understand the living environment of those affected. Usefulness and usability of digital technologies arise primarily from understanding the problem situation as well as the motivations and needs of users in their specific contexts of use. Thus, user acceptance must be ensured and consistently considered from the outset through continuous user research. Holtzblatt and Breyer (2014) refer in this context to Contextual Inquiry (CI)—a method that combines classical interview techniques and observational approaches. Context of use analyses help to understand the context and framework conditions in which a technology is to be used and to gain insights into the actual needs, requirements, and expectations of users.

To assess the usefulness of digital technologies for people with chronic illnesses, various instruments can be employed. These relate to different aspects of capturing or ensuring usefulness, such as acceptance and usability criteria, user experience, accessibility, and, increasingly in recent years, participation in the sense of actively involving those affected in development processes. The acceptance of digital technologies by users is a decisive factor for their success in chronic care. This is ensured by a positive user experience. Ensuring and reviewing user acceptance of digital technologies in chronic care is important at all times. The evaluation and assessment of user acceptance can, for example, be determined using the Technology Acceptance Model (*TAM*) (Holden and Karsh 2010) or the Unified Theory of Acceptance and Use of Technology (*UTAUT*) (Venkatesh et al. 2003). These instruments measure factors such as perceived usefulness and ease of use as well as social influences on the acceptance of digital technologies. The Health Information Technology Acceptance Model (*HITAM*) (Kim and Park 2012) is specifically designed to assess the acceptance of health technologies. The *TPB* (Theory of Planned Behaviour) (Ajzen 1991) can also be used to make statements about acceptance. With regard to the acceptance of digital technologies for people with chronic illnesses, the TPB can be used to understand how likely they are to adopt and use these technologies.

Depending on the specific context and objectives, other instruments or modified versions of the aforementioned instruments may also be used. It is important to select the appropriate instruments according to the specific requirements of the target group. In addition, acceptance is determined by other factors such as anxiety, technological self-efficacy, innovativeness, and trust (AlQudah et al. 2021). For high user acceptance, it is also advisable to actively involve the user group throughout all development phases of digital health technologies from the outset. This has a fundamental impact on the acceptance and adoption of the technology, as the active involvement of those affected brings their needs, requirements, and perspectives to the forefront of development and enables a user-centered and realistic design of technologies tailored to the specific challenges and life circumstances of these individuals. Furthermore, involvement promotes empowerment and self-determination, as those affected are given the opportunity to improve their own situation and participate in decisions that affect their lives.

User acceptance is also influenced by ease of use, which can be captured in the development process both through the usability of a technology and through the user experience. Usability is objectively measurable, whereas user experience is based on the subjective feelings that users have before and after using a technology. The evaluation of these criteria serves to identify potential weaknesses of the technology from the perspective of those affected and to improve the user experience. However, this is a complex task for people with chronic illnesses, as factors such as multimorbidity or heterogeneity must be taken into account. For this reason, a mixed-methods approach is particularly suitable to do justice to the complexity and individuality involved.

From a qualitative perspective, targeted information about the experiences and assessments of users with chronic illnesses can be collected, for example, through structured or semi-structured interviews and questionnaires. In addition, for individuals without cognitive impairments, standardized questionnaires can be used to assess usability. Standardized questionnaires such as the System Usability Scale (SUS) or the Post-Study System Usability Questionnaire (PSSUQ) serve to subjectively assess usability from the users' perspective. In the case of cognitive impairments, however, ethnographic methods such as observational studies play an important role. Furthermore, a professional assessment of usability can be provided by experts, offering valuable recommendations for improving the user experience. However, it should be noted that the lack of real-life experience means that the involvement of experts should only be considered as a supplement to the actual user group.

Regardless of the choice of instrument, continuous evaluation and adaptation of technologies to the needs of people with chronic illnesses within an iterative process is essential and makes a significant contribution to the development or selection of a solution that is actually needed, accepted, and ultimately used by those affected.

55.3 Instruments for Evaluating Effectiveness

Measuring the effectiveness of digital technologies in chronic care is a complex undertaking. A standardized assessment of their effectiveness is complicated by the multitude of digital possibilities. In addition, chronic diseases are often complex and multifaceted. They require long-term care that encompasses various aspects of patients' health and well-being. The effectiveness of digital technologies must therefore be measured using various parameters. These include, for example, health-related indicators such as quality of life or health status, behavioral indicators such as self-management, satisfaction, or health literacy, care-related indicators such as hospitalization rates or number of physician contacts, as well as system-related indicators such as technology adoption, technology use, or usability and accessibility (Zanaboni et al. 2018). Moreover, each patient has individual needs and life circumstances. What may be effective for one patient may not work for another. Therefore, digital technologies must be evaluated in terms of their adaptability to different patient profiles and needs.

Furthermore, evaluating the effectiveness of digital technologies often requires a long-term perspective. Digital technologies may prove effective over time, for example by improving patients' self-management skills or reducing hospitalizations. Overall, measuring the effectiveness of digital technologies in chronic care is a complex task that requires a comprehensive understanding of the technologies, disease patterns, and the individual needs of patients.

From a quantitative perspective, randomized controlled trials (RCTs), in which digital interventions are compared with standard treatments or other interventions, represent the status quo and are particularly suitable for efficacy studies in the context of chronic care (Zanaboni et al. 2018). RCTs allow for the assessment of effectiveness based on objective clinical outcomes. In addition, instruments for capturing patient-reported criteria can also be used. These include, for example, quality of life questionnaires, symptom scales, or cognitive tests to capture patients' subjective perceptions. Depending on the chronic disease, however, measurement using subjective rating scales is not always straightforward. Demonstrating the effectiveness of technology use in people with chronic illnesses can therefore be associated with a number of challenges. People with chronic illnesses form a heterogeneous group with different disease patterns, severities, and individual needs. The effectiveness of a technology can therefore vary from person to person. Measuring the effectiveness of a technology over a longer period can be challenging, as factors such as long-term compliance, changes in disease progression, and other external influences must be taken into account. Moreover, technologies for people with chronic illnesses often involve complex interventions that include various components, such as self-management tools, monitoring systems, and communication platforms. It is not trivial to consider the specific effect of each individual component in isolation and to assess the overall impact of the intervention. The effectiveness of a technology also depends heavily on contextual factors, such as the social environment or integration into existing healthcare provision. Furthermore, when using technologies in healthcare, ethical aspects and privacy protection, as well as data, are always of great importance. Demonstrating the effectiveness of a technology must be in line with legal and ethical frameworks. In addition, personal attitudes toward technology and motivation to use it also influence the effectiveness of a technology. It can be challenging, in addition to users, to motivate all other stakeholders involved in care to use the technology continuously and actively integrate it into their daily care routines.

Taking these challenges into account is crucial in order to assess the effectiveness of technology use in people with chronic illnesses and to ensure that the technology actually has a positive impact on the health and well-being of users.

55.4 Summary and Conclusion

Evaluating the usefulness and acceptance of digital technologies for people with chronic illnesses requires a holistic approach. It is important to consider both the specific chronic condition and the care arrangement. The choice of instruments depends on the specific objectives of the evaluation and the existing competencies of people with chronic illnesses. Flexible methodological and methodological approaches are needed to meet the complex needs of people with chronic illnesses. Due to the multitude of individual factors, it seems necessary to use qualitative approaches and to recognize them as equivalent in order to gain a comprehensive understanding of individual needs. In addition, participatory involvement of people with chronic illnesses at the stage of technology development can help ensure that the solutions developed are better tailored to their needs, increase their acceptance and adoption, and ultimately improve their quality of life.

References

Ajzen I (1991) The therory of planned behavior. Organ. Behav Hum Decis Process 50(2):179–211

AlQudah A, Al-Emran M, Shaalan K (2021) Technology acceptance in healthcare: a systematic review. Appl Sci 11(22):10537

Holden R, Karsh B-T (2010) The technology acceptance model: its past and its future in health care. J Biomed Inf 43(1):159–172

Holtzblatt K, Beyer H (2014) Contextual design. In: The Interaction Design Foundation IxDF. The encyclopedia of human-computer interaction, 2nd edn. Chapter 8.

Kim J, Park H-A (2012) Development of a health information technology acceptance model using consumers' health behavior intention. J Med Internet Res 14(5):e133

Venkatesh V, Morris M, Davis G, Davis F (2003) User acceptance of information technology: toward a unified view. MIS Q 27(3):425

Zanaboni P, Ngangue P, Mbemba G, Schopf T, Bergmo T, Gagnon M-P (2018) Methods to evaluate the effects of Internet-based digital health interventions for citizens: systematic review of reviews. J Med Internet Res 20(6):e10202

Part V

Implementation of Chronic Care

Implementation of Transdisciplinary Educational Concepts

56

Daniela Schmitz and Jan-Hendrik Ortloff

Contents

56.1 Fundamentals of a Transdisciplinary and Transprofessional Pedagogy

Transdisciplinary learning transcends traditional boundaries and includes the disciplines involved within the learning process. As a result of these processes, disciplinary theories and methods are integrated and reconfigured within joint teaching and research.

For instructors and learners to develop a transdisciplinary orientation and mindset, it is necessary to engage with values, norms, conceptual skills, and knowledge that go beyond the established disciplinary boundaries of the academic system. Budwig and Alexander (2020) point out that the implementation of transdisciplinary concepts is

D. Schmitz (✉) · J.-H. Ortloff
Department of human medicine, Witten/Herdecke University, Witten, Germany
e-mail: Daniela.Schmitz@uni-wh.de

J.-H Ortloff
e-mail: Jan-Hendrik.Ortloff@uni-wh.de

D. Schmitz et al. (eds.), *Chronic Care—Science and Practice*,
https://doi.org/10.1007/978-3-662-72298-5_56

hindered by the focus on disciplinary structures, training, and knowledge systems of instructors and learners.

Disciplinarily narrow programs must address goal conflicts that arise between disciplinary and transdisciplinary bodies of knowledge and methodological approaches. Furthermore, initiatives for transdisciplinary learning spaces are hampered by administrative and legal barriers, as the disciplinary positioning and the appropriate timing of transdisciplinary approaches remain unresolved. It is still unclear whether disciplinary grounding is first required to enable transdisciplinary thinking, or whether transdisciplinary learning opportunities should be offered as early as possible to avoid disciplinary narrowness (Vilsmayer 2021).

Transdisciplinary educational approaches address problems in various subject areas that cannot be solved within a single discipline and design learning arrangements with dialogic formats that incorporate different types of knowledge (Philip and Schmohl 2021). To achieve this, these learning arrangements must integrate diverse perspectives and include opportunities for participation. The learning processes are iterative and collaborative, characterized by continuous interaction, internal reflection, and engagement with external stakeholders.

Transprofessionality, on the other hand, describes collaboration among different professional groups that goes beyond disciplinary boundaries and unites specialized knowledge to develop comprehensive solutions to problems (Schmitz and Schmohl 2021). Transprofessional cooperation transcends traditional responsibilities and areas of competence, thereby challenging established hierarchies. A transprofessional didactics focuses on developing universal skills in communication, cooperation, and collaboration.

56.2 Framework Conditions for Transdisciplinary Didactic Concepts

Key framework conditions for transdisciplinary concepts are time, structures, and wicked problems. The time factor includes periods for developing and coordinating joint syllabi and curricula, as well as the preparation and implementation of teaching content by the participating faculties, instructors, and learners. It also includes time to assess prior knowledge and experience, as well as to reflect on transdisciplinary experiences. Regarding structures, Yeung (2021) points out that transdisciplinary learning is not a matter of hours or days, since after an event, learners return to their disciplinary structures and cannot apply the new, transdisciplinary knowledge there.

Wicked problems are characterized by multiple perspectives, unpredictability, and complexity, and are addressed through reflective practice (Daneshpour and Kwegyir-Afful 2022). They form the basis for transdisciplinary learning content such as Planetary Health, One Health, climate change, food security, public health, or social justice. Transdisciplinary didactic concepts often include agile approaches with broadly defined goals. Design-oriented approaches such as Design Based Research interlink the development of innovative solutions to practical educational problems with the generation of scientific knowledge (Euler 2021). Implementation is guided by the perspective of how desirable and yet-to-be-specified goals can be achieved with interventions that are still to be developed, rather than solely assessing the effectiveness of an intervention.

Approaches to transdisciplinary didactics involve expanded roles for participants and more intensive processes of discussion and reflection. The foundation for developing and implementing joint concepts is trust, understanding, respect, and a coordinated selection of disciplinary learning content (Velez et al. 2022).

Van der Voorde (2018) summarizes the challenges. Disciplinary technical languages must be adapted and methods aligned to reach consensus. The learning environment also plays a role, as institutions are organized along disciplinary lines, leading to institutional constraints. Career paths follow disciplinary logics, which means that inter- and transdisciplinary skills receive little recognition.

Transdisciplinary teaching requires knowledge of different disciplines and flexible structures, as well as effective transdisciplinary concepts that include longitudinal elements and reflection. In the literature, transprofessional education is understood as situations where learners from clinical professions learn together with learners from other professions. In contrast, transprofessional learning refers to situations where instructors from different professions engage in continuing education together. Both approaches aim, using the example of reflective practice, to close gaps between teaching activities and clinical care (Field et al. 2020).

A truly transdisciplinary didactic approach, implemented according to the requirements of this concept, requires reforms of existing curricula, knowledge systems, and institutional structures (Vilsmayer 2021). In addition, coordination with non-university partners and stakeholders from politics, business, culture, and civil society is necessary.

56.3 Designing Transdisciplinary Educational Concepts

Fundamentally, points of connection must be identified when different disciplines learn together. Suitable elements include those that facilitate learning through authentic situations and problems, or that aim to recognize patterns (McGregor 2017). In the long term, integration should be pursued that includes regular opportunities for reflection on learning experiences and challenges, so that acquired transdisciplinary skills can be applied.

In principle, the target group includes learners from all disciplines. The establishment of learning communities can be a way to implement this, enabling students to share influence, needs, events, and connections for joint learning (McGregor 2017). Planning requires knowledge of the target group, their interests, prior knowledge, previous experiences, and learning habits.

Teaching and learning objectives include skills in collaboration, communication, reflection, beliefs and attitudes, as well as metacognitive abilities. The integration of disciplinary perspectives and methods should be coordinated within the team, taking into account the target group. Learning formats can be designed to focus on individuals, processes, or groups. Suitable approaches include, among others:

- Service learning, which combines academic learning with student engagement
- Problem-based learning, which supports problem-solving based on rules and predefined steps
- Project-based learning through authentic projects with societal stakeholders
- Forms of research-based learning, in which students investigate problems based on their own questions
- Experiential learning, which engages with real-world problems
- Design thinking, as a creative and simultaneously analytical process that generates solutions from the perspective of future users
- Transformative learning, in which individual assumptions are critically reflected upon in order to change them
- Approaches from citizen science, understood as projects involving interested citizens, as well as in real-world laboratories or living labs, where innovations are tested under real conditions.

56.4 Guiding Questions for the Implementation of Transdisciplinary Educational Concepts

The starting point for approaches to implementing transdisciplinary didactic concepts is the question of how changes become routine from the perspective of those involved. Normalization Process Theory analyzes these processes of change on the path to new routines and explains why changes do or do not become routine.

Wood (2017) has specifically addressed change and the sustainable implementation of transformation in the education sector. He characterized changes that exist only in strategic plans and are described as successful in reports as *zombie innovations*, which never actually take effect in practice. For the implementation of transdisciplinary educational concepts, the guiding questions proposed by Wood have been thematically adapted and referenced in parentheses to the terms of Normalization Process Theory:

1. Individual goals and perceptions of meaning associated with the change (coherence): "What does implementing transdisciplinary concepts mean for me?" is the guiding question as a starting point. This can be broken down into further sub-questions:
   - What is new about transdisciplinary educational approaches for me?
   - What goals do I associate with it?
   - Does the implementation of transdisciplinary concepts have a clear objective?
   - Can I articulate the planned change?
   - Do we (in my work area, etc.) have a shared goal?
   - What potential benefits does implementing transdisciplinary educational concepts offer in our teaching area?

2. Involvement of those affected and stakeholders in the change (cognitive participation): The second step is shaped by the question of who will be involved in the implementation and in what form. Stakeholders can use the following guiding questions to structure the change conceptually:
   - Who is affected by the implementation of transdisciplinary didactic concepts?
   - Who does what with whom? Who needs to be informed, when, and how?
   - What do others expect from me? What do I expect from them?
   - What do the participants think transdisciplinary didactics should look like?
   - What forms of collaboration are necessary for this?
3. Planning and carrying out a joint implementation of the changes (collective action): This step addresses the question of how the transdisciplinary educational concepts can be implemented and how they are compatible with existing routines:
   - How can the transdisciplinary concepts be reconciled with daily work or other teaching concepts?
   - What competencies and resources do we and the learners need?
   - How are tasks for implementation distributed, assigned, and supported?
4. Reflection and evaluation of the change (reflexive monitoring): The final step of the change process addresses the question of how the change and its effects are evaluated:
   - What impact has the experienced implementation had on me?
   - By what standards can this be evaluated?
   - How do we reflect on these changes?
   - What consequences does it have for teaching practice in my area?

Through joint discussion and reflection on these questions within the team of the work area involved in the implementation, both facilitating and hindering aspects of the process can be identified and the implementation can be advanced. The catalog of questions can also be specified for particular topics and can be used in preparation for the implementation process, as a tool for individual reflection during practice, and within the teams involved.

References

Budwig N, Alexander JA (2020) A transdisciplinary approach to student learning and development in university settings. Front Psychol 11. https://doi.org/10.3389/fpsyg.2020.576250

Daneshpour H, Kwegyir-Afful E (2022) Analysing transdisciplinary education: a scoping review. Sci Educ 31:1047–1074

Euler D (2021) Gestaltungsorientierte Lehrforschung. In: Phlipp T, Schmohl T (eds) Handbuch Transdisziplinäre Didaktik. Transcript, Bielefeld, pp 119

Field J, Hervey T, Valachovic R (2020) ADEA-ADEE shaping the future of dental education III: from interprofessional education to transprofessional learning: reflections from dentistry, applied linguistics, and law. J Dent Educ 84(1):105–110

McGregor SLT (2017) Transdisciplinary pedagogy in higher education: transdisciplinary learning, learning cycles and habits of minds. In: Gibbs P (ed) Transdisciplinary higher education. A theoretical basis revealed in practice. Springer, Cham, pp 3–16
Phlipp T, Schmohl T (2021) Transdisziplinäre Didaktik. In: Phlipp T, Schmohl T (eds) Handbuch Transdisziplinäre Didaktik. Transcript, Bielefeld, pp 13–24
Schmitz D, Schmohl T (2021) Transprofessionalität. In: Phlipp T, Schmohl T (eds) Handbuch Transdisziplinäre Didaktik. Transcript, Bielefeld, pp 357–367
Velez AL, Hall RP, Lewis SN (2022) Designing transdisciplinarity: exploring institutional drivers and barriers to collaborative transdisciplinary teaching. J Public Aff Educ 28(2):138–155
Vilsmayer U (2021) Transdisziplinarität. In: Phlipp T, Schmohl T (eds) Handbuch Transdisziplinäre Didaktik. Transcript, Bielefeld, pp 333–346
van der Voorde M (2018) Universities: enhancing the education, research and innovation base. ERUDITIO 2(4):112–122
Wood P (2017) Overcoming the problem of embedding change. Manag Educ 31(1):33–38
Yeung E, Carlin L, Sandassie S (2021) Transdisciplinary training: what does it take to address today's "wicked problems"? Innov Educ 3:4

Research-Led Approaches to Chronic Care Science

57

Manfred Fiedler, Simone Hatebur and Daniela Schmitz

Contents

57.1 Challenges of Health Services Research in Chronic Diseases

Health services research in the context of chronic disease, due to the diverse contextual references in care, must fundamentally address the issue of complex interventions. Complex interventions are characterized by, first, the fact that individual interventions are

M. Fiedler (✉) · D. Schmitz
Department of human medicine, Witten/Herdecke University, Witten, Deutschland
e-mail: manfred.fiedler@uni-wh.de

D. Schmitz
e-mail: Daniela.Schmitz@uni-wh.de

S. Hatebur
Faculty of Health, Witten/Herdecke University, Witten, Deutschland
e-mail: simone.hatebur@uni-wh.de

D. Schmitz et al. (eds.), *Chronic Care—Science and Practice*,
https://doi.org/10.1007/978-3-662-72298-5_57

directly related to each other and mutually influence each other in terms of implementation and effect; second, that more than one professional group is usually involved in their implementation; and third, that the interaction with the environmental conditions of the respective care setting plays a major role.

In this context, a distinction must be made between the categorical approach and the non-categorical approach. This distinction is important with regard to the question, on the one hand, of which disease-specific factors are relevant in disease management and health interventions (categorical), and on the other hand, with regard to the environmental conditions in chronic diseases (non-categorical approach), which are of particular significance, as the disease situation for those affected becomes individually normalized in relation to their own life situation and thus also specifically typified.

The undoubtedly necessary disease-categorical research thus represents *only* one field of research, in which medicine, psychology, nursing, and therapy sciences are primarily involved. The non-categorical approach expands this research, especially by including the everyday/life-world context of chronic disease. The focus is on family research, neighborhood research, social ecology or social work, and health science subdisciplines such as social medicine, environmental psychology, or palliative care.

Inter-/transdisciplinary connections become apparent in both approaches. This is especially true in research on complex interventions. In particular, in the non-categorical approach, classical methods of evidence generation, such as randomized controlled trials (RCTs), can only be used to a limited extent. Qualitative methods such as ethnographic and biographical research, action-in-action research, or participant observation are of outstanding importance. With regard to the evaluation of complex interventions in the field of chronic care, it is therefore appropriate to speak of science-based effectiveness.

57.2 Inter-/Transdisciplinary Research Understanding

Inter- and transdisciplinary research can contribute to a broader gain in knowledge, but is often criticized for conceptual confusion, being expensive and superficial, and therefore requires supportive framework conditions.

Interdisciplinary research integrates theories, methods, and empirical data from different disciplines. The choice of the *right theories* and methods is made in interdisciplinary coordination. In this way, research questions on chronic care can be jointly investigated from two or more disciplines. In the context of competitive third-party funding, interdisciplinary research is often addressed in the areas of climate, environment, and health. By providing these resources, decisions are also made regarding the content, research questions, and problem definitions of research proposals to be submitted. Researchers can enroll in the predetermined topics and subsequently reconstruct the appropriateness of the subject matter (Arnold et al. 2014). In order to establish a common understanding of the problem, participants must, on the one hand, represent their own discipline and disciplinary perspective as well as reflect on their own disciplinary boundaries, and on the other hand, feed the results of interdisciplinary research back into their discipline. Interdisciplinary publications and qualifications also require disciplinary feedback, "because academic degrees and honors are usually awarded on a disciplinary basis [...] [and] disciplines define themselves, among other things, through the shared specialist literature with which members of the respective scientific community relate to each other" (Arnold et al. 2014, p. 116).

Transdisciplinary research encompasses research approaches that seek solutions to socially relevant problems by utilizing knowledge, methods, and expertise from different disciplines, as well as integrating non-university practice fields (Krainer 2021). According to Krainer, the choice of transdisciplinary research approaches appears necessary due to five requirements:

1. A removal of boundaries due to increasing societal complexity: Research questions on socially relevant issues cannot always be addressed along disciplinary and university (separate) faculty structures; they transcend these boundaries.
2. Social responsibility of science and the expected concrete contributions to solving socially relevant problems.
3. Transformative potential of science: Science questions its own capacity for shaping how it can influence societal processes without being politically instrumentalized and losing its neutrality and independence (Krainer 2021). The question of the benefit of transdisciplinary research must therefore be answered in terms of who benefits from transdisciplinary knowledge and who should benefit from it.
4. Cooperation and co-creation: Transdisciplinary researchers cooperate in their research with actors from civil society and co-create knowledge to solve socially relevant problems by integrating the respective rationalities, languages, and perspectives of the involved sciences as well as of practice. Research is not conducted about those affected, but with them. This requires an appropriate attitude on the part of researchers, enabling framework conditions, and suitable didactic concepts of cooperative learning, transdisciplinary competencies to communicate with different disciplines and practice partners, as well as co-creative action (see contribution 57).
5. Blurring the boundaries between science and practice: Due to the increasing academization of practice fields, science is no longer tied only to academic institutions. As a result of this blurring of boundaries, questions about areas of expertise must be clarified. In the context of transdisciplinary research, experts from science and practice come together; experts from practice possess the practice-relevant knowledge that science must first access (Krainer 2021). In addition, appropriate participation from practice is required.

A transdisciplinary understanding of research is shaped by these framework conditions. In addition to methodological and research-practical questions, this also includes transdisciplinary determinations of subject-appropriate theory development, which, as a possible result of transdisciplinary research, explains and understands complex phenomena.

The research approaches presented in the following sections can be applied within the framework of transdisciplinary research on chronic care.

57.3 Ethnographic Research Approaches in People with Chronic Illnesses

57.3.1 Living Labs—Real-World Laboratories

Living Labs (a term commonly used in the English-speaking world) and Real-World Laboratories (a coined term combining reality and laboratory) are research formats that implement transdisciplinary research and its objectives, linking them with transformative approaches and practical goals (as well as educational objectives; see Contribution 03) in order to bridge the gap between research and practice. They investigate challenges and problems of everyday social life to develop and test desirable societal solutions using scientific methods. Their core characteristics are research orientation, transformativity, transdisciplinarity & participation, civil society orientation, and their model character (Parodi and Steglich 2021). They are characterized by a diversity of several transdisciplinary projects under one roof, with a wide range of real-world experiments in various settings, in which solution approaches are empirically tested with the involvement of different stakeholders. In this context, further transdisciplinary tasks under this umbrella include monitoring new topics, integrating results between projects, and building long-term cooperation (Beecroft et al. 2018). For Real-World Laboratories to realize their potential, they require an adequate research design, which, according to Beecroft and others (2018), is guided by the following principles:

1. Ensuring problem and topic relevance based on the interests of stakeholders from business and practice as a foundation for collaboration
2. Designing spatial appropriateness, providing a suitable frame of reference for the participants in line with the objectives and topics
3. Ensuring temporal appropriateness for transformative research approaches as well as temporal alignment between research and other processes in practice, implementation, and reflection
4. Establishing appropriate stakeholder roles regarding the scope, extent, and intensity of stakeholder participation in activities within the Real-World Laboratory
5. Promoting an experimental-reflective working style, enabling learning by reflecting on activities and roles and maintaining a certain degree of flexibility

Research approaches to chronic care adopt these five design principles and must, in particular, find suitable designs for temporal and spatial aspects. This also involves questions of participation in the Real-World Laboratory: when and by whom is participation considered successful, what are the objects and goals of participation, how can participation be structured, and who should participate?

57.3.2 Participatory Research

The goal of participatory research is to collaboratively investigate and influence social reality together with the actors of that reality. Science and practice conduct research together and cooperate transdisciplinarily. As a combination of research design or study concept with a form of intervention, it can be classified as a variant of intervention research as well as action research. In North America, questions of participatory health research aimed at health promotion and improving unequal health opportunities are addressed through the approach of Community-Based Participatory Research. Stakeholders from the community are both the target group for the health system to be studied and professional actors. Implementing this research approach is time-consuming, faces criticism regarding the quality of research due to the involvement of laypersons, and requires building long-term partnerships with communities based on trust and a common ground. Merely informing about the planned research and obtaining consent to participate does not constitute participatory research. Participation can take various forms (involvement in the research process ranging from co-determination to partial or even full decision-making authority, including the associated empowerment and enabling).

Depending on the model, advisory or inclusive activities can also be considered participatory research. Fundamental questions for designing participation are: 1. who participates in the research, 2. in what or which processes is participation taking place, and 3. how and in what form does participation occur (from Unger 2012). Research approaches to chronic care must, for question 1, define sampling strategies for the target groups: affected individuals, relatives, as well as professionals closely involved in interactions and those shaping the framework conditions of care. For question 2, depending on the specific research question, roles and tasks in the research process must be selected, such as to what extent research partners can participate in the selection of data collection methods, in the analysis, and in the utilization of research. The answer to question three regarding research on chronic care depends, among other things, on the extent to which people with chronic illnesses are able and willing to participate in research in terms of time, content intensity, and workload.

57.3.3 Disease Course and Life Phase-Oriented Research

Research on the course of disease is of particular importance. This predominantly follows a categorical approach, such as in research on the severity levels of dementing illnesses. Disease course research aims to provide insights into the use of specific interventions and their impact on the respective disease phases. This applies not only to all progressively developing diseases but especially to those that are regularly fatal. These insights form the basis for decisions on when to switch the care concept to palliative care.

Life phase-oriented research aims to influence the onset and course of disease, taking biographical aspects into account. In relation to and identification of risk populations, life phase-specific interventions can be identified and evaluated for their appropriateness. Even if the research is usually not directly disease-related, epidemiology, for example, plays a significant role, particularly in the context of life phase-related social determinants and their importance for health promotion and the development of diseases.

57.3.4 Cultural Approach

The cultural approach, recognizing a broad understanding of the concept of culture, has increasingly become a subject of research in Germany as well. How do cultural norms (see Contribution 29) influence care arrangements? Issues such as discrimination, stigmatization, or abuse play a significant role. This involves more than just research on migration (see Contribution 28). Cultural diversity as a feature of modern societies requires research to address the self-definition of cultural, group-related affiliation as part of personal identity and the resulting different care relationships. For example, what is the significance of spirituality in coping with illness or in the end-of-life phase? What is the importance of respecting bodily awareness, shame, and intimacy in the context of professional intervention for the quality of life of people with chronic illnesses (quality of life research)? What does this mean for lifestyle research, neighborhood-/milieu-based care research, for example, in relation to the experience of illness and coping with disease?

References

Arnold M, Gaube V, Wieser B (2014) Interdisziplinär forschen. In: Dressel G, Berger W, Heimerl K, Winiwarter V (eds) Interdisziplinär und transdisziplinär forschen, Praktiken und Methoden. transcript, Bielefeld, pp 105–119

Beecroft R, Trenks H, Rhodius R, Benighaus C, Parodi O (2018) Reallabore als Rahmen transformativer und transdisziplinärer Forschung. Ziele und Designprinzipien. In: Defila R, Di Giulio A (eds) Transdisziplinär und transformativ forschen, Eine Methodensammlung. Springer VS, Wiesbaden-Heidelberg, pp 75–100

Krainer L (2021) Theoriebildung in transdisziplinärer Forschung. In: Schmohl T , Phlipp T. (eds) Handbuch Transdisziplinäre Didaktik. transcript, Bielefeld, pp 313–322

Parodi O, Steglich A (2021) Reallabor. In:Schmohl T , Phlipp T. (eds) Handbuch Transdisziplinäre Didaktik. transcript, Bielefeld, pp 255–266

Unger, Hella von (2012) Partizipative Gesundheitsforschung: Wer partizipiert woran? Forum Qualitative Sozialforschung/Forum: Qualitative Social Research, vol 13, No 1 (2012): Participatory Qualitative Research. https://doi.org/10.17169/fqs-13.1.1781

Practice-Led Challenges in Chronic Care Practice

58

Manfred Fiedler and Jan-Hendrik Ortloff

Contents

58.1 Ensuring Dignified Care and the Shortage of Skilled Professionals

The demands in the healthcare sector are complex and dynamic. This affects institutions in general as well as actors in the health professions in particular, as an increasing number of elderly people are being cared for by a decreasing number of younger people. According to the coordinated population projection, by 2040 approximately 25% of the population in Germany will be older than 67 years and 18% will be younger than 20 years (Statistisches Bundesamt 2023). Moreover, the shortage of available skilled professionals is of societal interest and political urgency, as on the one hand, more and more

M. Fiedler (✉) · J.-H. Ortloff
Department of human medicine, Witten/Herdecke University, Witten, Germany
e-mail: manfred.fiedler@uni-wh.de

J.-H. Ortloff
e-mail: Jan-Hendrik.Ortloff@uni-wh.de

D. Schmitz et al. (eds.), *Chronic Care—Science and Practice*,
https://doi.org/10.1007/978-3-662-72298-5_58

people are in need of care, while on the other hand, fewer professionals are available, whose professional responsibilities are increasingly broad (digital, coordinative, and cross-interface, etc.). This raises the question of how future-proof, dignified care can be ensured despite the shortage of skilled professionals. Even though there is currently no nationwide shortage of skilled professionals, in some regions and (healthcare) sectors, vacant positions cannot already be filled with suitable professionals. This is substantiated, among other things, by the Federal Employment Agency's statistical bottleneck analysis, which calculates shortages in numerous health professions based on categories such as vacancy duration, jobseeker-to-vacancy ratio, occupation-specific unemployment rate, exit rate from unemployment, changing proportion of foreign employees subject to social insurance, and development of median earnings (Federal Employment Agency n.d.). The causes of these shortages have for years been attributed to various factors, ranging from unfilled positions due to a lack of new recruits, to a high proportion of part-time employees, to the lack of attractiveness of the professions. However, the shortage of skilled professionals refers not only to the quantitative factors of unfilled positions, but also to the qualitative working conditions of the actors as well as the situation of those affected. Health professionals have direct contact with those affected, are involved in their situation, and perform emotional labor to manage the burdens arising from illness situations in care. For this reason, ensuring dignified care requires not only interpersonal skills but also sufficient time, material, and personnel resources, as well as quality standards that must be (co-)defined by the respective health professions themselves.

This is linked to the question of the development of professional fields, which is closely related to the discussion about the academization of health professions. A reorganization of professional fields is not simply an expansion of areas of action by taking on previously non-profession-specific tasks. This is also not effective, as the shortage of skilled professionals is not limited to individual occupational groups. A formally and substantively well-conceived academization can help to increase decision-making competence at interfaces, accelerate processes, and improve process quality as well as professional expertise in the original field. Studies such as those on Magnet Hospitals (Aiken et al. 2008) show that this can improve health outcomes and reduce mortality. Participation in this context therefore requires that these change processes take place in an interprofessional discourse from a shared transprofessional perspective.

58.2 Changing Multiprofessional and Interinstitutional Collaboration—Division of Labor Between Tradition and Coherent Care Needs

Divisions of labor present a future challenge for healthcare institutions. Rigid, established structures and hierarchies have not yet been overcome. The increasing managerial orientation that has taken place in institutions in recent years has initially led to a rise in the importance of management. Since healthcare is a personal service, from this perspective, healthcare professionals primarily represent a cost factor and only secondarily human capital. This functionalization has also contributed to an alienation from the field of activity (Becker 2016), and possibly even an alienation from the profession itself.

To accomplish the aforementioned changes, it requires, to put it simply, the competence, intellect, and heart of the professionals. In fact, modern organizational development is always participatory and non-hierarchical. With their high level of competence in practical fields, healthcare institutions are particularly challenged to implement innovative changes together with the affected professionals and within the field of practice, involving those affected. Management thus assumes more of a moderating, supportive role, as well as the task of creating an innovation-friendly, solution-oriented atmosphere that is not, or at least not solely, based on so-called economic constraints.

As early as the 1990s, the German (Enquete-Kommission Demographischer Wandel, 2004) called for better collaboration among the various care providers to address demographic challenges. With the Health Modernization Act of 2003, legislators made the first cautious step toward models of integrative care, which have since been followed by further legislative measures to establish them.

As important as legislative openness is, it is equally significant that, in view of increasing resource scarcity, institutions are capable of cooperation both internally and externally. Especially for the growing number of chronically ill people, it is essential that their care, which is interconnected both professionally and processually, is conceived in a networked manner and practiced as intra- and interinstitutional cooperation. For example, a study by the Center for Hospital Management found that patients in post-clinical rehabilitation were not fully treated, thereby limiting rehabilitation success (von Eiff 2011). The competitive behavior demanded by political frameworks is not only economically, but also in terms of treatment outcomes, not explicitly beneficial.

Cooperation particularly means appropriate communication. Especially for chronically ill people, who have an individual illness biography, the presence of such personal information—which includes more than just medical findings—is crucial for high-quality and continuous care, especially when a new institution becomes involved. Digital information channels such as the electronic patient record will be decisive here. However, the level of development varies greatly, as in practice, if digital media consist, for example, of a fax machine, this clearly indicates a need for improvement.

58.3 Adequate Framework Conditions for Care

The care of chronically ill people largely takes place in the living environment of those affected. Community-based care therefore has particular significance. However, this is countered by the fact that municipal institutions are very differently developed both nationally and internationally. Especially in Germany, the pandemic has revealed major deficits after years of austerity. Policymakers are called upon to specifically strengthen the health policy competencies of municipalities, especially since all other institutional actors in Germany have increasingly lost their connection to the municipal level. This is all the more true as additional challenges from climate change are approaching municipalities. The topic of environment and health (see contribution 52) is gaining increasing practical relevance, for example in terms of managing environment-related health crises, reducing health-relevant environmental emissions, and creating a sustainable healthy city.

Health policy is ostensibly guided by the realization that decades of market-based regulatory policy have not made the healthcare system more efficient or economical, as is the case when, for example, the end of the DRG system in hospitals is proclaimed (n.n. 2022). However, there is a risk that decades of market regulation policy thinking will also shape the new reform measures. For example, if the so-called ambulatory-sensitive services are considered a savings potential in hospital care, while at the same time outpatient specialist care is already operating at maximum capacity, then answers are being given where the posing of the question is unclear or which are guided by the wrong guiding concepts.

The requirements become even clearer for patients who move between outpatient, day-care, and inpatient care and who are also continuously dependent on various forms of therapeutic services that promote self-determination. For example, for psychiatric patients, sector-oriented health reforms are a relic of an outdated health policy paradigm.

The increase in the number of chronically ill people corresponds with a decrease in the potential for professional as well as family support services. The realization that a massive shortage of care capacities is imminent has not yet been sufficiently reflected in political reform thinking. The organizational separation of services, financial flows, and responsibilities is not only an obstacle to the future care of chronically ill people, but could in the worst case threaten care security for everyone in the future. The demand for the ability to cooperate and to think in networks therefore also applies to health policy and to the institutions responsible for system governance.

References

Aiken LH, Buchan J, Ball J, Rafferty AM (2008) Transformative impact of magnet designation: England case study. J Clin Nurs 17(24):3330–3337. https://doi.org/10.1111/j.1365-2702.2008.02640.x

Becker K (2016) Loyale Beschäftigte—Ein Auslaufmodell? Zum Wandel der Beschäftigtenorientierungen in der stationären Pflege unter marktzentrierten Arbeitsbedingungen. Pflege & Gesellschaft 21(2):145–159

Bundesagentur für Arbeit (o. J.) Engpassanalyse: Berichtsjahr 2022. https://statistik.arbeitsagentur.de/DE/Navigation/Statistiken/Interaktive-Statistiken/Fachkraeftebedarf/Engpassanalyse-Nav.html

von Eiff W (2011) Medizinische Rehabilitation: Kürzere Akut-Verweildauern erhöhen Aufwand in der Reha. Dtsch Ärztebl 108(21):1164–1166

Enquetekommission Demographischer Wandel (2004) Herausforderungen unserer älter werdenden Gesellschaft an den einzelnen und die Politik: Zwischenbericht (BT-Drucksache 12/7876) n.n (2022) DRG-Reform Lauterbach: Ohne Fallpauschalen sollen Kliniken raus aus dem Hamsterrad. Ärztezeitung. https://www.aerztezeitung.de/Wirtschaft/Lauterbach-Ohne-Fallpauschalen-raus-aus-dem-Hamsterrad-434656.html. Accessed 29 Sept 2023

Statistisches Bundesamt (2023) 15. koordinierte Bevölkerungsvorausberechnung: Annahen und ERgebnisse. https://www.destatis.de/DE/Themen/Gesellschaft-Umwelt/Bevoelkerung/Bevoelkerungsvorausberechnung/begleitheft.html

MIX
Papier aus verantwortungsvollen Quellen
Paper from responsible sources
FSC® C105338

If you have any concerns about our products,
you can contact us on
ProductSafety@springernature.com

In case Publisher is established outside the EU,
the EU authorized representative is:
Springer Nature Customer Service Center GmbH
Europaplatz 3, 69115 Heidelberg, Germany

Printed by Libri Plureos GmbH
in Hamburg, Germany